MECHANISM OF CISPLATIN RESISTANCE AND ITS CIRCUMVENTION

MECHANISM OF CISPLATIN RESISTANCE AND ITS CIRCUMVENTION

Yoshihiro Kikuchi (Ed.)

NOVA SCIENCE PUBLISHERS, INC.
Commack, NY
1998

Editorial Production: Susan Boriotti
Office Manager: Annette Hellinger
Graphics: Frank Grucci and John T'Lustachowski
Information Editor: Tatiana Shohov
Book Production: Donna Dennis, Patrick Devin, Christine Mathosian, Tammy Sauter and Diane Sharp
Circulation: Maryanne Schmidt
Marketing/Sales: Cathy DeGregory

Library of Congress Cataloging-in-Publication Data available upon request

ISBN 1-56072-548-6

6080 Jericho Turnpike, Suite 207
Commack, New York 11725
Tele. 516-499-3103 Fax 516-499-3146
e-mail: Novascil@aol.com
Novascience@earthlink.net
Web Site: http://www.nexusworld.com/nova

Printed in the United States of America

CONTENTS

PART I

CISPLATIN RESISTANCE AND GLUTATHIONE

CHAPTER 1

CISPLATIN RESISTANCE AND GLUTATHIONE

Norio Yoshiya and Kenichi Tanaka
Department of Obstetrics and Gynecology, School of Medicine, Niigata University, Niigata

Cisplatin (CDDP) is the major therapeutic agent in the treatment of ovarian cancer (1). In patients with the advanced disease CDDP-based combination chemotherapy has resulted in increased complete response rates, with some studies reporting prolonged overall survival compared to single agent therapy (2-4). However, the majority of patients with bulky disease are not cured, and the emergence of resistance is common consequence of therapy (3-6).

In order to elucidate the mechanisms underlying resistance to CDDP, various resistant cell lines have been established. Many observations on resistant cell lines have demonstrated that mechanisms of resistance to CDDP are multifactorial, including reduced drug accumulation (7), increased efflux of the drugs mediated by P-glycoprotein (8), enhancement of DNA repair (9) and acceleration of detoxification systems such as an increase in the gluthatione (GSH) (10) (see ref. 11,12 for review).

Buthionine sulfoximine (BSO) results in reduction of intracellular GSH levels by inhibiting gamma-glutamyl cysteine synthetase, which is the rate-limiting enzymes involved in the synthesis of this tripeptide (13). In this work, we have examined relationship between the cytotoxicity of various anticancer drugs and the GSH level in a CDDP-resistant human ovarian cancer cell line established in our laboratory.

MATERIALS AND METHODS

CELL LINES

The TYK cell line established in our laboratory was derived from a patients with undifferentiated carcinoma of the ovary. The TYK-R cell line, CDDP-resistant subline, was developed by culturing TYK with exposure to CDDP in escalating doses. Both cell lines were grown in tissue culture dishes in a humidified 5% CO_2 atmosphere at 37°C. They were maintained in medium consisting of Eagle's MEM supplemented with 10% fetal calf serum, 2 mM glutamine and 60 mg kanamycin/ml.

DRUGS AND CHEMICALS

CDDP, carboplatin (CBDCA) and etoposide (VP-16) were obtained from Bristol-Myers Squibb Co. Ltd. (Glycolato-0,0') diammineplatinum (II) (254-S) was obtained from Shionogi Chemical Co. Ltd. Camptothecin-11 (CPT-11) was obtained from Yakult Co. Ltd. 5-Fluorouracil (5-FU) and adriamycin (ADR) were obtained from Kyowa Hakko Kogyo Co. Ltd. BSO and 3-(4,5-dimethyl-thiazol-2-yl)-2,5-diphenyltetrazolium bromide (MTT) were obtained from Sigma.

GSH ASSAY

The total cellular GSH contents were determined by an enzymatic recycling method (14). The GSH content was expressed as mg per 10^7 cells.

CYTOTOXICITY ASSAY

The cytotoxicity of anticancer agents was evaluated by the MTT assay based on the method of Mosmann et al (15). Tumor cell suspensions adjusted to 1 x 10^5 cells/ml were distributed into 96-well plate (Corning Inc.) at a density of 1 x 10^4 cells/well with 0.1 ml of growth medium and plates were incubated at 37°C for 24h before the addition of the drug. Then, TYK and TYK-R cells were incubated for 96h continuously in various concentrations of anticancer drugs with or without BSO (final concentration 50 μM).

After an incubation period, MTT solution was added at 10 μl/well and allowed to react for 4h. The 100 ml supernatants were removed from each well after centrifugation for 10 min at 1000 rpm, and 150 ml of dimethylsulfoxide was added into each well. The plates were then agitated on a shaker for 5 min to dissolve the formazon grain. Absorbance of each well was determined by measuring the optimal density (OD) with an ELISA analyser (STL210) at a wave length of 577-630 nm. Data were collected in quadruplicate and the cytotoxicities were defined as the survival fraction of cells according to the following formula.

Survival rate (%) = [(OD of treated cells - OD of medium) / (OD of control cells - OD of medium)] x 100

The results were expressed as the mean of two experiments and 50% inhibition drug concentration (IC_{50}) was determined graphically from the dose-response curve.

RESULTS

DRUG SENSITIVITY

When compared with the parent TYK cell line, the TYK-R cell line showed 4.0, 4.3, 6.0, 1.9, 1.6 and 2.0-fold degree of resistance to CDDP, 254-S, CBDCA, VP-16, 5-FU and ADR, respectively. However, the IC_{50} value of CPT-11 was about the same between the two cell lines. (Table 1)

TOXICITY OF BSO

When the TYK cells were incubated with 50 mM BSO for 96h, the cell survival rate was 87.8%, while that in the TYK-R cells showed 92.4% (Table 2).

EFFECT OF BSO ON GSH CONTENT

The intracellular GSH level of TYK and TYK-R cells was 14.2 and 18.5 $\mu g/10^7$ cells, respectively. When both the cell lines were exposed for 48h to 50 μM BSO, the GSH level of TYK and TYK-R cells decreased from 14.2 $\mu g/10^7$ cells to 0.69 $\mu g/10^7$ cells (4.9%) and from 18,.5 $\mu g/10^7$ cells to 3.33 $\mu g/10^7$ cells (18.0%), respectively. (Table 3)

EFFECT OF BSO ON IC_{50} VALUES OF VARIOUS ANTICANCER DRUGS

When BSO was combined with anticancer drugs, the IC_{50} values of anticancer drugs were decreased. The degree of decrease in the TYK cells was 12% for CDDP, 26% for 254-S, 25% for CBDCA, 6% for CPT-11, 49% for VP-16, 37% for 5-FU and 30% for ADR, while that in the TYK-R cells was 6% for CDDP, 28% for 254-S, 8% for CBDCA 13% for VP-16, 40% for 5-FU; and 50% for ADR, respectively. However, IC_{50} value of CPT-11 in the TYK-R cells was not changed by BSO. (Table 4)

Table 1. IC_{50} values to various anticancer drugs of TYK and TYK-R

	IC_{50}(mg/ml)		Resistance
Drug	TYK	TYK-R	index*
CDDP	0.8	3.2	4.0
254-S	0.23	1.0	4.3
CBDCA	0.8	4.8	6.0
CPT-11	1.8	1.8	1.0
VP-16	0.78	1.5	1.9
5-FU	2.7	4.2	1.6
ADR	0.2	0.4	2.0

*(IC_{50} value of TYK-R)/(IC_{50} value of TYK)

Table 2. Effect of BSO on cell proliferation

Cell line/Drug	OD577	Survival rate (%)**
TYK		
Control	0.443 ± 0.058*	-
BSO(50mM)	0.394 ± 0.026	87.8
TYK-R		
Control	0.424 ± 0.046	-
BSO(50mM)	0.395 ± 0.017	92.4

*Mean ± SD (n=8)
**[(OD of treated cells - OD of medium control)/
(OD of control cells - OD of medium control)] x 100 (%)

Table 3. Intracellular content of total GSH

Cell line	GSH content ($mg/10^7$ cells) BSO(-)	BSO(50mM)	Decrease rate**
TYK	14.2 ± 0.53*	0.69 ± 0.05	4.9%
TYK-R	18.5 ± 0.61	3.33 ± 0.02	18.0%

*Mean ± SD (n=3)
**(GSH content with BSO/GSH content without BSO) x 100 (%)

Table 4. Effect of BSO on IC_{50} value of various anticancer drugs

Drug	TYK		TYK-R	
CDDP	0.7 /0.8*	(12%)**	3.0 /3.2	(6%)
254-S	0.17/0.23	(26%)	0.72/1.0	(28%)
CBDCA	0.6 /0.8	(25%)	4.4 /4.8	(8%)
CPT-11	1.7 /1.8	(6%)	1.8 /1.8	(0%)
VP-16	0.4 /0.78	(49%)	1.3 /1.5	(13%)
5-FU	1.7 /2.7	(37%)	2.5 /4.2	(40%)
ADR	0.14/0.2	(30%)	0.2 /0.4	(50%)

*Upper figure shows IC_{50} of drug with 50mM BSO and lower figure shows IC_{50} of drug alone.
**[1- (IC_{50} of drug with BSO / IC_{50} of drug alone)] x 100 (%)

DISCUSSION

We have developed a CDDP-resistant TYK-R subline by continuously exposuring the parent TYK cells to escalating doses of CDDP. When the IC_{50} of TYK-R was compared to that of the parent TYK, TYK-R cell line was about 4.0-fold resistance to CDDP. Similar resistance to 254-S and CBDCA was observed, suggesting cross-resistance to CDDP. These findings have also been made for other CDDP-resistant human ovarian cancer sublines (16-19). The TYK-R cell line also expressed less cross-resistance to VP-16, 5-FU and ADR. Similarly, the absence of cross-resistance to VP-16 are also known(19,20). Hamilton et al.(7) and Niimi et al. (20) reported 4-fold and 6.4-fold cross-resistance to ADR, respectively, while Hill et al. (19) reported the absence of cross-resistance to ADR. Although Niimi et al.(20) reported significant cross-resistance of CPT-11 to CDDP, there was no evidence of cross-resistance of CPT-11 to CDDP in the TYK-R cell line. Since CPT-11 was reported to be effective for patients with refractory tumor to previous chemotherapies including CDDP(21), further studies are needed to elucidate usefulness of treatment with CPT-11 for CDDP-resistant ovarian cancer patients.

It has been suggested that elevated intracellular GSH level is one of important features in human ovarian cancer cell lines with acquired or intrinsic resistance to CDDP(10). Although the manner in which GSH potentiates CDDP-resistance is unknown, it is possible that the GSH-mediated transport alterations, spontaneous or enzyme-catalyzed formation of inactive GSH-platinum conjugates, protection of DNA from the formation of potentially cytotoxic platinum adducts and elevation of DNA repair (16) are involved in the mechanisms. In the present study, the GSH level in the TYK-R cell line was significantly higher than that in the TYK cell line. Several studies have reported similar findings (7,17,19,20,22), Godwin et al.(23) have also reported that the increased degrees of resistance of human ovarian cancer cell lines to CDDP were closely correlated with increases in the intracellular GSH levels. On the other hand, Loh et al.(24) have reported that no increase of the intracellular GSH levels in ovarian cancer cell lines with 2 to 6-fold resistance to CDDP was observed. Thus, we examined the effects of GSH depletion by BSO, an inhibitor of g-glutamyl cysteine synthetase (γ-GCS), on the cytotoxicity of CDDP and other anticancer drugs. The intracellular GSH levels significantly decreased by 48h exposure of TYK and TYK-R cells to 50 μM BSO. Similar reports have been made by Hamilton et al.(7), Hill et al.(19) and Niimi et al.(20). Subsequently, treatment of TYK cell line with BSO (96h exposure to 50 μM BSO) resulted in decrease of the IC_{50} values to all tested drugs (from 6% for CPT-11 to 49% for VP-16), while in TYK-R cell line decrease of the IC50 values (from 6% for CDDP to 50% for ADR) was observed but not CPT-11 (Table 4). In the other CDDP-resistant ovarian cancer cell lines, Hamilton et al.(7), Andrews et al.(17), and Niimi et al.(20) have reported 77%, 43% and 75% decrease of the IC_{50} to CDDP by BSO (48h exposure to 25 μM BSO, 48h exposure to 50 μM BSO and 24 h exposure to 100 μM BSO), respectively. On the other hand, Hill et al.(19) have found no effect of BSO on the CDDP-induced cytotoxicity. Further studies are necessary to confirm the relationship between CDDP-resistance and GSH synthesis, and the clinical relevance to these observations remains to be established.

REFERENCES

1. Loehrer, P. J. and Einhorn, L. H.: *Cisplatin. Ann. Int. Med.*, 100: 704-713, 1984.
2. Omura, G., Bundy, B., Berek, J. S., Curry, S., Delbado, G. and Mortel,R.: A randomized trial of cyclophoshamide plus cisplatin with or without adriamycin in ovarian cancer: A Gynecologic Oncology Group Study. *J. Clin. Oncol.*, 7: 457-467, 1988.
3. Ozols, R. F., and Young, R. C.: Chemotherapy of ovarian cancer. *Semin. Oncol.,* 11: 251-263, 1984.
4. Thigpen, T. and Blessing, J. A.: Current therapy of ovarian carcinoma. An overview. *Semin. Oncol.*, 12 (Suppl.4): 47-52, 1985.
5. Louie, K. G., Ozols, R. F., Myers, C. E., Ostecha, Y., Jenkin, J., Howser, D. and Young, R. C.: Long-term results of a cisplatin containing combination chemotherapy regimen for the treatment of advanced ovarian carcinoma. *J. Clin. Oncol.*,4: 1579-1585, 1986.
6. Hainsworth, J. D., Grosh, W. W. and Burnett, L. S.: Advanced ovarian cancer: long-term results of treatment with intensive cisplatin-based chemotherapy of brief duration. *Ann. Int. Med.*, 108: 165-170, 1988.
7. Hamilton, T. C., Winker, M.A., Louie, K. G., Batist, G., Behrens, B.C., Tsuruo, T., Grotzinger K. R., Mckoy, W. M., Young, R. C. and Ozols, R. F.: Augmentation of adriamycin, melphalan, and cisplatin cytotoxicity in drug-resistant and -sensitive human ovarian cancer cell lines by buthionine sulfoximine mediated depletion. *Biochem. Pharmacol.,* 34: 2583-2586, 1985.
8. Bradley, G., Naik, M. and Ling. V.: P-glycoprotein expression in multi-drug-resistant human ovarian carcinoma cell lines. *Cancer Res.,*49: 2790-2796, 1989.
9. Zijlstra, J. G., DeVries, E. G. E. and Mulder, N. H.: Drug resistance in medical oncology. *Netherlands J. Med.*, 30: 85-93, 1987.
10. Meister, A. and Anderson, M. E. Glutathione. *Ann. Rev. Biochem.*, 52: 711-760, 1983.
11. DeGraeff, A, Slebos, R. J. and Rodenhuis, S. : Resistance to cisplatin and analogues: mechanisms and potential clinical simplication. *Cancer Chemother. Pharmacol.*,22: 325-332, 1988.
12. Andrews, P. A. and Howell, S. B.: Cellular pharmacology of cisplatin: perspectives on mechanisms of acquired resistance. *Cancer Cells*, 2: 35-43, 1990.

13. Huang, C. S., Moore, W. R. and Meister,A.: On the active site thiol of gamma-glutamyl cysteine synthetase; relationship to catalysis, inhibition and regulation. *Proc. Natl. Acad. Sci. USA.*, 85:2464-2468, 1988.
14. Tietze, F.: Enzymic method for quantitative determination of nanogram amounts of total and oxidized glutathione. *Anal. Biochem.*, 27: 502-522,1969.
15. Mosmann, T.: Rapid colorimetric assay for cellular growth and survival: Application to proliferation and cytotoxicity assays. *J. Immnol. Methods*, 65: 55-63,1983.
16. Behrens, B. C., Hamilton, T. C., Masuda, H., Grotzinger, K. R., Whang-Peng, J., Louie, K. G., Kuntsen,T., Mckoy, W. M., Young, R. C. and Ozols, R. F.: Characterization of a cis-diammine-dichloroplatinum (II)-resistant human ovarian cancer cell line and its use in evaluation of platinum analogues. *Cancer Res.*, 47: 414-418, 1987.
17. Andrews, P. A., Murphy, M. P and Howell, S. B.: Characterization of cisplatin-resistant COLO316 human ovarian carcinoma cells. *Eur. J. Cancer Clin. Oncol.*,25: 619-625,1989.
18. Kikuchi, Y., Iwano, I., Miyauchi, M., Kita, T., Sugita, M., Tenjin, Y. and Nagata, I.: Possible mechanism of resistance to cis-diamminedichloroplatinum(II) of human ovarian cancer cells. *Jpn. J. Cancer Res.*, 81: 701-706,1990.
19. Hill, B. T., Shellard, S. A., Hosking, L. K., Dempke, W. C. M., Fichtinger-Schepman, A. M. J., Tone, T., Scanlon, K. J. and Whelan, R. D. H.: Characterization of a cisplatin-resistant human ovarian carcinoma cell line expressing cross-resistance to 5-fluorouracil but collateral sensitivity to methotrexate. *Cancer Res.*, 52: 328-333, 1992.
20. Niimi, S., Nakagawa, K., Sugimoto, Y., Nishio, K., Fujiwara. Y., Yokoyama, S., Terashima,Y. and Saijo,N.: Mechanism of cross-resistance to a camptothecin analogue (CPT-11) in a human ovarian cancer cell line selected by cisplatin. *Cancer Res.,* 52: 328-333, 1992.
21. Research group of CPT-11 in gynecologic cancers: An early phase II study of CPT-11 for gynecologic cancers. *Jpn. J. Cancer Chemother.*, 18: 579-584, 1991.(in Japanese)
22. Zinkewich-Peotti, K. and Andrews, P. A.: Loss of cis-diamminedi-chloroplatinum(II) resistance in human ovarian carcinoma cells selected for rhodamine 123 resistance. *Cancer Res.*, 52: 1902-1906, 1992.
23. Godwin, A. K., Meister, A., O'Dwyer, P. J., Huang, C. S., Hamilton, T. C. and Anderson, M. E.: High resistance to cisplatin in human ovarian cancer cell lines is associated with marked increase of glutathione synthesis. *Proc. Natl. Acad. Sci. USA.* 89: 3070-3074, 1992.

24. Loh, S. Y., Kelland, M. L. R., Abel, G. and Harrap, K. R.: Reduced drug accumulation as a major mechanism of acquired resistance to cisplatin in a human ovarian carcinoma cell line: circumvention studies using novel platinum (II) and (IV) ammine/amine complexes. *Br. J. Cancer*,66: 1109-1115, 1992.

CHAPTER 2

CORRELATION BETWEEN CDDP RESISTANCE AND CELLULAR GLUTATHIONE CONTENT

Kazuya Kudoh. MD
Department of Obstetrics and Gynecology,
National Defense Medical College

INTRODUCTION

The intracellular glutathione(GSH) metabolic system is one of the most important mechanisms for drug detoxification in cancer cells(1). It is well known that many *in vitro* induced drug resistant cancer cells contain more intracellular GSH than the drug sensitive parent cells(1,2). We examined the correlation between the sensitivity to cis-diamminedichloroplatinum(II), (CDDP) or its analogues {diammine[1,1-cyclobutanedicarboxylato(2-1)-0,0'] platinum(II) (CBDCA) and (-)-(R)-2-aminomethylpyrrolidine (1,1-cyclobutanedicarboxylato) platinum(II) monohydrate (DWA2114R)} and intracellular GSH levels in human ovarian cancer cell lines (HRA, KK and MH) with different sensitivity to CDDP (3). In addition, we examined the changes of drug sensitivity when the GSH levels were changed by D,L-buthionine-S,R-sulfoximine (BSO; a specific inhibitor for GSH synthesis enzyme, Sigma Chemical Co., St. Louis, MO., U.S.A.) or cystine (a component of GSH molecule, Sigma Chemical Co., St. Louis, MO., U.S.A.) for detecting correlation between the CDDP resistance and the GSH content.

Sensitivity to CDDP or its Analogues (CBDCA and DWA2114R) and Cellular GSH Levels in the Human Ovarian Cancer Cells

Cells used were HRA, KK and MH cells (4-6) . HRA cells were derived from ascites of a patient with serous cystadenocarcinoma of the ovary who responded well to CDDP-based combination chemotherapy. KK and MH cells were also established from ascites of a patient with clear cell carcinoma of the ovary and with serous cystadenocarcinoma of the ovary, respectively who did not respond to CDDP-based combination chemotherapy. To examine the sensitivity to CDDP or its analogues in HRA, KK and MH cells, we determined the concentrations of these drugs required for 50% inhibition of HRA, KK and MH cell proliferation in vitro (IC_{50}), using a crystal violet staining method described by Saotome et al.(7). Intracellular GSH levels were measured by using enzyme recycling method published elsewhere(8). Table 1 shows results of the drug sensitivity tests and the cellular GSH levels. HRA cells were most sensitive to CDDP and followed by KK and MH cells. The resistance factors (IC_{50} ratios to HRA cells) of KK and MH were 2.93 and 3.66, respectively. Similarly, those to CBDCA and DWA2114R were 6.35 and 9.19 for KK cells, respectively and 6.70 and 6.78 for MH cells, suggesting cross-resistance to these drugs. When compared GSH contents in these cell lines, the CDDP-resistant cell lines (KK and MH) had higher GSH levels than the sensitive cell lines (HRA), ratios of GSH content of KK and MH to that of HRA showing 1.93 and 4.84 respectively.

2. Effects of BSO and Cystine on the Intracellular GSH Levels

BSO is the specific inhibitor for γ-glutamyl cysteine synthetase and has ability to lower the intracellular GSH levels(9,10). To determine the effects of BSO on the intracellular GSH levels of HRA, KK and MH cells, cells were incubated in the absence or presence of 10, 25 and 50μM BSO. When the cellular GSH levels were examined after the 24h incubation, the GSH depletion by BSO occurred most rapidly in KK cells with high GSH levels before

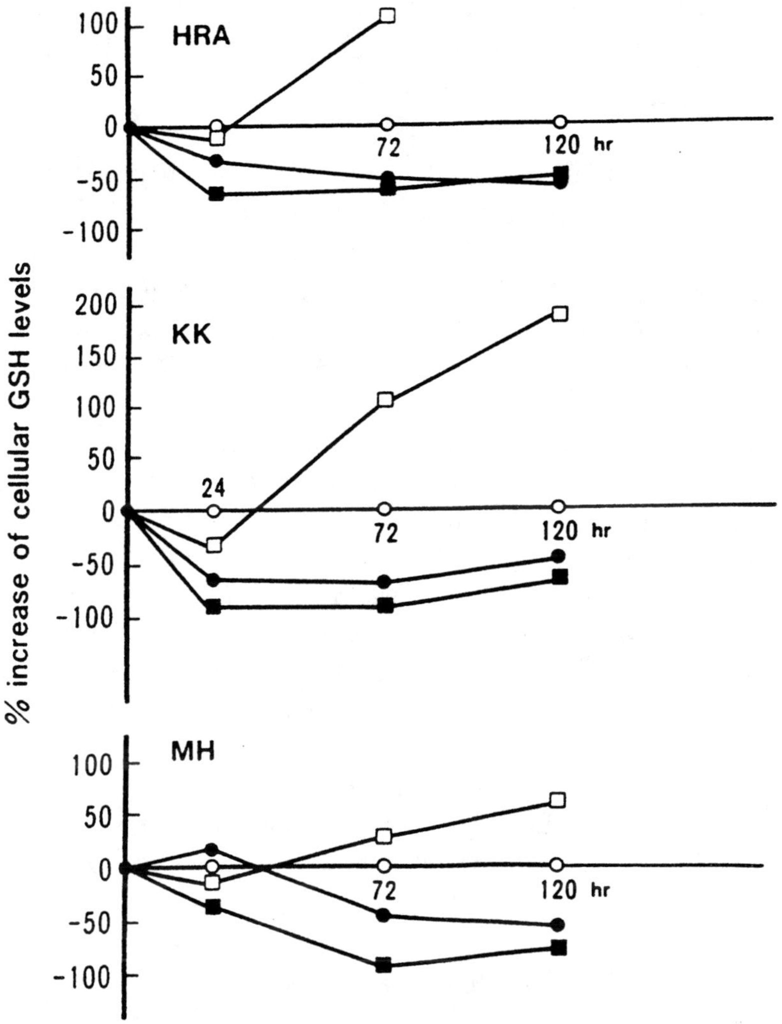

Fig.1 Effects of BSO or cystine on cellular GSH levels of ovarian cancer cells ○–○,Control; ●–●, BSO(1μM); □–□, cystine(25μM); ■–■ ,BSO(10μM).

incubation. When BSO was washed with fresh medium, the cellular GSH levels recovered to those of untreated cells after 48 h. If BSO was added after washing, the GSH levels remained depleted. The degree was more marked in KK and MH cells than in HRA cells. In addition, when these cell lines were exposed to 25μM cystine, the cellular GSH increased in a time-dependent fashion (Fig.1).

3. The Effects of BSO or Cystine on the CDDP Sensitivities of the Cancer Cells

Table 2 shows the effect of BSO or cystine on the CDDP sensitivities. In the CDDP-resistant cells (KK and MH), the GSH depletion by BSO resulted in sensitization to CDDP and its analogues. In MH cells the GSH elevation by cystine induced significant desensitization to CDDP, CBDCA and DWA2114R as shown in Fig.2, sensitivity of MH to DWA2114R was increased by BSO and decreased by cystine. On the other hand, in the CDDP sensitive HRA cells, BSO lowered rather than elevated the sensitivity to CBDCA and DWA2114R, and cystine elevated the sensitivity to CDDP and the analogues (Table2). Fig.3 shows the correlation between the drug sensitivity and the cellular GSH level. When the cellular GSH levels were changed by BSO or cystine, changes of the IC_{50} to CDDP and its analogues of the CDDP resistant KK and MH cells correlated with those of the cellular GSH levels while the IC_{50} values of the CDDP sensitive HRA cells remained unchanged.

From these results, we conclude that in the CDDP resistant (but not sensitive) cells, the cellular GSH levels are associated with CDDP sensitivity and depletion of GSH resulted in sensitization to CDDP and its analogues.

Discussion

The development of acquired resistance to CDDP represent a significant problem in the treatment of patients with cancer. Our results suggested that resistance to CDDP may be due in part to the elevated cellular GSH concentration. Similar observations have also been made by other investigators(11-14). CDDP can be inactivated by direct binding to the sulphydryl moiety of GSH, thereby preventing the drug from reaching the critical DNA.

Table 1 IC_{50} values of anticancer drugs and the cellular GSH levels of HRA, KK and MH cells

Drugs	HRA	KK	MH
CDDP	0.41[a]	1.20(2.93)[b]	1.50(3.66)
CBDCA	1.49	9.46(6.35)	9.99(6.70)
DWA2114R	1.22	11.21(9.19)	8.27(6.78)
GSH contents	33.4[c]	64.4(1.93)[d]	161.5(4.84)

a: Concentrations (μM) required for 50% inhibition of cell proliferation (IC_{50})
b: Ratio of IC_{50} of KK or MH cells to that of HRA cells
c: GSH concentrations (nmol/10^7 cells)
d: Ratio of GSH content in KK or MH cells to that in HRA cells.
Each value is the average from three experiments.

Table 2 Effects of BSO or cystine on drug sensitivity of ovarian cancer cells

			BSO		cystine	
cells	drugs	IC_{50}[a]	IC_{50}	IC_{50} ratio[b]	IC_{50}	IC_{50} ratio[c]
HRA	CDDP	0.41	0.31	75.6	0.36	89.1
	CBDCA	1.49	1.77	118.8	1.26	84.3
	DWA2114R	1.22	1.48	121.3	1.20	98.3.
KK	CDDP	1.20	0.83	69.2	1.11	92.8
	CBDCA	9.46	7.23	76.4	8.04	84.8
	DWA2114R	11.21	6.53	58.1	8.68	77.4.
MH	CDDP	1.50	1.19	79.5	1.70	113.4
	CBDCA	9.99	7.42	74.2	11.13	111.4
	DWA2114R	8.27	3.15	38.1	9.59	116.0

a: Concentrations (μM) required for 50% inhibition of cell proliferation. Contact time was 5 days.
b: Percent of IC_{50} in the presence of 10 μM BSO to IC_{50} in the absence of BSO
c: Percent of IC_{50} in the presence of 25 μM cystine to IC_{50} in the absence of cystine.
Each values is the average from three experiments.

Therefore, GSH depletion by BSO may be the potential novel strategies for overcoming the CDDP resistance. Some studies, however, have reported

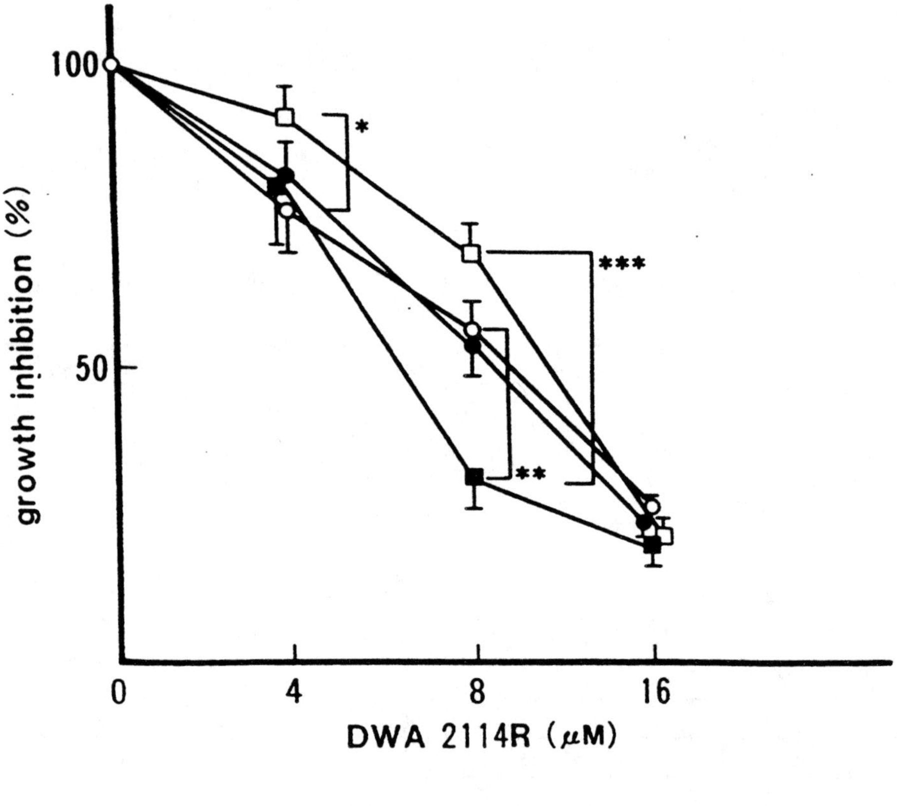

Fig. 2. Effects of BSO or cystine on MH cell growth inhibition by DWA2114R. Vertical bars shows Mean ±SD. ○–○,Control; ●–●, BSO(1μM); □–□, cystine(25μM); ■–■ ,BSO(10μM). *p<0.01, **p<0.002, *<p<0.001**

equal or hardly elevated levels of GSH in the CDDP sensitive and resistant cells(15), while other studies showed increased cellular GSH levels in the CDDP

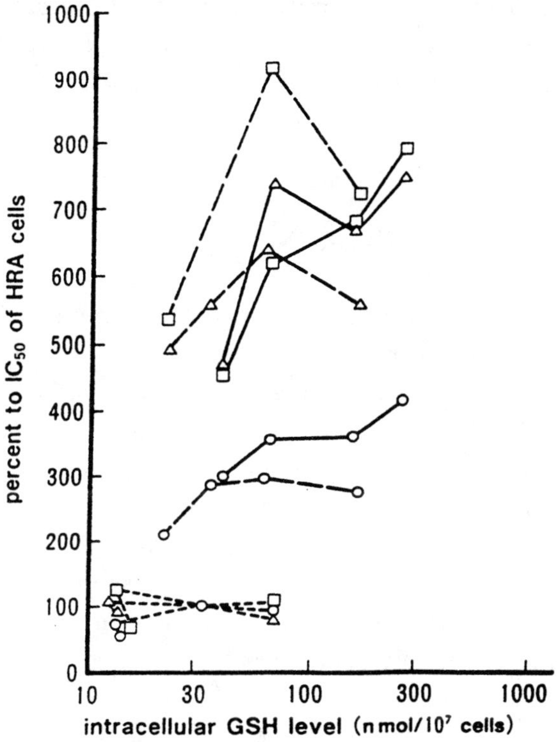

–O,Control; ●–●, BSO(1μM); □–□, cystine(25μM); ■–■ ,BSO(10μM).

Fig.3 Correlation between IC_{50} values to CDDP or it's analogues and intracellular GSH levels in human ovarian cancer cells. Each point shows average values from three separate experiments. Dotted lines, HRA; Interrupted lines, KK; Solid lines, MH. O ,CDDP; ▽,CBDCA; □,DWA2114R.

resistant cells without sensitization after GSH depletion with BSO(12,16). The mechanisms of CDDP resistance in most of cancer cells are multifactorial and the GSH metabolic system may be only one of various CDDP resistance mechanisms. Accordingly, in cancer cells which the CDDP-resistance seemed to be resulted in by high cellular GSH levels, depletion of GSH may induce sensitization to CDDP. However, our in vitro experiments of depletion of GSH demonstrated that BSO must be continuously administered to overcome CDDP resistance. Therefore, short-term depletion of GSH may not be sufficient to overcome resistance to CDDP. The clinical trials with BSO are on going(17). These results suggest that selection of patients in whom sensitization to CDDP by BSO will be expected may become the important issues for treatment with BSO.

REFERENCES

1. Godwin AK, Meister A, O'Dwyer PJ, Huang CS, Hamilton TC, Anderson ME. High resistance to cisplatin in human ovarian cancer cell lines is associated with marked increase of glutathione synthesis. *Proc Natl Acad Sci* USA 1992;89:3070-3074
2. Galivan J. Transport and metabolism of methotrexate in normal and resistant cultured rat hepatoma cells. *Cancer Res* 1979;39:735
3. Kamisango K, Matsumoto T, Akamatsu K, Morikawa K, Tashiro T, Koizumi K. Antitumor activity and cellular accumulation of a new platinum complex, (-)-(R)-2-aminomethylpyrrolidine(1,1-cyclobutanedicarboxylato) platinum(II) monohydrate, in cisplatin-sensitive and -resistant murine P388 leukemia cells. *Jpn J Cancer Res* 1992;83:304-311
4. Kikuchi Y, Kizawa I, Oomori K, Miyauchi M, Kita T, Sugita M, Tenjin Y. Establishment of a human ovarian cancer cell line capable of forming ascites in nude mice and effects of tranexamic acid on cell proliferation and ascites formation. *Cancer Res* 1987;47:592-596
5. Kikuchi Y, Hirata J, Kita T, Imaizumi E, Tode T, Nagata I. Enhancement of anti-proliferative effect of cis-diamminedichloroplatimum(II) by clomiphene and tamoxifen in human ovarian cancer cells. *Gynecol Oncol* 1993;49:365-372
6. Kudoh K, Kita T, Hirata J, Ishii K, Hiramatsu H, Kikuchi Y, Nagata I. Potentiation of cisplatin sensitivity of cisplatin-resistant human ovarian cancer cell lines by L-buthionine-S,R-sulfoximine. *Acta Obst Gynaec Jpn* 1994;46:525-532 (in Japanese)
7. Saotome K, Morita H, Umeda M. Cytotoxicity test with simplified crystal violet staining method using microtiter plates and its application to injection drugs. *Toxic In Vitro* 1989;3:317-321
8. Griffith OW. Determination of glutathione and glutathione disulfide using glutathione reductase and 2-vinyl pyridine. *Anal Biochem* 1980;106:207-212

9. Griffith OW, Meister A. Potent and specific inhibition of glutathione synthesis by buthionine sulfoximine (S-n-butyl homocysteine sulfoximine). *J Biol Chem* 1979;254:7558-7560
10. Griffith OW. Mechanism of action, metabolism, and toxicity of buthionine sulfoximine and its higher homologs, potent inhibitors of glutathione synthesis. *J Biol Chem* 1982;257:13704-13712
11. Hamilton TC, Winker MA, Louie KG, Batist G, Behrens BC, Tsuruo T, Grotzinger KR, McKoy NM, Young RC, Ozols RF. Augumentation of adryamycin, melpharan and cicplatin cytotoxicity in drug-resistant and sensitive human ovarian carcinoma cell lines by buthionine sulfoximine mediated glutahtione depletion. *Biochem Pharmacol* 1985;34:2583-2586
12. Richon VM, Schulte N, Eastman A. Mltiple mechanisms of resistance to cis-diamminedichloroplatinum(II) in murine leukemia L1210 cells. *Cancer Res* 1987;47:2056-2061
13. Hormos RA, Andrews PA, Murphy MP, Burns CP. Glutathione depletion reverse cisplatin resistance in murine L1210 leukemia cells. *Cancer Lett* 1987;34:9-13
14. Meijer C, Mulder NH, Hospers GAP, Uges DRA, deVries EGE. The role of glutathione in resistance to cisplatin in a human small cell lung cancer cell line. *Brit J Cancer* 1990;62:72-77
15. Begleiter A, Johnston JB. DNA cross-linking by 3'-(3-cyano-4-morpholinyl)-3'-deaminoadriamycin in HT-29 human colon carcinoma cells in vitro. *Biochem Biophys Res Commun* 1985;131:336-338
16. Andrews PA, Shiefer MA, Murphy MP, Howell SB. Enhanced potentiation of cisplatin cytotoxicity in human ovarian carcinoma cells by prolonged glutathione depletion. *Chem Biol Interact* 1988;65:51-58
17. Ozols RF. Roles of chemotherapy in the future treatment of ovarian cancer. *Acta Obstet Gynecol Scand Suppl* 1992;155:55-60

CHAPTER 3

INTRACELLULAR GLUTATHIONE LEVELS REGULATE PLATINUM-RESISTANCE IN OVARIAN CANCER CELL LINES

Kinya Hamaguchi, MD
Department of Obstetrics and Gynecology, Kurume University School of Medicine

We have previously reported a panel of human ovarian cancer cell lines with a wide range of cisplatin resistance developed in vitro by exposure to cisplatin. A panel of 5 platinum-resistant cell lines called C-series; C30, C50, C80, C100 and C200 exhibit primary resistance to cisplatin ranging 290- to 424-fold when compared to A2780, a parental cell line. These cells have increased GSH levels (13-to 42-fold) as compared with A2780 cell. Recently, we obtained revertant platinum-resistant variants(Rs) in a drug-free environment (*i.e.*, without cisplatin) for long periods of time (*i.e.*, at least 2 years). C30R and C200R increased sensitivity to cisplatin ranging from 2- to 3-fold, compared to the primary sensitivity of C30 and C 200 cells. In addition, the levels of GSH in the partial revertant cells (C30R and C200R) decreased in a range of one-half and one-fourth of those observed in C30 and C200 cells. These results substantiated the role of increased cellular GSH levels in the platinum-resistant phenotype. Moreover, cisplatin accumulation and platinum-DNA adducts in C30R and C200R cells increased to 1.5- and 2.0- fold of those in C30 and C200 cells in addition to an increase of the CDDP sensitivity. In addition, we utilized other human ovarian cancer cell lines; OVCAR5, derived from untreated ovarian cancer patient, and OVCAR10, derived from cisplatin/carboplatin-refractory ovarian cancer patient in order to determine whether the kinetic changes of GSH levels induced by cisplatin challenge may have an impact on cisplatin resistance. It is noteworthy that OVCAR10 showed of 4-fold increase while OVCAR5 showed a decrease of GSH levels at 24 hrs, as compared to each initial level. In conclusion, both the role of initial GSH steady state concentration *per se* and the kinetic changes induced by cisplatin challenge may be possible factors determining cellular response to cisplatin in the development of cisplatin resistance.

INTRODUCTION

Platinum complexes are the primary agents used in the treatment of ovarian cancer, yielding response rates of 40-60% (1) (2). However, long-term survival of these patients has not, thus far, paralleled favorable response rates(3). Majority of these patients relapse after responding to initial chemotherapy and die of their chemo-refractory disease. The primary factor that has limited success of chemotherapy in ovarian cancer is the emergence of drug resistance in the tumor cell population, leading subsequent death. One approach with the potential to improve the treatment for ovarian cancer is to identify the mechanisms responsible for the complex resistance phenotype observed clinically and exploit pharmacological approaches to prevent the emergence of drug resistance or to reverse the phenotype when it occurs.

Resistance to platinum agents is multifactorial including [1] decreased cell-associated drug, [2] altered drug inactivation, and [3] increased DNA damage tolerance or repair (4,5). Of these mechanisms, increased drug inactivation, mediated by glutathione (GSH), is a crucial mechanism with potential to contribute to primary cisplatin resistance in ovarian cancer. We and others have shown that increased GSH levels are associated with increased resistance to cisplatin in some ovarian cancer cell lines, and other human tumor cell lines (6-9). Interestingly, a strong correlation has been demonstrated between GSH levels and resistance to platinum drugs in a panel of ovarian cancer cell lines. Buthionine sulfoximine (BSO), an inhibitor of γ-gulutamylcysteine synthetase (GCS) which catalyzes the rate-limiting step in GSH biosynthesis and results in reduced cellular glutathione levels, has been synthesized. Hamilton *et al.* (6) observed that treatment of cisplatin-sensitive and -resistant ovarian cancer cell lines with BSO resulted in a 70-90% reduction in intracellular GSH levels and a 1.8-to 4.3-fold increase in cisplatin cytotoxicity. These results has prompted clinical trials of BSO in combination with melphalan against drug-refractory cancer patients indicationg that this combination may be administered with lower toxicity while effectively lowering GSH levels in normal tissues and tumor cells.

In the present work, we further examined GSH synthesis including its kinetic changes induced by cisplatin challenge in cisplatin-resistant human ovarian cancer cell lines.

MATERIAL AND METHODS

All cell lines used in this experiments are summarized in Table 1. All cell lines were maintained as previously reported (10). Cytotoxicity was determined by tetrazolium reduction (MTT) assay, as previously described (11). Briefly, cytotoxicity was based on MTT assay staining 72 hrs after drug treatment. Percent survival was determined as relative percents to untreated control values (percent survival = staining units for treated cells / staining units of untreated control ¥ 100). Intracellular glutathione (GSH) levels and glutathione S-transferase activity (GST) were determined as previously described (10). Cells were exposed to cisplatin for 4 hrs before harvesting. Cell-associated platinum was measured by atomic absorption spectrometry (AAS). Briefly, cells harvested by trypsinization were incubated for 48 hrs in 0.5 ml concentrated nitric acid at the room temperature. Aliquots of the resulting clear, yellow solution were analyzed directly by AAS. Approximately 125 μg of each purified DNA sample after removal of contaminating RNA was extracted with phenol/iso-amyl alcohol, re-precipitated with ethanol and resuspended in 130 ml of 5% HCl. The absorbance at 260 nm was measured in the resulting hydrolysate and the platinum content was determined by AAS. Details were described previously (12). Total cellular RNA was isolated from the cell lines by a one step guanidinium isothiocyanate-phenol chloroform extraction procedure. Total RNA (16μg/per lane) was denatured in 50% formamide containing 7.4% formaldehyde and separated by electrophoresis on an agarose gel and blotted. Expression of γ-glutamyl transpeptidase (13) was analyzed by northern blot analysis. In order to examine the kinetic changes of cellular GSH, cells were treated with cisplatin continuously for 24 hrs, and each cell was collected at 0, 3, 6, 12, and 24 hrs for GSH determination.

RESULTS

RELATIONSHIP BETWEEN PLATINUM-RESISTANCE AND GSH LEVELS

C-series are the platinum-resistant variants derived from A2780 after nearly continuous exposure to the indicated concentrations of cisplatin-i.e., C30 = 30 μM; C200 = 200 μM. as shown in Table 1. C30 exhibited marked increase in resistance (273-fold) to cisplatin. C200 was more than 400-fold higher than that of A2780. There was good correlation between the magnitude of resistance and the increase of cellular GSH; a plot of fold-resistance against cellular GSH was essentially linear (r = 0.94) (11). C200 had about a 50-fold increase in cellular GSH. Revertant platinum-resistant

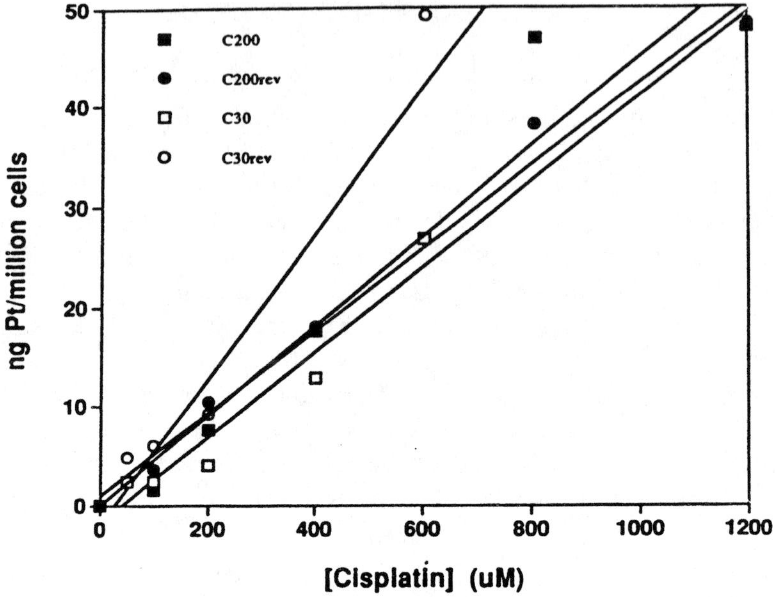

Fig.1. Cell-associated platinum of C30, C200 and each revertant platinum-variants (Rs) measured by atomic absorption spectrometry (AAS). Cells were exposed to various concentrations of cisplatin indicated for 4 hrs before harvest.

variants of C30 and C200; C30R and C200R, obtained in a drug-free environment for at least 2 years exhibited about a 2-fold and 3-fold decrease in platinum resistance, respectively. These revertant-cell lines showed about a 2-fold and 4 fold decrease in cellular GSH. No difference in GST activity was observed among parental and platinum-resistant variants. These data are shown in Table 2.

Cell-associated Cisplatin and Pt-DNA Adducts in Revertants

Cells were exposed to cisplatin for 4 hrs at increasing concentrations (Fig.1 and 2). At a point of 600 μM of cisplatin, C30R had a 2 fold increase in platinum-accumulation, although not significantly observed in C200R (Fig.1). Likewise, C30R had about 2-fold increase in Pt-DNA adduct, while C200R had a 1.5 fold increase at a point of 800 μM of cisplatin (Fig.2).

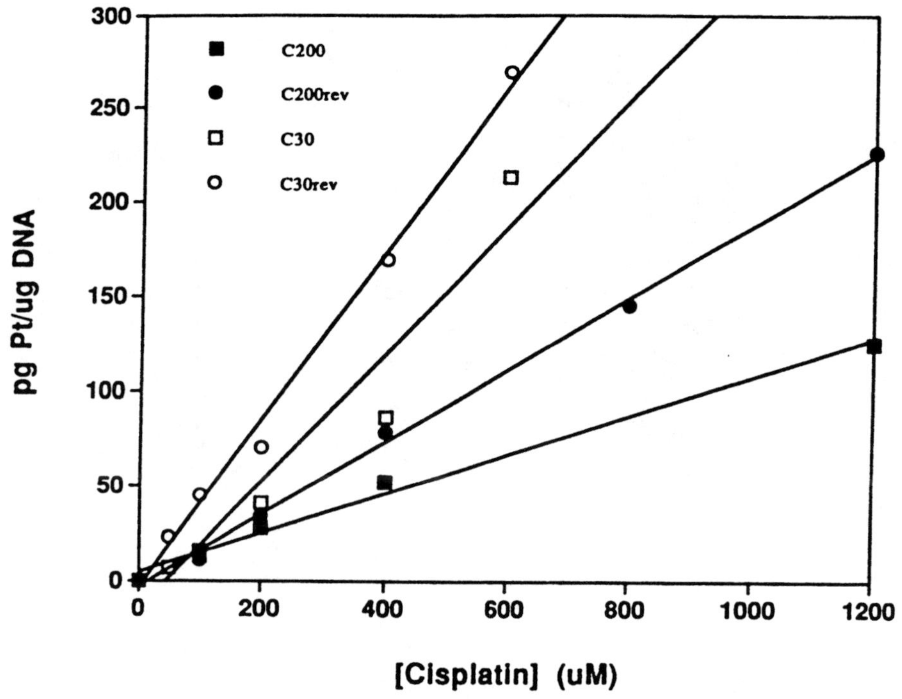

Fig.2. Pt-DNA adduct of C30, C200 and each Rs measured by AAS.

γ-GLUTAMYL TRANSPEPTIDASE (GT) EXPRESSION IN REVERTANTS

To evaluate an alternative pathway involved in regulation of cellular GSH, we examined expression levels of the γ-GT mRNA of revertants and parental platinum-resistant variants in Fig.3. As previously reported (10), C200 showed a dramatic increase (40-fold) in γ-GT steady state mRNA levels. C30R, C80R (2-fold decrease in platinum-resistance and cellular GSH, although not described in this work), and C200R showed a marked decrease with a range of 3- to 10-fold in the expression of γ-GT, in an association with a similar decrease in platinum-resistance.

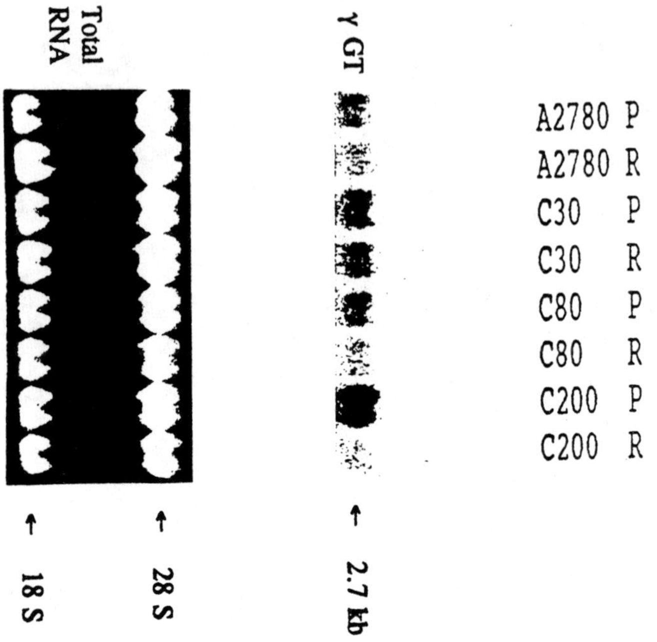

Fig. 3. Expression of γ -glutamyl transpeptidase(GT) genes by Northern blot analysis in C-series and each Rs. A2780 is a parental cell line and A2780R is essentially the same. C80 and C80R (highly resistant variants between C30 and C200) were also examined.

THE KINETIC CHANGES OF CELLULAR GSH CHALLENGED BY EXPOSURE TO CISPLATIN

OVCAR10 was about a 30-fold higher than OVCAR5 in platinum-resistance by MTT assay (data not shown), reflecting treatment status when established (Table 1). However, OVCAR5 an OVCAR10 cells had similar cellular GSH levels, respectively. In order to elucidate the mechanism involved in platinum-resistance between these cell lines, we examined the kinetic changes of cellular GSH challenged by cisplatin exposure (Fig.4). Cells were exposed to 100 μM cisplatin for 24 hrs, continuously, and harvested at 5 points during treatment. Very interestingly, OVCAR5, a cisplatin sensitive cell line, showed a rapid 2-fold increase of GSH within 6 hours, as compared to initial 3 hrs, subsequently showing a gradual decrease toward 24 hrs of treatment. On the other hand, OVCAR10, a cisplatin-resistant cell line, exhibited a dramatic increase in cellular GSH, resulted in 4-fold increase at 24 hrs.

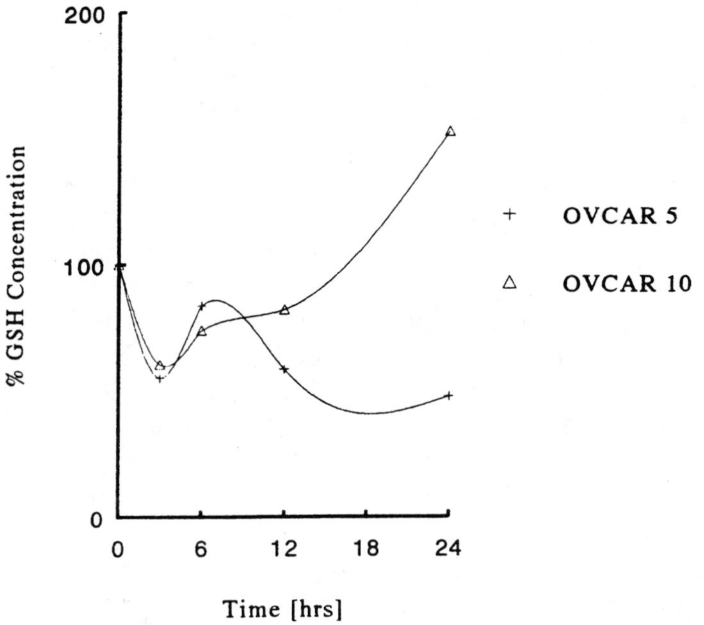

Fig. 4. The kinetic changes of cellular GSH of OVCAR5 and OVCAR10 cells. Cells were continuously exposed to cisplatin for 24 hrs. Cells were harvested at 0, 3, 6 and 24 hrs for GSH determination. Percent GSH concentrations were calculated by initial GSH level of each cell line. Each point was means of triplicate determinations.

DISCUSSION

The manner in which glutathione (GSH) potentiates cisplatin resistance is unknown. Possibilities include GSH-mediated transport alternation, formation of GSH-platinum conjugate, and participation in DNA repair (4). As shown in Table 2, there was a strong correlation between GSH levels and resistance to cisplatin in a panel of cisplatin-resistant ovarian cancer cell lines. Moreover, it has been first demonstrated that reversal of cisplatin resistance is associated with decreased GSH levels in revertant cell lines. This is the strong data suggesting the direct contribution of cellular GSH levels to the platinum-resistant phenotype. These accumulated data led to clinical study demonstrating that the simple measurement of GSH in peripheral-blood erythrocyte might allow prediction of the probable response to chemotherapy and identification of individuals who might benefit by GSH depletion(14).

Increased -cisplatin accumulation and -platinum-DNA adducts was shown to be associated with increase in cisplatin cytotoxicity in some extent. Recently, some studies have suggested a role for increased DNA repair activity as a factor in the cisplatin resistance (15-18). Platinum agents react with cellular DNA to form both intra- and inter- strand crosslinks, which interfere with the DNA replication(19). The adducts formed by the reaction of platinum with DNA are thought to be ultimately responsible for the cytotoxic effect of the drug. Moreover, increased expression of the ERCC-1 excision repair gene has been detected in cisplatin resistant cells (data no shown). Our laboratory recently reported that ERCC-1 expression levels may have a role in clinical cisplatin resistance, utilizing tumor tissues from 26 ovarian cancer patiens(20). Some efforts to restore cisplatin sensitivity to resistant ovarian cancer cells using DNA repair inhibitors such as aphidicolin, and inhibitor of DNA polymerase α and γ have been done, indicating association of these DNA repair inhibitors with enhanced cisplatin cytotoxicity(21). Moreover, quenching of cisplatin-DNA monoadducts by GSH may also occur in cells to prevent the formation of crosslink(22). Thus, investigation on DNA repair inhibition is a potential strategy for reversal and detection of cisplatin resistance. Expression of γ-glutamyl transpeptidase(GT) decreased with decrease of cisplatin resistance. The regulation of cellular GSH depends upon not only the ability of γ-glutamylcystein synthetase (GCS), a rate-limiting enzyme catalyzing the initial step of GSH synthesis, but also the availability of cysteine moieties whose derivation from extracellular glutathione and transport into the cell involves in the activity of γ-GT (13). These results strongly support that GSH synthesis directly contribute to acquired cisplatin resistance and modulation of GSH levels may be a notable strategy for the reversal of cisplatin resistance. Thus, clinical trials of BSO plus melphalan have been shown to result in lowering effects of GSH levels in normal tissues and tumor cells of cancer patients with low toxicity (23).

In addition, the kinetic changes of GSH by cisplatin appears quite interesting. As shown in Fig.4, ovarian cancer cell lines with the consistent steady-state GSH levels showed the differencial kinetic changes of GSH by cisplatin treatment. In fact, OVCAR10, cell lines derived from platinum-refractory ovarian cancer patients, showed marked increase in GSH levels, whereas OVCAR5, a sensitive cell line, from untreated patient showed decrease in GSH levels. This preliminary result implied that potential activity of GSH synthesis may play an important role in clinical cisplatin resistance. Other laboratories reported that the GSH level of a sensitive ovarian cancer cell line decreased while that of a resistant ovarian cancer cell line increased, when exposed clinically relevant dose of adriamycin, indicating that changes in cellular GSH concentration during treatment may be an important indicator of tumor cell response to adriamycin(24). These data are consistent with our data shown in Fig.4. Further investigation revealed elevated GSH levels in human ovarian tumors following induction chemotherapy, suggesting an association with the clinical development of acquired

Table 1. Human ovarian cancer cell lines

Cell line	Treatment[a]	Comment
A2780	Untreated	-
C30, C200		Platinum-resistant variants obtained after continuous exposure of A2780 to the indicated concentrations of cisplatin (30μM or 200 μM). C30=30μM: C200=200 μM.
OVCAR5	Untreated	-
OVCAR10	CDDP, CBDCA	Progressive disease CDDP-based regimen, high-dose CDDP (200mg/m^2), and high-dose CBDCA (800mg/m^2).

[a]Treatment status when established.

Table 2. GSH levels in platinum-resistant and its revertant-human ovarian cancer cell lines

	IC_{50} [a] (Fold-resistant)		GSH[b] (Fold GSH increase)		GST Activity[c]
Cell line	Parental	Revertant	Parental	Revertant	Parental
A2780	0.37(1)	0.34(1)	1.4(1)	1.6(1)	1.3
C30	101(273)	45(132)	27.8(20)	16.5(11)	1.1
C200	150(450)	47(138)	63.1(49)	19.1(12)	1.1

[a]Cytotoxicity was determined by MTT assay continuously exposed for 72 hrs. The IC_{50} is concentration of cisplatin (μM) which inhibited growth by 50%. [b]Total glutathione [GSH+1/2 glutathione (GSSG)] is shown as nmol per 10^6 cells. [c]Glutathione S-transferase (GST) activity with 1-chloro-2, 4-dinitrobenzene is reported as nmol/min per 10^6 cells.

resistance to alkylating agents (25). This clinical data, which are in agreement with in vitro data on cultured ovarian cancer cells including our present data, implies that kinetic changes of GSH levels may be a determinant of cellular and clinical response to chemotherapy.

In conclusion, further investigation on GSH synthesis may reveal mechanisms of complex cisplatin resistance, and may contribute to find out effective strategies to overcome clinical cisplatin-resistance.

ACKNOWLEDGMENTS

The author thanks Drs Yakushiji, Godwin, Jonnson, Ozols, and Hamilton for critical discussions.

REFERENCES

1. Ozols, R.F. Chemotherapy for advanced epithelial ovarian cancer. *Hematol. Oncol. Clin. North Am.*, 6: 879-894, 1992.
2. Advanced Ovarian Cancer Trialists Group. Chemotherapy in advanced ovarian cancer: an overview of randomized clinical trials. *Br. Med. J.*, 303: 884-893, 1991.
3. Ozols, R.F., and Young, R.C. Chemotherapy of ovarian cancer *Semin. Oncol.*, 11: 251-263, 1984.
4. Johnson, S.W., Ozols, R. F., Hamilton, T. C. Mechanisms of drug resistance in ovarian cancer. *Cancer*, 71: 644-649, 1993.
5. Friedlander, M.L. Drug resistance in ovarian cancer. *Int. J. Gynecol. Cancer*, 1: 2-9, 1992.
6. Hamilton, T.C., Winker, M.A., Louie, K. G., Batist, G., Behrens, B.C., Tsuruo, T., Grotzinger K.R., Mckoy, W.M., Winker, M.A., Young, R. C. and Ozols, R. F. Augmentation of adriamycin, melphalan, and cisplatin cytotoxicity in drug resistant and sensitive human ovarian cancer cell lines by buthionine sulfoximine mediated depletion. *Biochem. Pharmacol.* 34: 2583-2586, 1985.
7. Lewis. A.D., Hayes, J.D., Wolf, C. R. Glutathione and glutathione-dependent enzymes in ovarian adenocarcinoma cell lines derived from a patient before and after the onset of drug resistance: intrinsic differences and cell cycle effects. *Carcinogenesis*. 9: 1283-1287, 1988.
8. Misty, P., Kelland, L. R, Able. G., Sidhar, S. and Harrap, K. R. The relationships between glutathione, glutathione S-transferase and cytotoxicity of platinum drugs and melphalan in eight human ovarian cancer cell lines. *Br. J. cancer* 65: 215-220, 1991.

9. Batist, G. Serial determination of glutathione levels and glutathione-related enzyme activities in human tumor cells in vitro. *Biochem. Pharmacol.* 31: 2257-2259, 1986.
10. Godwin, A. K., Meister, A., O'Dwyer, P. J., Huang, C.S., Hamilton, T. C. and Anderson, M. E. High resistance to cisplatin in human ovarian cancer cell lines is associated with marked increase of glutathione synthesis. *Proc. Natl. Acad. Sci.* USA. 89: 3070-3074, 1992.
11. Hamaguchi, K., Godwin, A.K., Yakushiji, M., O'Dwyer, P.J., Ozols, R.F. and Hamilton, T.C. Cross-resistance to diverse drugs is associated with primary cisplatin resistance in ovarian cancer cell lines. *Cancer Res.* 53: 5225-5232, 1993.
12. Johnson, S.W., Perez, R.P., Godwin, A. K., Yeung, A.T., Handel, L.M., Ozols, R. F. and Hamilton, T.C. Role of platinum-DNA adduct formation and removal in cisplatin resistance in human ovarian cancer cell lines. *Biochem. Pharmacol.* 47: 689-697, 1994.
13. Meister, A. Novel Drugs that affect glutathione metabolism. In: Woolley, P.V. III, Tew, K.D., editors. *Mechanisms of drug resistance in neoplastic cells.* San Diego: Academic Press, pp. 99-126, 1988.
14. Hercbergse, A., Brok-Simoni, F., Holtzman, F., Bar-am, J., Leith, J.T. and Brenner, H.J. Erythrocyte glutathione and tumor response to chemotherapy. *The Lancet.* 339: 10874-1076, 1992.
15. Lai, G.M., Ozols, R.F., Smyth, J.F., Young, R. C. and Hamilton, T.C. Enhanced DNA repair and resistance to cisplatin in human ovarian cancer. *Biochem. Pharmacol.* 37: 4597-4600, 1988.
16. Masuda, H., Ozols, R.F., Lai, G.M., Fojo, A., Rothenberg, A. and Hamilton, T.C., Increased DNA repair as a mechanism of acquired resistance to cis-diamminedichloroplatinum (II) in human ovarian cancer cell lines. *Cancer Res.* 48: 5713-5716. 1988.
17. Masuda, H., Tanaka, T., Kusaka, I. Increased removal of DNA-bound platinum in a human ovarian cancer cell line resistant to cis-diamminedichloroplatinum (II). *Cancer Res.* 50: 1863-1866, 1990.
18. Eastman, A. The formation, isolation and characterization of DNA adducts produced by anticancer platinum complex. *Pharmaco. Ther.* 34: 181-192, 1987.
19. Parker, P. J., Eastman, A., Bostick-Burton, F. and Reed, E. Acquired cisplatin resistance in human ovarian cancer cells is associated with enhanced repair of cisplatin-DNA lesions and reduced drug accumulation. *J. Clin. Invest.* 87: 772-777, 1991.
20. Dabholkar, M., Bostick-Burton, F., Weber, C., Bohr, V.A., Egwugagu, C. and Reed E. ERCC1 and ERCC2 expression in malignant tissues from ovarian cancer patients. *J. Natl Cancer Inst.* 84: 1512-1517, 1992.
21. Kalz, E. J., Andrews, P.A. and Howell, S.B. The effect of DNA polymerase inhibitors on the cytotoxicity of cisplatin in human ovarian carcinoma cells. *Cancer Commun.* 2: 159-164, 1990.

22. Lai, G.M., Ozols, R.F., Young, R.C. and Hamilton, T.C. Effects of glutathione on DNA repair in cisplatin-resistant ovarian cancer cell lines. *J. Natl. Cancer Inst.* 81: 535-539, 1989.
23. O'Dwyer, P.J., Hamilton, T.C., Young, R.C., Carp, N. Tew, K.D., Paravic, K. and Ozols, R.F. Depletion of glutathione in normal and malignant human cells in vivo by buthionine sulfoximine: clinical and biochemical results. *J. Natl. Cancer Inst.* 84; 264-267, 1992.
24. Lee, F. Y. F., Siemann,m D.W. and Sutherland, R.M. Changes in cellular glutathione content during adriamycin treatment in human ovarian cancer- a possible indicator of chemosensitivity. *Br. J. Cancer*. 60: 291-298, 1989.
25. Britten, R.A., Green, J.A. and Warenius, H.M. Cellular glutathione (GSH) and gultathione S-transferase (GST) activity in human ovarian tumor biopsies following exposure to alkylating agents. *I J. Radiation Oncology Biol.* 24: 527-531, 1992.

CHAPTER 4

EFFECTS OF ANTIESTROGEN BINDING SITE LIGAND, N,N-DIETHYL-2-[4-(PHENYL-METHYL)PHENOXY]ETHANAMINE-HCL ON ANTITUMOR ACTIVITY OF CIS-DIAMMINE-DICHLOROPLATINUM(II) IN HUMAN OVARIAN CANCER CELL BEARING NUDE MICE

Hisakazu Hiramatsu*, Yoshihiro Kikuchi, Kenji Yamamoto, Kazuya Kudoh,Junko Hirata, Tsunekazu Kita, Ichiro Nagata[1],and Lorne J. Brandes[2]

[1]Department of Obstetrics and Gynecology, National Defense Medical College, Namiki 3-2, Tokorozawa, Saitama 359,Japan; and [2]Department of Internal Medicine and Pharmacology & Therapeutics, Faculty of Medicine, University of Manitoba, The Manitoba Institute of Cell Biology, 100 Olivia Street, Winnipeg, Manitoba, Canada R3E 0V9

SUMMARY

Tamoxifen has several estrogen receptor independent antitumor effects. Some of them are thought to be through inhibition of protein kinase C (PKC), or through binding to antiestrogen binding site. N,N-Diethyl-2-[(4-phenylmethyl)-phenoxy]ethanamine-HCl.(DPPE) is a novel synthetic ligand, which binds to the microsomal antiestrogen binding site. Brandes et al. have demonstrated that DPPE enhances antiproliferative effects of doxorubicin and 5-fluorouracil on the

* Correspondence to Hisakazu Hiramatsu, M.D., Department of Obstetrics and Gynecology, National Defense Medical College, Namiki 3-2, Tokorozawa, Saitama 359, Japan

tumor growth in tumor-bearing mice. In this study we attempted to enhance antitumor activity of *cis*-diamminedichloroplatinum(II) (CDDP) by DPPE in nude mice bearing human ovarian cancer cells. Regarding the effect on the tumor growth,a synergistic effect by combinations of high doses(25 and 50 mg/kg) of DPPE with CDDP was obtained without any significant prolongation of the survival time because of adverse side effects. On the other hand, when low doses(5 and 10 mg/kg) of DPPE were combined with CDDP, a significant prolongation of the survival time was obtained without a significant inhibitory effect on the tumor growth.

Keywords:
N,N-Diethyl-2-[(4-phenylmethyl)phenoxy]ethanamine-HCl; Antiestrogen binding site ligand-*Cis*-Diamminedichloroplatinum(II); Ovarian cancer cells.

INTRODUCTION

In 1984, Brandes and Hermonat synthesized a paradiphenylmethane derivative,N,N-diethyl-2-[4-(phenylmethyl)phenoxy]ethanamine-HCl.(DPPE) (1), in an attempt to find a ligand selective for the microsomal antiestrogen binding site(AEBS) (2), but not the estrogen receptor (3). The chemical structure of DPPE resembles the prototype AEBS ligand,tamoxifen(TAM) and classical histamine(H_1)-antagonists such as phenyltoloxamine and diphenhydramine (Fig.1).

Binding studies using [^{3}H]tamoxifen revealed that AEBS exists in rat brain membranes, rat liver, chicken liver, and MCF-7 cell line (4). In rat liver microsomes, DPPE competes potently for AEBS labelled by [^{3}H]tamoxifen and for an equal number of low affinity sites labelled by [^{3}H]histamine (5). Based on these studies, Brandes et al. (6) have demonstrated that AEBS is a histamine binding site with low(μM) affinity different from classical H_1, H_2 histamine receptors. And they named AEBS H_{IC} receptor to denote their intracellular location.

Through binding to the H_{IC}, intracellular histamine regulates cell proliferation. DPPE modulates the growth of transformed or malignant cells with a bell-shaped dose-response curve. At low doses (1 to 4 mg/kg), DPPE accelerates tumor growth in rodents (7), while as the doses of DPPE is increased

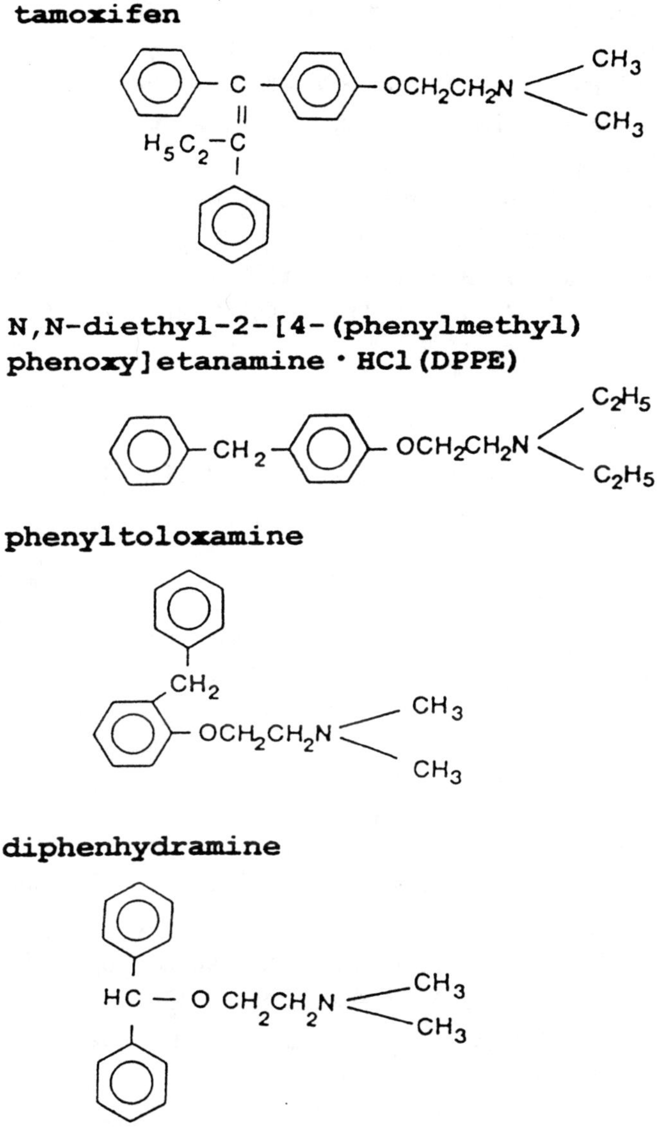

Fig.1. Chemical structures of tamoxifen, N,N-diethyl-2-[4-(phenylmethyl)phenoxy]ethanamine.HCl (DPPE), phenyltoloxamine and diphenhydramine.

the growth promotion decreases, and high doses of DPPE were antiproliferative/cytotoxic to 40 of 40 murine or human cancer cell lines tested in the National Cancer Institute screening panel (8). In tumor-bearing mice, DPPE(4 to 50 mg/kg) significantly potentiates the cytotoxicity of antineoplastic drugs such as doxorubicin and 5-fluorouracil to C-3 fibrosarcoma and B16 melanoma cells (9).

Cis-diamminedichloroplatinum (II) (CDDP) is a key drug in the treatment of ovarian cancer, but emergence of the drug resistance is common and the survival rate still seems to be unsatisfactory. Thus in this study we attempted to determine combined effects of DPPE with CDDP in vivo, using a human ovarian cancer cell line.

Materials and Methods

Chemicals

CDDP was obtained from Bristol-Myers Squibb Co. Ltd. (Tokyo, Japan). DPPE was kindly supplied by Dr. Lorne J. Brandes.These drugs were dissolved and diluted with medium or saline to the desired concentrations prior to use.

Cells

KF cells were established from tissue of a patient with serous cystadenocarcinoma of the ovary in 1982 [9]. The cells were incubated in RPMI 1640 medium supplemented with 10% fetal calf serum, 2 mM glutamine, 100 units penicillin/ml and 100 μg streptomycin/ml (GIBCO, Grand Island, NY) in 5% CO^2 at 37°C. The medium was changed every 3 days, and the cells were passaged when they reached confluence.

Nude Mice

About 6-week-old female BALB/c nude mice were obtained from Japan Clea Laboratories, Tokyo, Japan, and maintained in a pathogen-free environment. They were inspected daily and tumor growth was determined with a caliper.

When necessary, they were killed and dissected. The tumor tissues were fixed in formalin for histological examination. The larger tumors (more than 2cm in diameter) contained a larger necrotic area in the center. Distant metastases were not observed during the experimental period. Unless treated, all mice with tumor died of tumor burden within 150 days of tumor inoculation.

IN VIVO TREATMENT

To determine the effect of CDDP and DPPE on the tumor growth and the survival time, 5×10^5 KF cells were inoculated s.c. into the right flank of nude mice. From 7 days after tumor inoculation, treatment with CDDP and DPPE was initiated as follows: Group 1 (n=6), medium alone was administered i.p. once a week for 6 weeks; group 2 (n=6), 2 mg/kg CDDP alone was administered i.p. once a week for 6 weeks; group 3 (n=8), 5 mg/kg DPPE alone was administered i.p. once a week for 6 weeks; group 4 (n=7), 10 mg/kg DPPE alone was administered i.p. once a week for 6 weeks; group 5 (n=7), 25 mg/kg DPPE alone was administered i.p. once a week for 6 weeks; group 6 (n=7), 50 mg/kg DPPE alone was administered i.p. once a week for 6 weeks; group 7 (n=9), 2 mg/kg CDDP and 5 mg/kg DPPE were simultaneously administered i.p. once a week for 6 weeks; group 8 (n=9), 2 mg/kg CDDP and 10 mg/kg DPPE were simultaneously administered i.p. once a week for 6 weeks; group 9 (n=7), 2 mg/kg CDDP and 25 mg/kg DPPE were simultaneously administered i.p. once a week for 6 weeks; group 10 (n=7), 2 mg/kg CDDP and 50 mg/kg DPPE were simultaneously administered i.p. once a week for 6 weeks. At the time of tumor inoculation, every group contained 10 mice, but 7 days after tumor inoculation mice without tumor were excluded. Each injection was given in a 0.15 ml volume. The tumor growth was determined by the measurement of diameters of the tumor nodule in two dimensions with a caliper once a week. Tumor volume (cm^3) was calculated according to the following formula: $4\pi/3 \times (r_1 + r_2)^3 /8$, where r_1 is the longitudinal radius and r_2 is the transverse radius. Blood from a tail vein was collected into hematocrit tubes every two weeks and the hematocrit values and body weight were recorded for monitoring the side effects of drugs.

RESULTS

As shown in Table 1, 10-50 mg/kg DPPE alone did not seem to have any effect on the tumor growth and the survival, while 5 mg/kg DPPE tended to enhance rather than inhibit the tumor growth. Regarding the effect on the tumor growth, combinations of high doses (25 and 50 mg/kg) of DPPE with CDDP inhibited significantly more markedly the tumor growth compared to not only CDDP alone but also DPPE alone, showing a synergistic effect (Fig.2). However, the combinations of high doses of DPPE with CDDP failed to result in a significant prolongation of the survival time compared to CDDP or DPPE alone, because of adverse side effects as confirmed by monitoring the hematocrit

Table 1. Effects of DPPE and CDDP on the tumor growth, the mean survival time, the hematocrit and the body weight

Treatment	Tumor volume(cm^3	Survival time(days)	Hematocrit(%)	Body weight(g)
Untreated	4.57±0.47	78.7±18.0	53.4±1.0	23.1±1.0
CDDP(2mg/kg) alone	5.20±0.46	94.8±17.9	50.1±2.0	22.1±1.1
DPPE(5mg/kg) alone	6.18±1.17	87.1±32.0	52.1±1.5	21.8±1.6
DPPE(10mg/kg) alone	4.86±1.82	72.1±24.9	53.1±1.9	22.5±0.5
DPPE(25mg/kg) alone	4.06±1.74	66.9±25.4	51.9±0.8	20.5±1.0
DPPE(50mg/kg) alone	4.64±1.77	66.7±23.3	49.8±2.5	19.4±1.5
CDDP+DPPE(5 mg/kg)	5.55±1.88	116.8±10.3*	51.7±1.7	20.5±2.1
CDDP+DPPE(1 0mg/kg)	4.77±1.29	127.1±9.5*	50.7±2.0	20.5±2.1
CDDP+DPPE (25mg/kg)	1.12±0.81*	97.3±27.5	45.1±3.7*	18.5±1.2*
CDDP+DPPE (50mg/kg)	1.73±0.75*	98.9±32.7	43.9±3.9*	18.0±1.7*

Tumor volume, hematocrit and body weight were measured at 49 days after tumor inoculation. Results are the mean SD. *p<0.05, compared to untreated and CDDP alone.

and the body weight (Table 1). On the other hand, when low doses (5 and 10 mg/kg) of DPPE were combined with CDDP, the survival time was significantly prolonged without any significant side effect regardless of failure to inhibit the tumor growth.

DISCUSSION

Tamoxifen therapy benefits not only pre-menopausal estrogen receptor-positive breast cancer patients but also post-menopausal estrogen receptor-negative ones. Tamoxifen is also starting to be used with some success in the treatment of other cancers, including malignant gliomas, malignant melanoma and hepatocellular carcinoma (4). Some of the estrogen receptor-independent responses of cancer cells to tamoxifen may be attributed to interactions of tamoxifen with cellular membranes and binding of tamoxifen to microsomal AEBS. We have demonstrated that tamoxifen and clomiphene can potentiate antitumor activity of CDDP in the estrogen receptor-negative ovarian cancer cells by enhancing the CDDP uptake (10) and by inhibition of translocation of the protein kinase C activity from cytosol to cytoplasmic membrane (11). The chemosensitizing effect of tamoxifen on CDDP may also be attributed to binding to AEBS. In the recent study, we have proved that DPPE has a marked antiproliferative effect on various estrogen receptor-negative human ovarian cancer cell lines in vitro(12). The IC_{50} values of these cell lines to DPPE seemed to be similar to that reported for MCF-7 cells (6). It has been reported that both L1210 leukemia and colon 26 adenocarcinoma cells were more efficiently killed by combinations of L-histidinol and CDDP (13).Similarly,DPPE has also been shown to increase therapeutic index of antineoplastic drugs but not CDDP in mice (9).

Thus, we investigated the effect of AEBS ligand, DPPE alone on the tumor growth in vivo and whether DPPE can augment antitumor activity of CDDP. Ten to 50 mg/kg DPPE alone did not seem to have any effect on the tumor growth, while 5 mg/kg DPPE tended to enhance rather than inhibit the tumor growth. Brandes et al.(14) have ascertained that DPPE promotes the tumor growth at low dose and inhibit it at high dose, showing a bell-shaped dose-response curve. They assumed that potency to bind AEBS (H_{IC}) may correlate with tumor growth-promoting activity. Similarly, it is well known that some H_1-

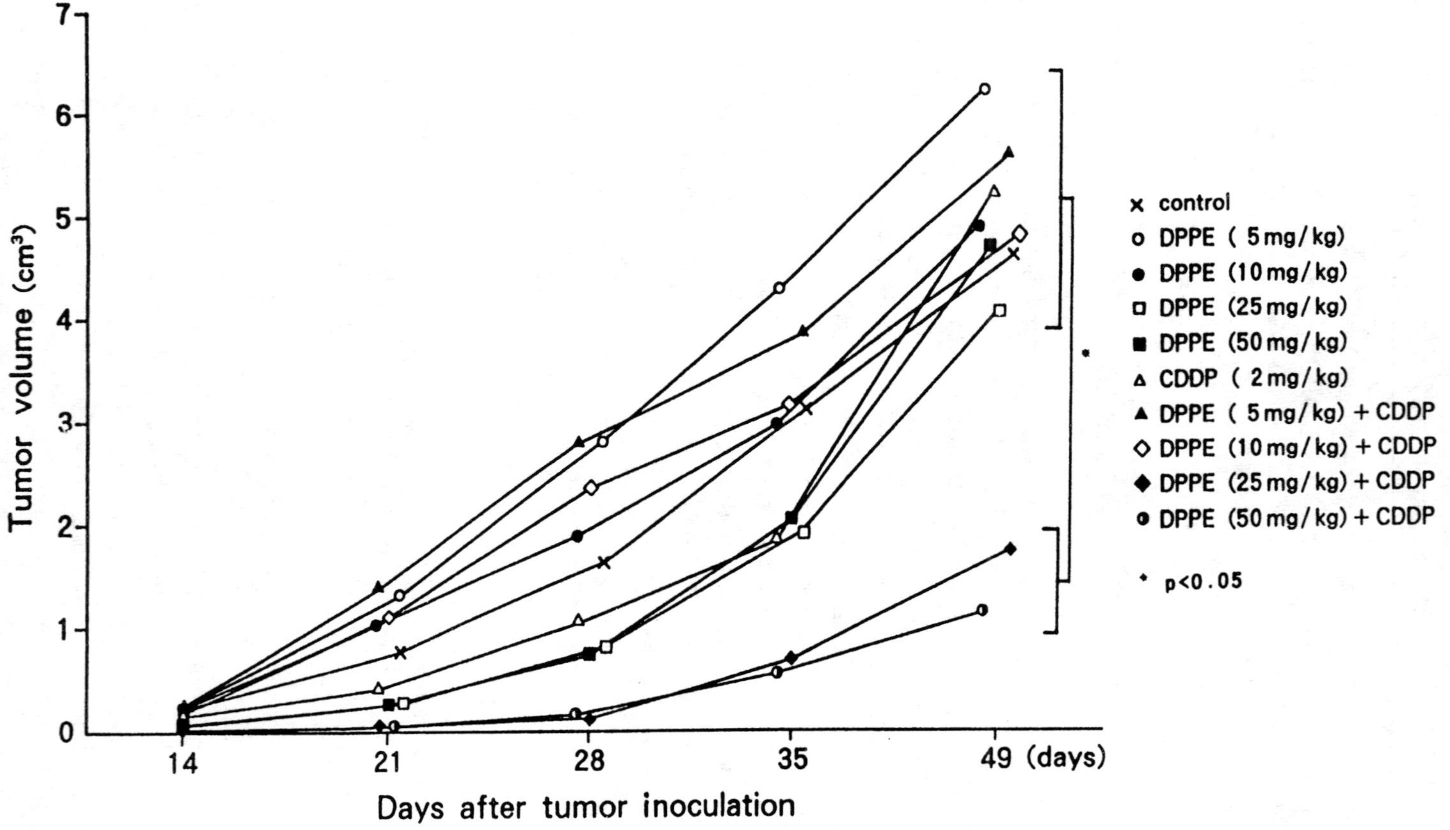

Fig.2. Effects of DPPE and CDDP on the tumor growth of KF cells inoculated into nude mice. *P<0.05 (Mann-Whitney U-test), compared to control, DPPE alone (low and high doses), CDDP alone and combinations of low doses DPPE with CDDP.

antihistamines enhance tumor growth at low dose(15). The tumor growth curve was not affected even if CDDP was combined with low doses (5 or 10 mg/kg) DPPE. However, when CDDP was combined with high doses (25 and 50 mg/kg) DPPE, the tumor growth was significantly more markedly inhibited than that in mice treated with CDDP alone and high doses DPPE alone. These results show synergistic effects of CDDP and high doses DPPE on the tumor growth. However, such combinations of high doses DPPE with CDDP did not result in a significant prolongation of the survival time, compared to CDDP alone because of adverse side effects as confirmed by monitoring the hematocrit and the body weight. A significant prolongation of the survival time was obtained by combinations of low doses (5 and 10 mg/kg) DPPE with CDDP.

Recently, Brandes et al. (8) have demonstrated that the maximally tolerated dose of DPPE in humans is 240 mg/m² when administered by intravenous infusion over 1 to 2 hours, following preclinical toxicologic studies in rodents. Although preliminary, the results of clinical phase I/II trial of DPPE combined with various single chemotherapy drugs in humans with advanced refractory cancer showed that, of 48 patients, 16 (33%) progressed, 12 (25%) stabilized, 12 (25%) improved, and eight (17%) responded (one complete and seven partial remissions). Our results show that about human equivalent-doses (5mg/kg or 10mg/kg in mice) of DPPE combined with CDDP is most effective in a nude mouse model.

REFERENCES

1. Brandes, L.J., Hermonat, M.W. A diphenylmethane derivative specific for the antiestrogen binding site in rat liver microsomes. *Biochem Biophys Res Commun* 1984,123:724-728.
2. Brandes, L.J. A diphenylmethane derivative selective for the antiestrogen binding site may help define its biological role. *Biochem Biophys Res Commun* 1984,123:244-249.
3. Sutherland, R.L., Murphy, L.C., Foo, M.S., Green, M.D., Whybourne,A.M., Krozowski,Z.S. High affinity antiestrogen binding site distinct from the estrogen receptor. *Nature* 1980,288:273-275.
4. Wiseman, H., Tamoxifen*: Molecular Basis of Use in Cancer Treatment and Prevention* John Wiley & Sons Ltd. 1994

5. Brandes, L.J., Macdonald, L.M., Bogdanovic, R.P. Evidence that the antiestrogen binding site is a histamine or histamine-like receptor. *Biochem Biophys Res Commun* 1985,126:905-910.
6. Brandes, L.J., Bogdanovic, R.P., Cawker, M.D., Labella, F.S. Histamine and growth: Interaction of antiestrogen binding site ligands with a novel histamine site that may be associated with calcium channels. *Cancer Res* 1987,47:4025-4031.
7. Brandes, L.J., Beecroft, W.A., Hogg, G.R. Stimulation of in vivo tumor growth and phorbol ester-induced inflammation by N,N-diethyl-2-[4-(phenylmethyl)phenoxy]-ethanamine HCl, a potent ligand for intracellular histamine receptors. *Biochem Biophys Res Commun* 1991,179:1297-1304.
8. Brandes, L.J., Simons, K.J., Bracken, S.P., Warrington, R.C. Results of a clinical trial in humans with refractory cancer of the intracellular histamine antagonist, N,N-diethyl-2-[4-(phenylmethyl)phenoxy]ethanamine-HCl, in com-bination with various single antineoplastic agents. *J Clin Oncol* 1994,12:1281-1290.
9. Brandes, L.J., Labella, F.S., Warrington, R.C. Increased therapeutic index of antineoplastic drugs in combination with intracellular histamine antagonists. *J Natl Cancer Inst* 1991,83:1329-1336.
10. Kikuchi, Y., Hirata, J., Kita, T., Imaizumi, E., Tode, T., Nagata, I. Enhancement of antiproliferative effect of cis-Diamminedichloroplatinum(II) by clomiphene and tamoxifen in human ovarian cancer cells. *Gynecol Oncol* 1993,49:365-372
11. Ishii, K., Kita, T., Kudoh, K., Hisano, A., Hirata, J., Imaizumi, E., Tode, T., Kikuchi,Y., Nagata,I. Circumvention of cisplatin resistant ovarian cancer cells by antiestrogens. *Acta Obst Gynaec Jpn* 1995,47:19-26
12. Kudoh, K., Kikuchi, Y., Hiramatsu, H., Hirata, J., Yamamoto, K., Kita, T., Nagata,I., Brandes,L.J. Enhancement of antitumor activity of cis-Diamminedichloroplatinum(II) by N,N-diethyl-2-[4-(phenylmethyl)-phenoxy]ethanamine-HCl in human ovarian cancer cells. *Oncol. Report*, in press.
13. Edelstein, M.B. Infused L-histidinol and cisplatin: Schedule, specificity, and proliferation dependence. *J Natl Cancer Inst* 1989,81:298-301.
14. Brandes, L.J., Labella, F.S. Identification of intracellular histamine receptors (H_{IC}) that regulate cell proliferation. *Adv Biosci* 1993,89:31-41.

15. Brandes, L.J., Warrington, R.C., Arron, R.J., Bogdanovic, R.P., Fang, W., Queen, G.M., Stein, D.A., Tong, J., Zaborniak, C.L.F., Labella, F.S. Enhanced cancer growth in mice administered daily human-equivalent doses of some H_1-antihistamines: Predictive in vitro correlates. *J Natl Cancer Inst* 1994,86:770-774.

CHAPTER 5

CIRCUMVENTION OF CIS-DIAMMINEDICHLOROPLATINUM(II) RESISTANCE BY ANTIESTROGENS*

Kenji Ishii, M.D.[1], Tsunekazu Kita, M.D., Kazuya Kudo, M.D., Junko Hirata, Ph.D., Eiji Imaizumi, M.D., Takehiko Tode, M.D., Yoshihiro Kikuchi, M.D. and Ichiro Nagata, M.D.

Department of Obstetrics and Gynecology, National Defense Medical College, Namiki 3-2, Tokorozawa, Saitama 359, Japan

Keywords; Ovarian cancer cells, Antiestrogens, cis-Diammine-dichloroplatinum(II), Chemosensitizing effect, Protein kinase C activity

ABSTRACT

Antiestrogens (AEs) have been considered to elicit antitumor effects via estrogen receptor(ER). However, recent reports have demonstrated that AEs had antitumor effect even in the cases without ER, and that AEs made various biological behaviors such as chemosensitizing effect. Therefore, we investigated the possibility of circumvention of cis-diamminedichloroplatinum(II) (CDDP) resistance by AEs using 5 ovarian cancer cell lines designated KF, MH, KK, KFra and KFrb. KF and MH were derived from serous cystadenocarcinomas of

---

* The abbreviations used are: CDDP, cis-Diamminedichloroplatinum(II); AE, antiestrogen; IC_{50}, concentrations of agents required for 50% inhibition of cell proliferation; CLO, clomiphene; TAM, tamoxifen; TOR,toremifene; PKC, protein kinase C; ER, estrogen receptor.

[1] To whom requests for reprints should be addressed.

the ovary and KK from a clear cell carcinoma. KFra and KFrb CDDP-resistant cell lines were established by continuous exposure of the KF cells to escalating doses of CDDP. MCF-7 cell line derived from breast cancer was used as an ER positive control cell line.

With regard to concentrations of agents required for 50% inhibition of cell proliferation (IC_{50}), clomiphene (CLO) had most potent antiproliferative effect among AEs used, and followed by tamoxifen (TAM) and toremifene (TOR) with the similar effect. KFra cell line which showed highest CDDP resistance among 5 ovarian cancer cell lines used was most sensitive to AEs, especially to CLO. In the study of combined administration of CDDP and AEs, 1μM of CLO, TAM and TOR significantly reduced the IC_{50} of CDDP to KFrb, KK and MCF-7 cell lines, to KF, KFra and MCF-7 cell lines and to KFra, KK and MCF-7 cell lines, respectively. Isoborographic analysis of CDDP and CLO revealed that CLO to KFra cells in combination with CDDP was synergistic at high dose, while it was antagonistic at low dose. On the other hand, CLO to KK cells was additive at any dose and CLO to MCF-7 cells was synergistic at any dose. To elucidate such mechanisms of chemosensitizing effects of AEs, we measured the protein kinase C (PKC) activity in the cytosolic and membrane fraction of the KFrb cell line cultured for 24 hr in the absence or presence of AEs. Although 1μM of AEs stimulated the cytosolic PKC activity, AEs inhibited the cytosolic PKC activity dose-dependently between 5μM and 50μM. Similarly, although AEs also inhibited the membrane PKC activity, the inhibitory effect appeared to be more marked than that on the cytosolic PKC activity.

In conclusion, three kinds of AEs had chemosensitizing effect to CDDP in ER negative ovarian cancer cell lines. The mechanism of the chemosensitizing effect to CDDP may be partly involved in the inhibition of translocation of the PKC activity from cytosol to cytoplasmic membrane caused by AEs.

INTRODUCTION

We have many opportunities of performing cis-diamminedichloroplatinum(II) (CDDP)-based combination chemotherapy in clinical management of solid tumors. However, we often meet with the patients who have the resistance to CDDP in the initial treatment or in the course of continual treatment. On the other hand, antiestrogens (AEs) as antitumor drugs mainly have been used for breast cancer or endometrial cancer of uterus (1-3). Although AEs have been considered to elicit antitumor effects via estrogen receptor (ER), recent reports have demonstrated that AEs had antitumor effect not only to ER-positive but also to ER-negative tumors, showing chemosensitizing effect to various antitumor drugs (7,8). Therefore we investigated the possibility of circumvention of CDDP resistance by chemosensitizing effect of AEs to various ovarian cancer cell lines.

MATERIALS AND METHODS

CHEMICALS.

CDDP was obtained from Bristol Myers Squibb Co. Ltd., Tokyo, Japan. Clomiphene (CLO) and tamoxifen (TAM) were from Sigma Chemical Company, St.Louis, MO., USA and toremiphene (TOR) was from Nippon Kayaku Co. Ltd., Tokyo, Japan. Fig.1 showes the structual formulas of the AEs. They were dissolved in absolute ethanol prior to use and diluted in RPMI 1640 to desired concentrations. Final concentrations of ethanol containing CLO,TAM or TOR were adjusted with RPMI 1640 to be less than 1.25% of ethanol which did not affect the cell proliferation.

CELL CULTURE.

KF and MH cells were established from tissue of patients with serous cystadenocarcinoma of the ovary. KK cells were established from ascites of a patient with clear cell carcinoma of the ovary. CDDP-resistant KFra and KFrb cell lines were established by continuous exposure of KF cells to escalating doses of CDDP in vitro. ER-positive MCF-7 cells derived from human breast cancer were used for comparison with these cells. These cell lines were incubated in RPMI 1640 medium supplemented with 10% fetal bovine serum, 2 μM glutamine, 100 units penicillin/ml and 100mg streptomycin/ml (Grand Island Biological Co., Grand Island, NY) in 5% CO_2 at 37°C. The medium was changed every 3 days, and the cells were passaged when they reached confluence.

INHIBITION OF CANCER CELL PROLIFERATION BY CDDP OR AE ALONE.

To examine concentrations of CDDP required for 50% inhibition of KF, KFra, KFrb, MH, KK and MCF-7 cell proliferation in vitro (IC_{50}), 1.5×10^3 cells

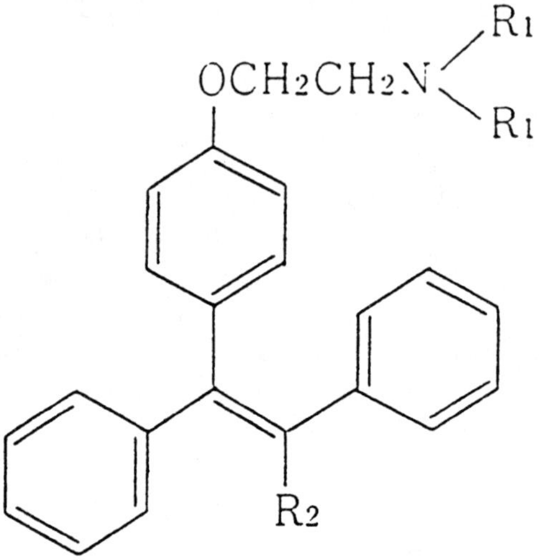

	CLO	TAM	TOR
R1:	-CH2CH3	-CH3	-CH3
R2:	-Cl	-CH2CH3	-CH2CH2Cl

Fig. 1. Structual formulas of CLO, TAM and TOR. These triphenylethylene antiestrogenic compounds were used as citrate.

for KF, KFra and KFrb, 3.0×10^3 cells for KK and MH and 2.0×10^3 cells for MCF-7 cells were seeded into 96-well flat-bottomed microtitre-plates (Becton-Dickinson Co., Mountain View, CA., USA). These cells were all in the logarithmic phase of growth. After 24 hr incubation to allow cell attachment, the medium was removed and replaced with fresh medium containing varying concentrations of CDDP. After additional 5 days' culture, the cell numbers in each well were determined by crystal violet staining method (9). Briefly, an equal volume of 10% formalin phosphate-buffered saline containing 0.2% crystal violet was added into each well and left in room temperature for 30 min. After washing twice with distilled water and drying in room temperature, absorbance at 590nm of stained cells in each well was measured by an automatic microtiter plate reader (Multiscan MCC/340, Titertek Co.). Average absorbance of the control wells in the absence of anticancer drugs was regarded as 100%, and the percentage cell growth in each well was calculated. The IC_{50} was obtained from graphical plots. The degree of resistance to CDDP was compared using IC_{50} value. Similarly, the IC_{50} values by CLO, TAM and TOR alone were determined by 5 days' exposure of each cells to these drugs. The AEs were dissolved in absolute ethanol and then diluted in RPMI 1640 to the desired concentration. Control wells received only ethanol. The final ethanol concentration was 1.25% (V/V) or less.

INHIBITION OF CANCER CELL PROLIFERATION BY COMBINATION WITH CDDP AND AE.

The combined effects of 1μM of AEs (CLO, TAM or TOR) to CDDP were also examined by determining effects of AE on the IC_{50} value of CDDP alone. These effects were expressed as dose-modifying factor (DMF). DMF was calculated as (IC_{50} of CDDP alone)/(IC_{50} of CDDP in the presence of 1 μM of AE). Similarly, various concentrations of AEs were tested and cytotoxic effects of CDDP and AEs were analysed by isobologram of IC_{50}.

PKC ASSAY IN CELLS.

The 10^7 KFrb cells were suspended in 1ml of 20 μM Tris/HCl (pH 7.5) buffer containing 5 μM EDTA, 10 μM EGTA, 0.3% (W/V) b-mercaptoethanol, 10 μM benzamidine and 50 mg/ml phenylmethylsuphoxyl fluoride to prevent protein degradation. The cell suspension was sonicated for 30 sec using a W-225 sonicator (Heat Systems-Ultrasonics, Inc., Farmingdale, NY) and centrifuged at 105,000 g for 1 hr. The resultant supernatant was used for cytosolic PKC assay. The cell pellet was suspended again in the Tris/HCl buffer with 1% TritonX-100 and sonicated for 15 sec. After gentle mixing for 1 hr, it was centrifuged as described above. The resultant supernatant was used for membrane PKC assay. All procedure described above was carried out at 4°C. The enzyme activity was determined by using PKC enzyme assay kit (Amersham International plc, Amersham, UK). The assay is a modification of a mixed micelle assay, activating enzyme with phorbol 12-myristate 13 acetate. One unit of PKC is defined as the ammount of enzyme which catalyze the transfer of 1 pmol phospate from ATP to histone per min at 30°C.

Table 1 IC50 (μM) of CDDP or AEs alone to various established cancer cell lines

Cell line	CDDP	Clomiphene	Tamoxifen	Toremifene
KF	0.44*	1.40	10.0	10.4
KFra	1.77	0.56	2.40	6.20
KFrb	0.49	1.13	3.20	10.7
MH	0.88	10.8	19.0	18.0
KK	0.78	5.80	26.0	24.0
MCF-7	2.03	7.60	11.0	4.40

* Average value from three repeated experiments.
Contact time was 5 days

Table 2 Effect of CLO on CDDP cytotoxicity

Cell line	Relative resistance	Cisplatin IC_{50} (μM) CDDP	Cisplatin IC_{50} (μM) CDDP+CLO(1μM)	P[a]	DMF[b]
KF	1	0.44±0.02[c]	0.33±0.10	n.s.	-
KFra	4.0	1.77±0.05	-	-	-
KFrb	1.1	0.49±0.05	0.23±0.02	<0.005	2.13
MH	2.0	0.88±0.05	0.86±0.11	n.s.	-
KK	1.7	0.78±0.04	0.40±0.08	<0.001	1.95
MCF-7	4.6	2.03±0.47	0.71±0.11	<0.02	2.86

[a] Student' *t* test
[b] Dose-modifying factor (IC_{50}CDDP/IC_{50}CDDP+CLO)
[c] Mean±S.D. from quadruplicate cultures n.s.;not significant

RESULTS

Effect of CDDP or AE alone on cancer cell growth. As shown in Table 1, sensitivity of KF cells to CDDP was highest among 6 cancer cell lines examined in this study, showing the IC_{50} of 0.44 μM. The IC_{50} of KFrb, MH and KK cells was 0.49, 0.88 and 0.78, respectively. The IC_{50} values of KFra and MCF-7 cells were about 4- and 4.6-fold higher than those of KF cells, respectively. As a whole, CLO had most potent antiproliferative effect among three AEs examined in this study and was followed by TAM and TOR with the similar effect. The degree of CDDP sensitivity was not correlated with the degree of AEs sensitivity. KFra cell line which showed highest CDDP resistance among 5 ovarian cancer cell lines used was most sensitive to AEs, especially to CLO.

COMBINED EFFECTS OF CDDP AND AES ON CANCER CELL GROWTH.

The combined effects of 1 μM of CLO to CDDP are shown in Table 2. KFra cells were too sensitive to CLO to observe combined effects of 1 μM CLO to CDDP. In the other cell lines, 1 μM CLO could reduce the IC_{50} of CDDP, especially in KFrb, KK and MCF-7 cell lines. Their DMF on CDDP cytotoxicity by 1 μM CLO was 2.13, 1.95 and 2.86, respectively. Similarly, the combined effects of 1 μM TAM to CDDP are shown in Table 3. Except for KFrb, 1 μM TAM could reduce the IC_{50} of CDDP in all cell lines and significantly in KF, KFra and MCF-7 cell lines. Their DMF was 2.59, 2.53 and 4.32, respectively. The combined effects of 1 μM TOR to CDDP are shown in Table 4. One μM TOR could significantly reduce the IC_{50} of CDDP in KFra, KK and MCF-7 cell lines. Their DMF was 1.90, 2.89 and 2.67, respectively.

Figure 2. shows isobologram for IC_{50} according to equi-effective dose-fraction formula produced by CDDP and CLO in KFra, KK and MCF-7 cell lines. In KFra cell line, concentrations of 0.4-0.5 μM CLO showed synergistic cytotoxicity to CDDP. In KK cell line, the isobolographic plots were on the line which connected IC_{50} of CDDP alone (0.78 μM) and that of CLO alone (5.80 μM), indicating additive effects between CDDP and CLO on cell cytotoxicity. On the other hand, in MCF-7 cell lines CLO seemed to have synergistic effects to CDDP. Similarly, TAM or TOR also had additive or synergistic effects to CDDP with regard to cell citotoxicity (data not shown).

EFFECT OF AES ON PKC ACTIVITY.

Fig.3 showes the PKC activity in cytosolic and membrane fraction of the KFrb cell line after incubating for 24 hr in the absence or presence of AEs. Results were expressed as percent to the PKC activity in the absence of AEs. The

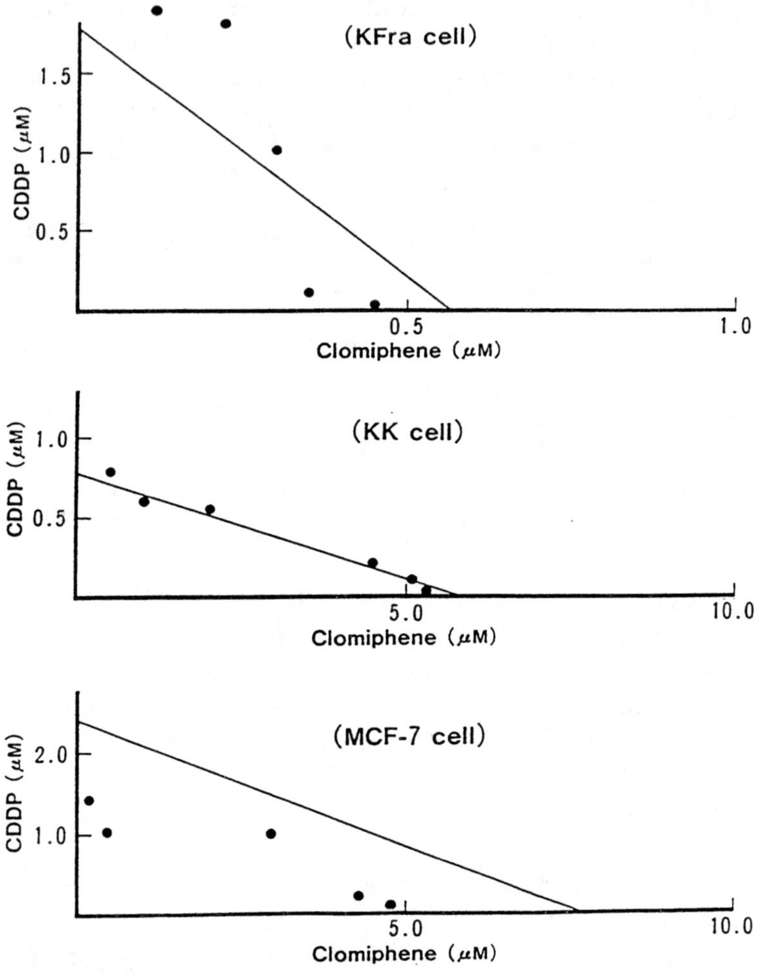

Fig. 2. Isobologram for IC_{50} according to equi-effective dose-fraction formula produced by CDDP and CLO.

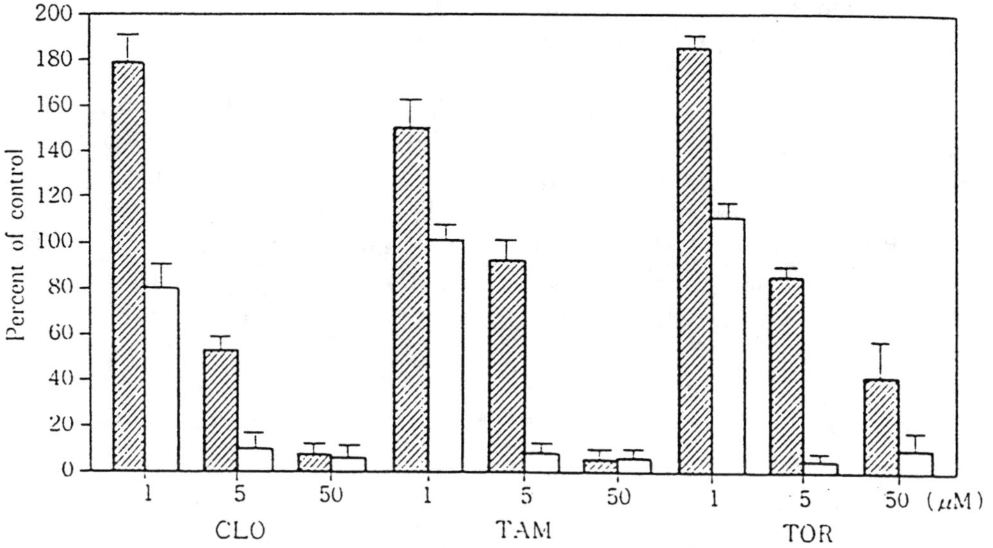

Fig. 3. Effects of CLO, and TOR on PKC activities in KFrb cells.

cytosolic PKC activity membrane PKC activity

The PKC activities in cytosolic and membrane fraction of the KFrb cell line cultured for 24 hr in the presence of various concentrations of AEs are presented. Results are shown as percent to the PKC activity in the absence ofAEs. Vertical bars are the mean±S.D. from quadruplicate cultures. When the KFrb cells were not exposured to AEs, the PKC activity was 693.9 pmoles/min/mg protein in cytosolic fraction and 83.3 pmoles/min/mg protein in membrane fraction.

PKC activity in the absence of AEs was 693.9 pmoles/min/mg protein in cytosolic fraction and 83.3 pmoles/min/mg protein in membrane fraction, respectively. Although 1 μM AEs stimulated the cytosolic PKC activity, 5 μM and 50 μM AEs inhibited the cytosolic PKC activity in a dose-dependent manner. The inhibitory effect of AEs on the membrane PKC activity was greater than that on the cytosolic PKC activity.

DISCUSSION

AEs as antitumor drugs have been mainly used for breast cancer or endometrial cancer of uterus (1-3). TAM has been shown to be clinical use as antitumor drug and TOR, the analogue of it, also has been expected the antitumor effect. Although these AEs have been considered to elicit antitumor effects via ER (10-12), recent reports have demonstrated that AEs had antitumor activities even to the ER negative tumors (4-6) and various biological behaviors such as chemosensitizing effect (7,8). In Table 1, CLO, TAM and TOR were shown to have potent antitumor activities not only to ER-positive MCF-7 cells but also to ER-negative KF, KFra, KFrb, MH and KK cells. It is possible that AEs elicit antitumor effects not only via ER but also via antiestrogen binding sites (13-15). In addition, it is well-known that AEs has the inhibitory effect of PKC activity (16-18), antagonistic effect to calmodulin (19,20), inducing effect to transforming growth factor b (21,22), inhibitory effects on insulin-like growth

Table 3 Effect of TAM on CDDP cytotoxicity

Cell line	Relative resistance	Cisplatin IC50 (μM) CDDP	CDDP+ TAM (1μM)	P[a]	DMF[b]
KF	1	0.44±0.02[c]	1.77±0.05	<0.002	2.59
KFra	4.0	1.77±0.05	0.70±0.08	<0.001	2.53
KFrb	1.1	0.49±0.05	0.73±0.14	n.s.	-
MH	2.0	0.88±0.05	0.69±0.21	n.s.	-
KK	1.7	0.78±0.04	0.54±0.45	n.s.	-
MCF-7	4.6	2.03±0.47	0.47±0.24	<0.05	4.32

[a] Student' t test. [b] Dose-modifying factor (IC_{50}CDDP/IC_{50}CDDP+TAM)

[c] Mean±S.D. from quadruplicate cultures n.s.;not significant

Table 4 Effect of TOR on CDDP cytotoxicity

Cell line	Relative resistance	Cisplatin IC50 (μM) CDDP	CDDP+ TOR (1μM)	P[a]	DMF[b]
KF	1	0.44±0.02[c]	0.45±0.21	n.s.	-
KFra	4.0	1.77±0.05	0.93±0.11	<0.002	1.90
KFrb	1.1	0.49±0.05	0.70±0.35	n.s.	-
MH	2.0	0.88±0.05	0.89±0.13	n.s.	-
KK	1.7	0.78±0.04	0.27±0.05	<0.002	2.89
MCF-7	4.6	2.03±0.47	0.76±0.20	<0.05	2.67

[a]Student' t test. [b] Dose-modifying factor (IC_{50}CDDP/IC_{50}CDDP+TOR)

[c]Mean±S.D. from quadruplicate cultures n.s.;not significant

factor-I and epidermal growth factor (23), inhibitory effects on natural killer activity (24) and chemosensitizing effects to doxorubicin and CDDP (7,8). Therefore, we have investigated the possibility of circumvention of CDDP resistance by chemosensitizing effect of AEs on ER-negative 5 ovarian cancer cell lines and ER-positive breast cancer cell line. CLO had most potent antiproliferative effect among three AEs examined in this study and 1 μM CLO had significant chemosensitizing effects to CDDP on KFrb and KK cells. CLO has been reported to have severe side effects such as hyperstimulation and carcinogenesis (development of low potential malignancy) of ovary. However, it is difficult to obtain serum concentration of 1 μM CLO in clinical dose. On the other hand, TAM and TOR as antitumor drugs have been used clinically for treatment of breast cancer. Although TOR have mild side effects such as hot flush, it is noteworthy that TOR can be used without severe side effects such as described above (10,11,25,26). In addition, it has been reported that serum concentration of TOR can rise up to 1.4 μM by oral administration of 120 mg and 5.1 μM by oral administration of 480mg (27). Therefore, serum concentration of 1 μM TOR which we examined in this study will be clinically attainable.

The mechanism of chemosensitizing effects of AEs is not fully understood. As shown in Fig.2, the interaction between CDDP and CLO was varied with their concentration and the kind of target cells. In some cases they interacted in antagonistic fashion. Various interaction between CDDP and AEs were also observed in the study used TAM or TOR (data not shown). All three kinds of AEs had synergistic antitumor activities to CDDP at any concentration in ER-positive MCF-7 cells and antagonistic effects at extremely low concentration in KFra cells. These data will give some clues to know the mechanism of chemosensitizing effects of AEs on CDDP. It has been already reported that AEs have inhibitory effect on PKC activity (16-18) and the drug which inhibits PKC activity stimulates antiproliferative activity of CDDP (26). Therefore, we assume that the inhibition of PKC activity by AEs might be one of the mechanisms of chemosensitizing effects on CDDP. Kikuchi et al. have already reported the inhibition of cytosolic PKC activity by AEs in KF, KK, MH and MCF-7 cell lines (29). In this study, we examined the translocation of PKC activity from cytosolic fraction to membrane fraction by using KFrb cells. It is well-known that PKC translocates from the cytosol to the membrane by exogenous stimulation and subsequently the ratio of cytosolic PKC activity to membrane PKC activity changes (30). Although total PKC activity was dose-dependently inhibited at more than 1 μM of AEs concentration, cytosolic PKC activity was stimulated rather than inhibited by 1 μM AEs. These effects are consistent with the previous report by Kikuchi et al. (29). When the cells were incubated in the absence of AEs, the ratio of cytosolic PKC activity to membrane PKC activity was 8.4. The ratio of cytosolic PKC activity to membrane PKC activity after exposure to CLO was 18.9 at 1 μM, 47.8 at 5 μM and 12.3 at 50 μM. Similarly, that after exposure to TAM was 12.8 at 1 μM, 94.7 at 5 μM and 7.2 at 50 μM and that after exposure to TOR was 14.9 at 1 μM, 168.1 at 5 μM and 4.0 at 50 μM. These data demonstrate that PKC translocation from cytosol to membrane is inhibited by 1-5 μM of AEs. This may be one of the mechanisms of chemosensitizing effect of AEs on CDDP.

In summary, three kinds of AEs had chemosensitizing effects to CDDP in ER negative ovarian cancer cell lines. The mechanism of the chemosensitizing effect to CDDP may be partly implied by the inhibition of translocation of the PKC activity from cytosol to cytoplasmic membrane induced by AEs.

REFERENCES

1. Izuo M. New drugs in endocrine treatment of breast cancer. *Folia endocrinol* 1992;68:538-849 (in Japanese)
2. Kanoh H, Hosono T, Matsui Y, Okudaira Y. Growth of endometrial cancer and hormone. *Jpn J Cancer Chemother* 1989;16:3696-3703
3. Nomura Y. Recent progress of endocrine therapy for breast cancer. *Jpn J Canc Chemotherapy* 1992;19:783-789 (in Japanease)
4. Baum M, Brinkley DM, Dossett JA, McPherson K, Patterson JS, Rubens RD, Smiddy FG, Stoll BA, Wilson A, Richards D, Ellis SH. *Controlled trial of tamoxifen as single adjuvant agent in management of early breast cancer.* 1985;i:836-840
5. Breast Cancer Trials Committee, Scottish Cancer Trials Office. Adjuvant tamoxifen in the management of operable breast cancer: The scottish trial. *Lancet* 1987;ii:171-175
6. Maruyama S, Koga K, Kuroiwa S, Ekimoto H. Growth inhibitory effect of toremifene (NK622), a new antiestrogenic drug and its metabolite on human breast cancer cells in the presence of growth factor. *J Jpn Soc Cancer* Ther 1993;28:826-834 (in Japanese)
7. Mäenpää J, Spilä P, Kangas L, Karnani P, Grönroos M. Chemosensitizing effect of an antiestrogen, toremifene on ovarian cancer. *Gynecol Oncol* 1992;46:292-297

8. McClay EF, Albright KD, Jones JA, Christen RD, Howell SB. Tamoxifen modulation of cisplatin sensitivity in human malignant melanoma cells. *Cancer Res* 1993;53:1571-1576
9. Saotome K, Morita H, Umeda M. Cytotoxicity test with simplified crystal violet staining method using microtitre plates and its application to injection drugs. *Toxic in Vitro* 1989;3:317-321
10. Kallio S, Kangas L, Blanco G, Johansson R, Karjalainen A, Perilaä M, Pippo I, Sundquist H, Södervall M, Toivola R. A new triphenylethylene compound,Fc-1157a. Hormonal effects. *Cancer Chemother Pharmacol* 1986;17:103-108
11. Kangas L, Nieminen AL, Blanco G, Grönroos M, Kallio S, Karjalainen A, Perilaä M, Södervall M, Toivola R. A new triphenylethylene compound, Fc-1157a áU.Antitumor effects. *Cancer Chemother Pharmacol* 1986;17:109-113
12. Kangas L. Agonistic and antagonistic effects of antiestrogens in different target organs. *Acta Oncol* 1992;31:143-146
13. Ebbs SR, Roberts JV, Baum M. Alternative mechanism of action of "anti-oestrogens" in breast cancer. *Lancet* 1987;ii:621
14. Lin L,Hwang PL. Antiproliferative effects of oxygenated sterols: positive correlation with binding affinities for the antiestrogen- binding sites. *Biochim Biophys Acta* 1991;1082:177-184
15. Pavlik EJ, Nelson K, Srinivasan S, Powell DE, Kenady DE, DePriest PD, Gallion HH, van Nagell JR. Resistance to tamoxifen with persisting sensitivity to estrogen: Possible mediation by excessive antiestrogen binding site activity. *Cancer Res* 1992;52:4106-4112
16. Su HD, Mazzei GJ, Vogler WR, Kuo JF. Effect of tamoxifen,a nonsteroidal antiestrogen, on phospholipid/calcium-dependent protein kinase and phosphorylation of its endogenous substrate proteins from the rat brain and ovary. *Biochem Pharmacol* 1985;34:3649-3653
17. O'Brian CA, Liskamp RM, Solomon DM, Weinstein IB. Inhibition of protein kinase C by tamoxifen. *Cancer Res* 1985;45:2462-2465
18. O'Brian CA, Liskamp RM, Solomon DH, Weinstein IB. Triphenylethylenes: a new class of protein kinase C inhibitors. *J Natl Cancer Inst* 1986;76: 1243-1246
19. Lam HYP. Tamoxifen is a calmodulin antagonist in the activation of cAMP-phosphodiesterase. *Biochem Biophys Res Commun* 1984;118:27-32
20. Gulino A, Barrera G, Vacca A, Farina A, Ferretti C, Screpanti I, Dianzani MU, Frati L. Calmodulin antagonism and growth-inhibiting activity of triphenylethylene antiestrogens in MCF-7 human breast cancer cells. *Cancer Res* 1986;46:6274-6278

21. Coletta AA, Wakefield LM, Howell FV, van Roozendaal KE, Danielpour D, Ebbs SR, Sporn MB, Baum M. Anti-estopgens induce the secretion of active transforming growth factor beta from human fetal fibroblasts. *Br J Cancer* 1990;62:405-409
22. Kanabbe C, Zugmaier G, Schmahl M, Dietel M, Lippman ME, Dickson RB. Induction of transforming growth factor b by the antiestrogens droloxifene, tamoxifen, and toremifene in MCF-7 cells. *Am J Clin Oncol* 1991;14(Suppl.2):15-20
23. Freiss G, Prebois C, Rochefort H, Vignon F. Anti-steroidal and anti- growth factor activities of anti-estrogens. *J Steroid Biochem Molec Miol* 1990; 37: 777-781
24. Robinson E, Rubin D, Mekori T, Segal R, Pollack S. In vivo modulation of natural killer cell activity by tamoxifen in patients with bilateral primary breast cancer. *Cancer Immunol Immunother* 1993;37:209-212
25. Valavaara R, Pyrhönen S, Heikkinen M, Rissanen P, Blanco G, Thölix E, Nordman E, Taskinen P, Holsti L, Hajba A. Toremifen,a new antiestrogenic compound, for treatment of advanced breast cancer. Phase II study. *Eur J Cancer Clin Oncol* 1988;24:785-790
26. Mäenpää J, Spilä P, Hajba A. Toremifene for recurrent and advanced endometrial carcinoma. *Eur J Cancer* 1992;28A:1768
27. Watanabe N, Koyama M. (unpublished)
28. Hofmann J, Doppler W, Jakob A, Maly K, Posch L, Überall F, Grunicke H. Enhancement of the antiproliferative effect of cis-diamminedichloro-platinum(II) and nitrogen mustard by inhibitors of protein kinase C. *Int J Cancer* 1988;42:382-388
29. Kikuchi Y, Hirata J, Kita T, Imaizumi E, Tode T, Nagata I. Enhancement of antiproliferative effect of cis-diamminedichloroplatinum(II) by clomiphene and tamoxifen in human ovarian cancer cells. *Gynecol Oncol* 1993;49:365-372
30. Chambers TC, McAvoy EM, Jacobs JW, Eilon G. Protein kinase C phospholates P-glycoprotein in multidrug resistant human KB cartinoma cells. *J Biol Chem* 1990;256:7679-7686

PART II

CIRCUMVENTION OF CDDP RESISTANCE

CHAPTER 6

ENHANCEMENT OF ANTITUMOR ACTIVITY OF CISPLATIN BY CALMODULIN ANTAGONISTS AND SURAMIN

Yoshihiro Kikuchi and Junko Hirata
Department of Obstetrics and Gynecology, National Defense Medical College, Namiki 3-2, Tokorozawa, Saitama 359, Japan

INTRODUCTION

It is well documented that calcium and/or calmodulin play significant roles in DNA synthesis and cell proliferation (1, 2). Accordingly, drugs that inhibit the function of calmodulin also arrest cell proliferation (3-7). Recently, it has been reported that calmodulin inhibitors decrease the binding of epidermal growth factor (EGF) to transformed, but not normal, human fibroblasts (8). We have also demonstrated that binding of EGF to human ovarian cancer cells was significantly inhibited by calmodulin antagonists (9) and combinations of calmodulin antagonists and anticancer drug resulted in adjuvant effects with regard to the inhibition of tumor cell proliferation in vitro (6). Similarly, suramin inhibits the cellular binding of growth factors such as EGF (10) and the cellular proliferation of several human tumor cells in vitro (11-14).

Since the discovery of the antineoplastic effects of cisplatin (CDDP) by Rosenberg et al (15), cisplatin-based combination chemotherapy has been undertaken for ovarian cancer patients and improvement in the survival and response rates have been reported (16-18). However, the initial response is often followed by a relapse due to either intrinsic or acquired drug resistance. In order to develop strategies for overcoming this resistance more insight into its origin is needed. Thus, we have attempted to enhance the anticancer effects of cisplatin by calmodulin antagonists (W-7 and W-5) and suramin.

ENHANCEMENT OF ANTINEOPLASTIC EFFECT OF CISPLATIN BY CALMODULIN ANTAGONISTS.

Fig. 1 shows effects of calmodulin antagonists (W-5 and W-7) on proliferation of two kinds of human cell lines, designated HR and KF, derived from serous cystadenocarcinoma of the ovary. Although both W-5 and W-7 inhibited their proliferation in vitro, the degree of inhibition was more marked with W-5 rather than with W-7. The mechanism which W-5, a chlorine-deficient analogue of W-7 that interacts with calmodulin only weakly, inhibits cell proliferation to more extent compared to W-7 remains unclear.

It is well-known that calmodulin antagonists can affect cellular accumulation of anticancer drugs by impairing calcium fluxes and stabilizing membranes (19). Accordingly, we attempted to determine effects of calmodulin antagonists on the cellular accumulation of cisplatin using KF and the cisplatin-resistant (KFr) cells which was induced by continuous exposure of KF cells to escalating doses of cisplatin. The degree of cisplatin resistance of the KFr cells was about 3.7-fold higher than that of the parent KF cells, with regard to the concentration of cisplatin required for 50% inhibition of cell proliferation (IC_{50}). As shown in Fig. 2, when KF and KFr cells were incubated with 10 mg/ml cisplatin for 4 hr, cisplatin-content in the KF cells was significantly higher than that in the KFr cells. If KF cells were incubated in the presence of 5 mg/ml W-7 (but not W-5), the cellular cisplatin-content was significantly higher than that of cells treated with cisplatin alone. In the presence of W-7 or W-5, cisplatin uptake by KFr cells significantly increased to the level comparable to that by KF cells treated with cisplatin alone. Such an increase of cisplatin uptake seemed to enhance inhibitory effects of cisplatin on KFr cell proliferation in vitro. As shown in Fig. 3, 1 or 2 mg/ml W-7 showed a significant adjuvant effect in the presence of 0.5 mg/ml cisplatin with regard to inhibition of cell proliferation in vitro, while 1 mg/ml W-5 had no significant effects in the presence of any concentration of cisplatin used.

In addition, we have demonstrated that cisplatin uptake by the KF tumor grown in nude mice was significantly higher than that by the KFr tumor 4 hr after cisplatin administration, like the in vitro experiment (Fig. 4). When cisplatin and calmodulin antagonists were simultaneously administered, the cisplatin uptake by both KF and KFr tumors was significantly increased, compared to that when cisplatin alone was administered. Enhancing effects of calmodulin antagonists on cisplatin uptake by the KFr tumor were more marked than those on uptake by the KF tumor. The cisplatin uptake by the KFr tumor was increased to about

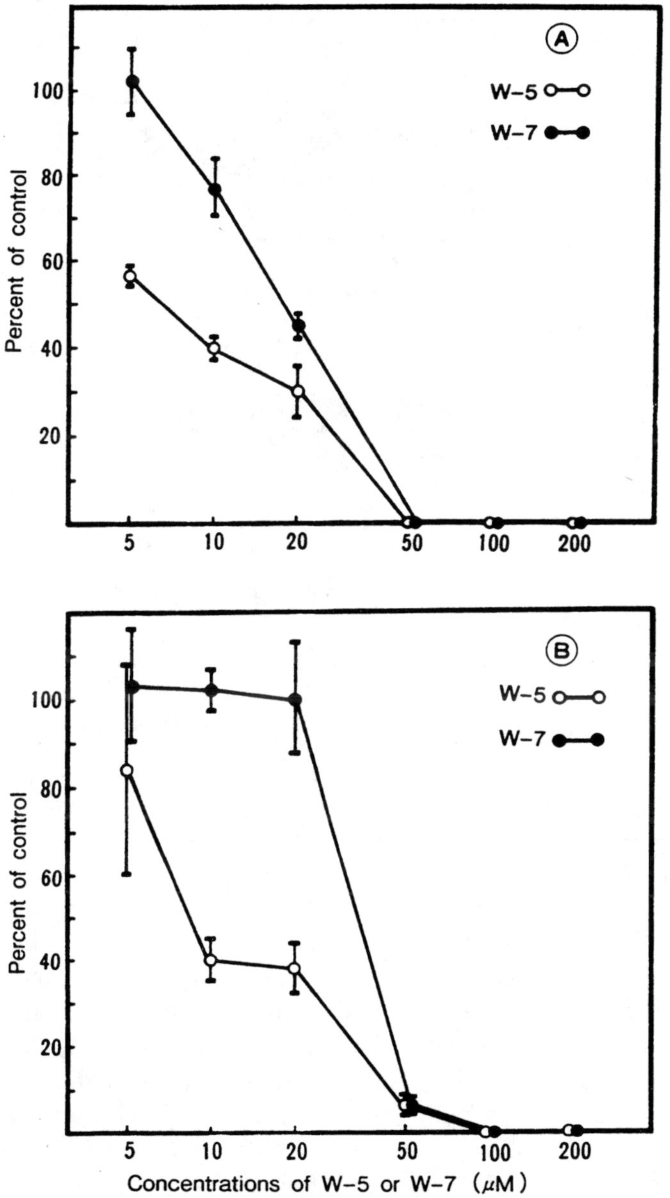

Fig. 1. Inhibition of HR and KF cell proliferation by W-5 and W-7. A; HR cell line, B; KF cell line. Exposure time to W-5 and W-7 was 3 days. Bars show the mean ± SD from 3 experimental cultures.

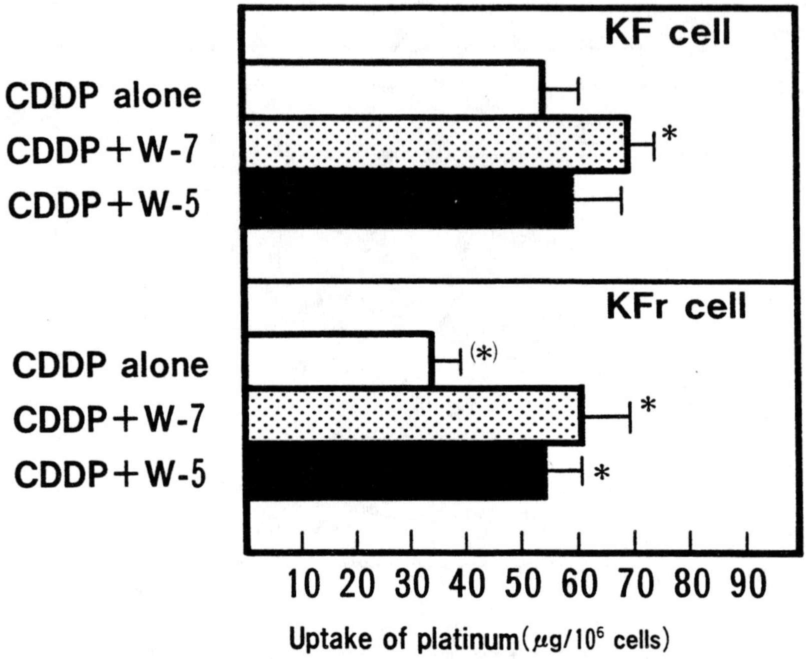

Fig. 2. Effects of W-7 and W-5 on the uptake of cisplatin by KF and KFr cells. Bars show the mean ± SD. (*)p<0.05, compared to KF cells. *p<0.01, compared to cisplatin alone.

2.5-fold by W-5 and about 3.0-fold by W-7. Since W-5 has been reported to have weaker actions as a calmodulin antagonist than W-7 (20), the degree of effect on cisplatin accumulation by W-5 was less than that by W-7. Thus, we attempted to potentiate the antineoplastic effects of cisplatin by combination with W-7 in nude mice bearing human ovarian carcinoma (KFr) cells. KFr (5 x 10^5) cells were inoculated s.c. to right flank of nude mice. After 7 days of tumor inoculation, 2 mg/kg cisplatin and 15 mg/kg W-7 were administered i.p. every week for 6 weeks. Each group consisted of 10 mice. All mice developed palpable tumor on Day 14. Tumor volumes and the survival time in a W-7 alone treated group were not different from those in an untreated group. When treatment with W-7 was followed by cisplatin, the tumor growth was similar to that in a cisplatin alone treated group and subsequently the survival time was not significantly prolonged, compared to that not only in a cisplatin alone treated group but also in an untreated group. However, 2 of 10 mice in a W→7 cisplatin treated group were survived more than 100 days with tumor. If treatment with cisplatin was followed by W-7, the tumor growth was markedly inhibited after 21 days of tumor inoculation and the

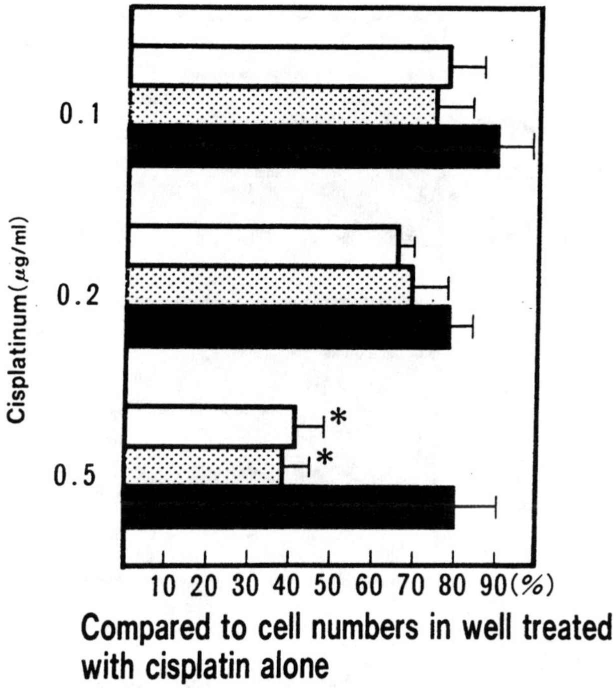

Fig. 3. Circumvention by calmodulin antagonists of cisplatin resistance of KFr cells. Each point is presented as the percentage of the cell number in the well treated with cisplatin alone. Bars show the mean ± SD.□ , W-7 (1mg/ml); ■ , W-7 (2mg/ml); □ , W-5 (1mg/ml). *p<0.01, compared to cisplatin alone.

survival time was significantly prolonged, compared to that not only in an untreated group but also in a cisplatin alone treated group. Five of 10 mice in a cisplatinÆW-7 treated group survived more than 100 days (2 mice without tumor and 3 mice with tumor) (Fig. 5). We previously reported that a combination of cisplatin and calmodulin antagonists (W-7 and W-5) resulted in enhancement of its antitumor effects only when treatment with cisplatin was followed by treatment with calmodulin antagonists (21). In the present study, it is noteworthy that similar results could be obtained using cisplatin-resistant KFr cells. Recently, we observed that exposure of cisplatin-resistant (but not sensitive) cells to cisplatin resulted in a marked increase of the cellular glutathione (GSH) (22). It has also been reported that calmodulin antagonists caused a marked inhibition in recovery from bleomycin induced potentially lethal damage of cells by preventing the repair of damaged DNA (23). Similarly, it is possible that W-7 disturbs the repair process of DNA damaged by cisplatin. In addition, a newly synthesized calmodulin antagonist (W-7) have been reported to

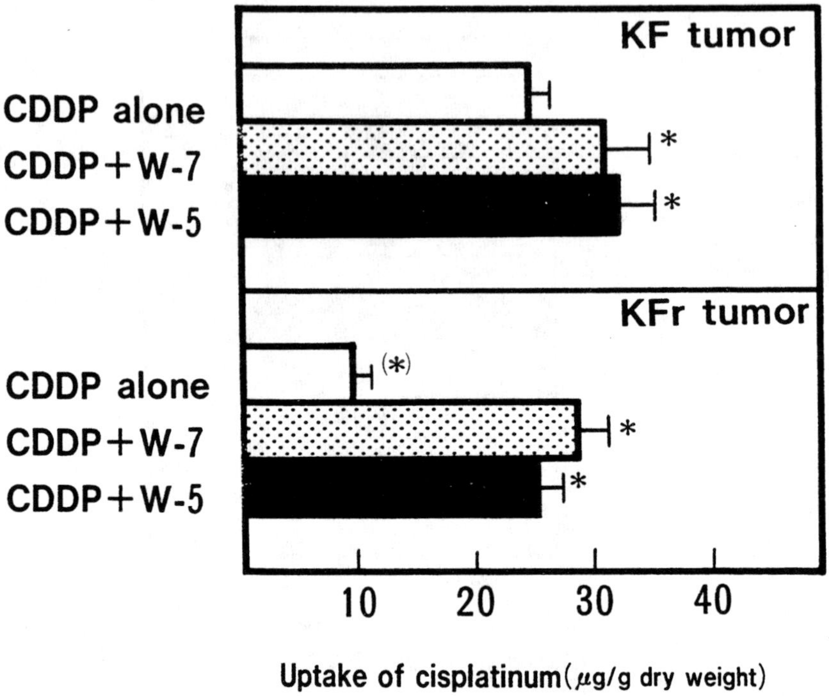

Fig. 4. Effects of W-7 and W-5 on the uptake of cisplatin by the KFr tumor. Bars show the mean ± SD. (*)p<0.05, compared to KF tumor. *p<0.05, compared to tumors treated with cisplatin alone.

enhance the antitumor activity of anticancer drugs by inhibiting GSH synthetase activity (24). Therefore, these observations provide a new strategy for enhancement of sensitivity of cancer cells to cisplatin and circumvention to its resistance.

ENHANCEMENT OF ANTITUMOR ACTIVITY OF CISPLATIN BY SURAMIN

Suramin is a polysulfonated compound originally developed nearly 75 years ago for use as a trypanocidal agent. Recent studies indicate that suramin can also disrupt mammalian cell function, notably by blocking growth factor receptor interactions and by inhibiting the activity of enzymes that are critical for cell growth and proliferation. In preclinical studies, suramin has been shown to exert an antiproliferative effect on a variety of human cancer cell lines grown in vitro (25-27). The principal

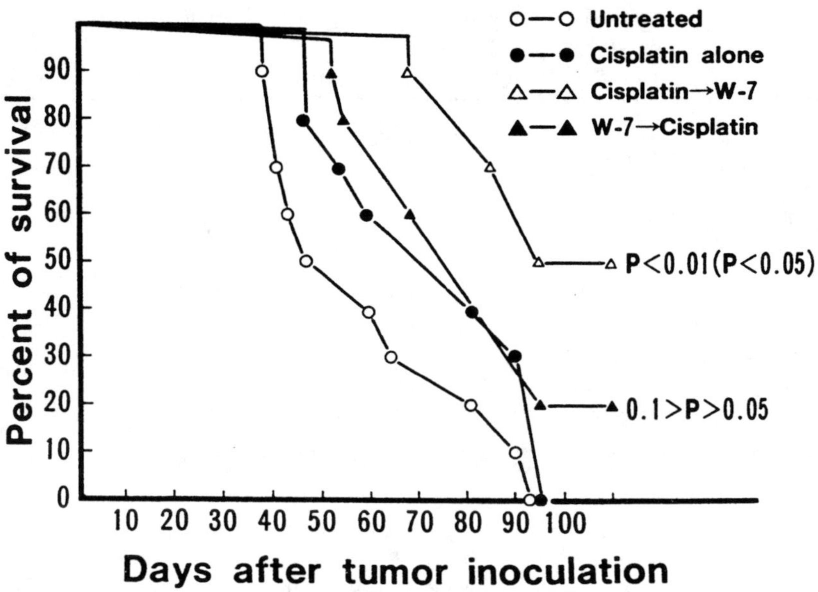

Fig. 5. Effect of combination of cisplatin and calmodulin antagonist (W-7) on survival time of nude mice bearing cisplatin-resistant human ovarian carcinoma (KFr) cells. Each group consisted of 10 mice. After 7 days of tumor inoculation, 2 mg/kg cisplatin and 15 mg/kg W-7 were administered i.p. every week for 6 weeks. The statistical analysis was by Wilcoxon test. P, when compared to untreated control. P in parenthesis, when compared to cisplatin alone.

mechanism through which suramin acts has been considered to be probably via interference with the interaction of growth factors and their receptors, and as a result in their signal transduction pathways (10, 28-31). Since in vitro data about the activity of suramin on tumor cells were obtained in a variety of experimental conditions, we have evaluated the cytotoxic effect of suramin on several kinds of human ovarian cancer cell lines and investigated the relation between drug efficacy and cellular EGFR content.

Nine cell lines derived from 5 different human ovarian cancers were tested for the cytotoxic activity of suramin (Table 1). KF, HRA and MH cell lines were established from serous cystadenocarcinoma of the ovary (32-34). KK and TYK cells were derived from clear cell carcinoma and undifferentiated carcinoma of the ovary, respectively (34, 35). KFra, KFrb and KFrc were CDDP-resistant cell lines induced by continuous exposure of the parent KF cells to escalating doses of CDDP. TYK/R is also an acquired CDDP-resistant cell line induced similarly from the parent TYK cell line. MH and KK cell lines were assumed to be intrinsically CDDP-resistant because of these cell lines derived from the

Table 1. Suramin cytotoxicity and EGFR expression

Cells	IC_{50} to CDDP(μM)	IC_{50} to suramin(μM)	EGF bound*	Kd (pmol)
KF	0.38†	29	n.d.††	
KFra	1.28	28	n.d.	
KFrb	1.05	34	n.d.	
KFrc	1.31	34	n.d.	
HRA	0.21	26	n.d.	
KK	0.76	225	319.0	58.1
MH	3.20	125	231.6	46.2
TYK	0.31	13	63.6	60.1
TYK/R	0.92	29	161.7	212.2

KF, HRA, and TYK; CDDP sensitive cell lines. KFra, KFrb, KFrc, KK, MH, and TYK/R; CDDP resistant cell lines. *pg/10^6cells. †Contact time was 5 days. ††not detectable.

tumor of patients who did not respond to initial CDDP-based chemotherapy. As shown in Table 1, KF, KFra, KFrb, KFrc and HRA cells did not have detectable EGF-binding sites. However, presence or absence of EGF-binding sites did not seem to be associated with the sensitivity to CDDP. In cell lines with measurable levels of EGF-binding sites, there seemed to be some correlation between amount of EGF-binding sites and the corresponding suramin IC_{50} values. However, the presence of EGFR in our cell lines was not necessary condition for the manifestation of suramin cytotoxicity, because cells without detectable levels of this growth factor receptor were also sensitive to this drug effect. These observations are consistent with previous reports (14, 25). Cellular binding of EGF measured by Scatchard analysis was similar to data reported by others. Wan et al. (36) reported Kd values ranging between 0.08 and 0.19 nmol/l. Olivier et al. (25) demonstrated that two families of EGF binding sites per lineage were characterized for six of 18 cell lines; for twelve others, only a single family was detectable. In the other report, EGF was detectable for Scatchard analysis as a single class of high-affinity binding sites in 66% of the ovarian tumor analysed (37). Our human ovarian cancer cell lines with EGFR had similar Kd values as a single family of sites (Table 1). As shown in Fig. 6, suramin inhibited EGF binding in a dose-dependent manner in 4 cell lines with detectable EGFR. Although the degree of the inhibition was similar among MH, TYK and TYK/R cell lines, that in KK cell line was remarkably weak. However, such an inhibition by suramin did not seem to be directly associated with suramin cytotoxicity, suggesting that the mode of action of suramin on tumor-cell proliferation is not only dependent on inhibition of EGF-binding.

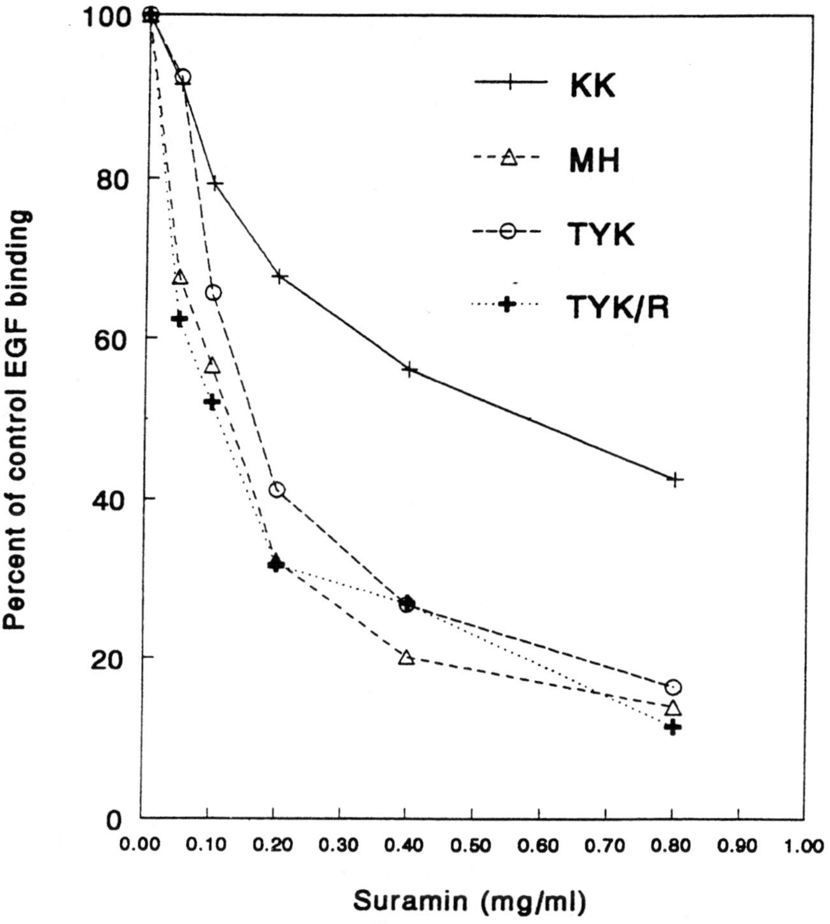

Fig. 6. Inhibition of EGF binding by suramin. Concentrations of suramin required for 50% inhibition of EGF binding (IC_{50}) were 588, 122, 164 and 109 1mg/ml for KK, MH, TYK and TYK/R cells, respectively.

Thus, to elucidate other mechanisms of antitumor effects by suramin, we examined the cellular PKC activity in the cell line with or without detectable EGFR. As shown in Fig. 7, the cytosolic PKC activity of KF cells was inhibited in a dose-dependent manner between 50 and 400 mM suramin, while the membrane PKC activity was not inhibited. In MH cells with detectable EGFR, 100 mM suramin stimulated rather than inhibited the cytosolic PKC activity, whereas the membrane PKC activity was stimulated in a dose-dependent manner to about 1.6-fold level of untreated MH cells by 400 mM suramin. Recently, it has been reported

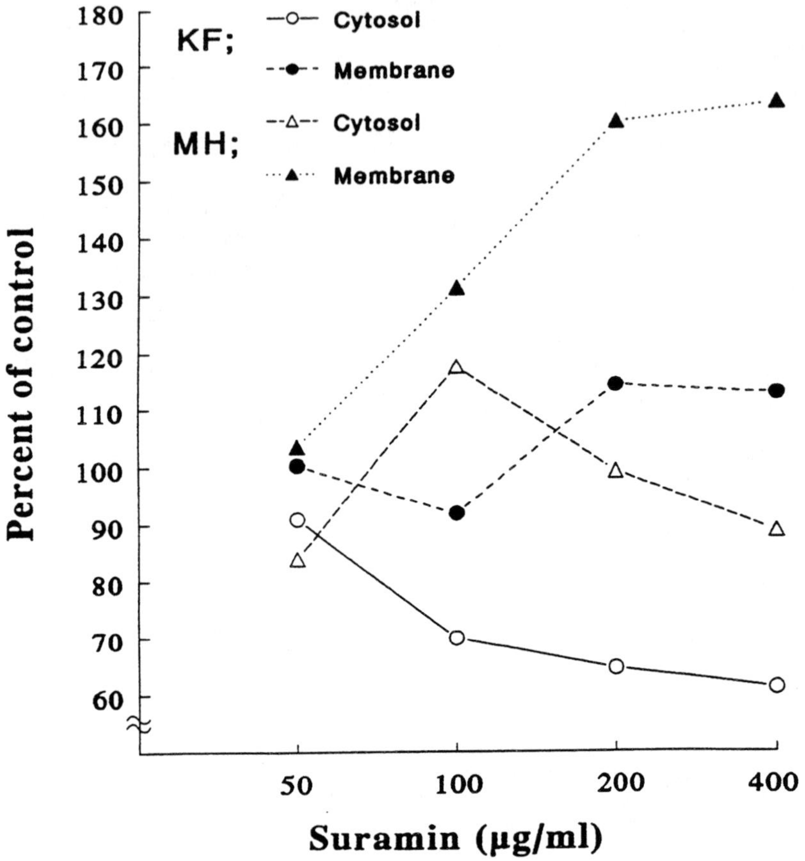

Fig. 7. Effects of suramin on the cytosol and membrane PKC activities in the KF and MH cells. Logarithmically growing cells were pre-incubated with concentrations of suramin indicated for 24 hr before assaying for PKC activity. Results were expressed as percent of PKC activity before exposure to suramin.

that PKC inhibitors, such as staurosporine or calphostin C, prevent TPA-induced differentiation but not cell growth arrest (38). These data suggest that the two events are mediated by different pathways; a possible interpretation is that the activation of one or more PKC isoforms mediates the induction of differentiation, whereas the down-regulation of the same or different isoforms mediates the growth arrest. Therefore, it is possible that cytosolic PKC plays a role in the cell proliferation while membrane PKC is related to the cell differentiation. Our observations suggest that inhibition of the KF cell proliferation by suramin is mainly mediated via inhibition of the cytosolic PKC, while that of the MH cell

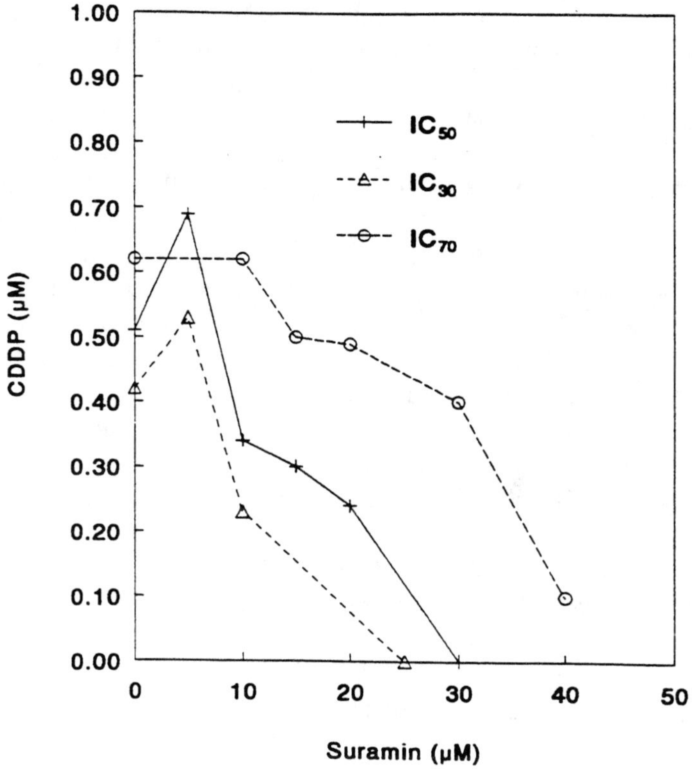

Fig. 8. Isobologram to CDDP and suramin of KF cells. After continuous exposure for 5 days, cytotoxicity of CDDP and suramin on KF cells was determined by using a crystal violet staining method as described previously (42). The IC30 IC_{50}, and IC70 of CDDP and suramin were obtained from graphical plots and the isobologram was depicted.

proliferation is mediated via inhibition of the EGF-binding. Although data were not shown, suramin inhibited not only internalization of EGFR in the cell lines with EGFR but also the EGFR tyrosin kinase in a dose-dependent manner (39).

In addition, we previously reported that down-regulation of the cellular PKC by TPA elevates the sensitivity of KF cells to CDDP (40). Therefore, we attempted to determine whether inhibition of the cellular PKC by suramin can enhance antiproliferative effects of CDDP, using KF cells without EGFR. We have demonstrated that suramin inhibited KF cell proliferation in a dose-dependent manner and blocked the cell cycles in the G2-M phase (41). As shown in Fig. 8, analyses of isobologram to CDDP and suramin of KF cells revealed that the effect of suramin on antiproliferative activity of CDDP was additive and somewhat synergistic according to the method described by Chou and Talalay (42). Based on these in vitro results, we examined effects of suramin on the growth of KF tumor heterotransplanted into nude mice. As shown in Table 2, complete inhibition of the tumor formation was observed when CDDP and suramin were combined. However, suramin did not inhibit the tumor growth after the formation of palpable tumor. These results suggest that suramin play an inhibitory role in the process of tumor formation or tumor progression. It is well-known that suramin has multiple potential mechanisms of action as a novel antineoplastic agent (43). Suramin has activity against hormonal refractory prostate cancer (44) and clearly merits further studies. However, a preliminary report showed no evidence of response to advanced platinum-resistant ovarian cancer (455). Of great interest would be a trial of i.p. suramin in refractory ovarian cancer. It is most likely that very high levels of suramin can be attained with little or no systemic toxicity. Furthermore, malignant cells can frequently be withdrawn via paracentesis and treated prior to therapy; this may guide or help to individualize drug dosing. Phase I trials are eagerly expected.

CONCLUSIONS

With respect to calmodulin inhibitors, we have demonstrated that the survival of ovarian tumor bearing nude mice can be prolonged by treatment with naphthalene disulfonamides after CDDP. Trifluoperazine, in vitro, increased CDDP cytotoxicity in both sensitive human ovarian carcinoma cells and two sublines with different degrees of resistance to CDDP (46).

Regarding suramin, there can be little doubt of the ability of suramin to affect cellular biology and physiology. However, at the present time, it is probably not prudent to claim that the drug exerts its antiproliferative properties by any single mechanism. The specific mechanism of cellular growth inhibition (e.g., blockade of growth factor-receptor binding) is probably highly tissue type dependent. Furthermore, critical determinants of the mechanism, such as rates of drug intracellular internalization and subcellular compartmentalization, are currently poorly understood. Whether the drug itself will eventually become part of the therapeutic armamentarium is also not clear, although the initial trials are encouraging.

CDDP resistance as find with clinic will be multifactorial. Interactions between several mechanisms identified in vitro such as signal transduction alterations, oncogenic expression and activities of DNA repair enzymes

Table 2. Effect of CDDP and suramin on tumor formation in nude mice

Treatment	Weeks after tumor inoculation								
	2	3	4	5	6	7	8	9	10
Untreated	2/10*	4/10	8/10	8/10	8/10	8/10	8/10	7/ 9	7/9
CDDP (2mg/kg)	1/10	1/10	3/10	4/10	6/10	7/10	7/10	7/10	8/10
Suramin (5mg/kg)	0/10	1/10	1/10	3/10	5/10	5/10	5/10	5/10	5/10
Suramin (10mg/kg)	0/10	0/10	1/10	1/10	3/10	3/10	3/10	3/10	3/10
CDDP→suramin (5mg/kg)	0/10	0/10	1/10	1/10	1/10	2/10	2/10	2/10	2/10
CDDP→suramin (10mg/kg)	0/10	0/10	0/10	0/10	0/10†	0/10†	0/10†	0/10†	0/10†
Suramin(5mg/kg) →CDDP	0/10	0/10	0/10	0/10	0/10†	0/10†	0/10†	0/10†	0/10†
Suramin(10mg/kg) →CDDP	0/10	0/10	0/10	0/10	0/10†	0/10†	0/10†	0/10†	0/10†

*Left and right figures show the number of nude mice with tumor and the total in each group, respectively.

†$P<0.05$ (χ^2 test and contingency table analysis), compared to untreated, CDDP-treated, and suramin (5mg/kg)-treated groups.

have been suggested (47). Further research to establish the identity of such resistance cascades in vitro should be an objective for further research. Finding the in vitro connection between resistance mechanisms might facilitate cancer treatment in more than one way. A cascade will indicate a starting point in the development of resistance, an early event that might serve as a focus for the detection of tumor unresponsiveness. In contrast, patient material will probably show all stages of resistance development in one tumor. In summary, for modulation of CDDP resistance in the clinic a growing number of potentially useful agents emerges from the laboratory bench, including suramin and calmodulin inhibitors. The impact of the known, potentially useful modulators on response and survival is eagerly awaited.

REFERENCES

1. Duraham ACH, and Walton JM.: Calcium ions and the control of proliferation in normal and cancer cells. *Biosci Rep*, 2: 15-30, 1982.
2. Whitfield JF, Boynton AL, MacManus JP, Rixon RH, Siroska M, Tsang B, Walker PR, and Swierenga SHH.: The roles of calcium and cyclic AMP in cell proliferation. *Ann NY Acad Sci*, 339: 216-240, 1980.
3. Chafouleas JGR, Bolton WE, Hidaka H, Boyd AE, and Means AR.: Calmodulin and the cell cycle: Involvement in regulation of cell-cycle progression. *Cell* 28: 41-50, 1982.
4. Ito H, and Hidaka H.: Antitumor effect of a calmodulin antagonist on the growth of solid sarcoma-180. Cancer Lett, 19: 215-220. 1983.
5. Wei JW. Hickie RA, and Klaasen DJ.: Inhibition of human breast cancer colon formation by anticalmodulin agents, trifluoperazine, W-7 and W-13. *Cancer Chemother Pharmacol*, 11: 86-90, 1983.
6. Kikuchi Y, Iwano I, and Kato K.: Effects of calmodulin antagonists on human ovarian cancer cell proliferation in vitro. Biochem Biophys Res Commun, 123: 385-392, 1984.
7. Lee GL, and Hait WN.: Inhibition of growth of C6 astrocytoma cells by inhibitors of calmodulin. *Life Sci*, 36: 347-354, 1985.
8. Bodine PV, and Tupper JT.: Calmodulin antagonists decrease the binding of epidermal growth factor to transformed, but not to normal, human fibroblasts. *Biochem J*, 218: 629-632, 1984.
9. Kikuchi Y, Miyauchi M, and Nagata I.: Inhibition of human ovarian cancer cell proliferation by calmodulin inhibitors and the possible mechanism. *Gynecol Oncol*, 35: 156-158, 1989.

10. Coffey RJ Jr, Leof EB, Shipley GD, and Moses HL.: Suramin inhibition of growth factor receptor binding and mitogenicity in AKR-2B cells. J *Cell Physiol*, 132: 143-148, 1987.
11. Danesi R, LaRocca RV, Stein CA, Neckers L, and Myers CE.: Effect of suramin on the human glioma cell line U706T. *Proc AACR*, 30: 578, 1989.
12. Ewing MW, LaRocca RV, Stein CA, Myers CE, and Linehan WM.: Effect of suramin on proliferation of human prostate carcinoma. *Proc AACR*, 30:310, 1989.
13. Clark J, Chu M, and Calabresi P.: Growth inhibition of colon cancer cells by genistein and suramin. *Proc AACR*, 30: 557, 1989.
14. Bergh J.: Suramin is a potent inhibitor of the cell proliferation in human non-small cell lung cancer cell lines. Proc ASCO, 8: 55, 1989.
15. Rosenberg B, VanCamp L, Trosko JE, and Monsour VH.: Platinum compounds: a new class of potent antitumor agents. *Nature* 222: 385-386, 1969.
16. Ehrlich CE, Einhorn L, Stehman FB, and Blessing J.: Treatment of advanced epithelial ovarian cancer using cisplatin, adriamycin, and cytoxan. *Clin Obstet Gynecol*, 10: 325-335, 1983.
17. Vogl SE, Pagano M, Kaplan BH, Greenwald E, Arseneau J, and Bennett B.: Cisplatin based combination chemotherapy for advanced ovarian cancer. High overall response rate with curative potential only in women with small tumor burdens. Cancer 51:2024-2030, 1983.
18. Piver MS.: Ovarian carcinoma. A decade of progress. Cancer 54: 2706-2715, 1984.
19. Weiss B, Prozialeck WC, and Wallace TL.: Interaction of drugs with calmodulin: Biochemical, pharmacological and clinical implications. *Biochem Pharmacol*, 31: 2217-2226, 1982.
20. Hidaka H, Sasaki Y, Tanaka T, Endo T, Ohno S, Fujii Y, and Nagata T.: N- (6 - aminohexyl) - 5 - chloro - 1 - naphthalenedisulfonamide, a calmodulin antagonist, inhibits cell proliferation. *Proc Natl Acad Sci* USA, 78: 4354-4357, 1981.
21. Kikuchi Y, Oomori K, Kizawa I, Hirata J, Kita T, Miyauchi M, and Kato K.: Enhancement of antineoplastic effects of cisplatin by calmodulin antagonists in nude mice bearing human ovarian carcinoma. *Cancer Res*, 47: 6459-6461, 1987.
22. Kudoh K, Kikuchi Y, Hirata J, Kita T, Hiramatsu H, Tode T, and Nagata I.: A role of glutathione in resistance mechanisms to cis-diaminnedichloroplatinum (II) in human ovarian cancer cell lines in vitro. *Oncol Reports* 2: 763-768, 1995.
23. Chafouleas JG, Bolton WE, and Means AR.: Potentiation of bleomycin lethality by anticalmodulin drugs: a role for calmodulin in DNA repair. *Science* 224: 1346-1348, 1984.

24. Maeda O, Terasawa M, Ishikawa T, Oguchi H, Mizuno K, Kawai M, Kikkawa F, Tomoda Y, and Hidaka H.: A newly synthesized bifunctional inhibitor, W-77, enhances adriamycin activity against human ovarian carcinoma cells. *Cancer Res*, 53: 2051-2056, 1990.
25. Olivier S, Formento P, Fischel JL, Etinne MC, and Milano G.: Epidermal growth factor receptor expression and suramin cytotoxicity in vitro. *Eur J Cancer* 26: 867-871, 1990.
26. Berns EMJJ, Schuurmans ALG, Bolt J, Lamb DJ, Foekens JA, and Mulder E.: Antiproliferative effects of suramin on androgen responsive tumor cells. *Eur J Cancer* 26: 470-474, 1990.
27. Foekens JA, Sieuwerts AM, Stuurman-Smeets EMF, Dorssers LCJ, Berns EMJJ, and Klijn JGM.: Pleiotropic actions of suramin on the proliferation of human breast-cancer cells in vitro. *Int J Cancer* 51: 439-444, 1992.
28. Hosang M.: Suramin binds to platelet-derived growth factor and inhibits its biological activity. J Cell Biochem, 29: 265-273, 1985.
29. Sato Y, and Rifkin DB.: Autocrine activities of basic fibroblastic growth factor: regulation of endothelial cell movement, plasminogen activator synthesis, and DNA synthesis. *J Cell Biol*, 107: 1199-1205., 1988.
30. Betsholtz C, Johnsson A, Heldin C-H, and Westermark B.: Efficient reversion of simian sarcoma virus-transformation and inhibition of growth factor-induced mitogenesis by suramin. *Proc Natl Acad Sci* USA, 83:6440-6444, 1986.
31. Pollak M, and Richard M.: Suramin blockade of insulin like growth factor 1-stimulated proliferation of human osteosarcoma cells. *J Natl Cancer Inst*, 82: 1349-1352, 1990.
32. Kikuchi Y, Miyauchi M, Kizawa I, Oomori K, and Kato K.: Establishment of a cisplatin-resistant human ovarian cancer cell line. *J Natl Cancer Inst*, 77:
33. Kikuchi Y, Kizawa I, Oomori K, Miyauchi M, Kita T, Sugita M, Tenjin Y, and Kato K.: Establishment of a human ovarian cancer cell line capable of forming ascites in nude mice and effects of tranexamic acid on cell proliferation and ascites formation. *Cancer Res*, 47: 592-596, 1987.
34. Kikuchi Y, Hirata J, Kita T, Imaizumi E, Tode T, and Nagata I.: Enhancement of antiproliferative effect of cis-diammine-dichloroplatinum (II) by clomiphene and tamoxifen in human ovarian cancer cells. *Gynecol Oncol*, 4: 365-372, 1993.
35. Yoshiya N.: Establishment of a cell line from human ovarian cancer (undifferentiated carcinoma of FIGO classification) and analysis of its cell-biological characteristics and sensitivity to anticancer drugs. *Acta Obstet Gynaec Jpn*, 38: 1747-1753, 1986 (in Japanese).

36. Wan CW, McKnight MK, Brattain DE, Brattain MG, and Yeoman LC.: Different epidermal growth factor growth responses and receptor levels in human colon carcinoma cell lines. *Cancer Lett*, 43: 139-143, 1988.
37. Henzen-Logmans SC, Berns EMJJ, Klijn JGM, van der Burg MEL, and Foekens JA.: Epidermal growth factor receptor in ovarian tumors: correlation of immunohistochemistry with ligand binding assay. *Br J Cancer* 66: 1015-1021, 1992.
38. Bouché M, Zappeli F, Palimeni M, Adamo S, Westel WC, Senni MI, and Molinaro M.: Rapid activation and down-regulation of protein kinase Ca in 12-O-tetradecanoylphorbol-13-acetate reduced differentiation of human rhabdomyosarcoma cells. *Cell Growth Differentiation* 5: 845-852, 1995.
39. Hirata J.: Personal communication.
40. Hirata J, Kikuchi Y, Kita T, Imaizumi E, Tode T, Ishii K, Kudoh K, and Nagata I.: Modulation of sensitivity of human ovarian cancer cells to cis-diamminedichloroplatinum (II) by 12-O-tetradecanoylphorbol-13-acetate and D,L-buthionine-S,R-sulphoximine. *Int J Cancer* 55:521-527, 1993.
41. Kikuchi Y, Hirata J, Hisano A, Tode T, Kita T, and Nagata I.: Complete inhibition of human ovarian cancer xenografs in nude mice by suramin and cis-diamminedichloroplatinum (II). *Gynecol Oncol*, 58: 11-15. 1995.
42. Chou T-C, and Talalay P.: Quantitative analysis of dose-effect relationships: The combined effects of multiple drugs or enzyme inhibitors. *Adv Enzyme Regul*, 22:27-55, 1984.
43. Stein CA.: Suramin: A novel antineoplastic agent with multiple potential mechanisms of action. *Cancer Res*, 53: 2239-2248, 1993.
44. Eisenberger MA, Reyno LM, Jodrell DI, Sinibaldi VJ, Tkaczuk KH, Sridhara R, Zuhowski EG, Lowitt MH, Jacobs SC, and Egorin MJ.: Suramin, an active drug for prostate cancer: Interim ovservations in a phase I trial. *J Natl Cancer Inst*, 85:611-621, 1993.
45. Reed E, Cosper M, LaRocca R, Bostick-Bruton F, and Myers C.: Suramin in advanced platinum-resistant ovarian cancer. *Eur J Cancer* 28A: 864-866, 1992.
46. Perez RP, Handel LM, Schilder RJ, Ozols RF, and Hamilton TC.: Potentiation of cisplatin cytotoxicity by trifluoperazine, a calmodulin inhibitor. *Proc AACR*, 31:403, 1990.
47. Timmer-Bosscha H, Mulder NH, and de Vries EGE.: Modulation of cis-diamminedichloroplatinum (II) resistance: a review. *Br J Cancer* 66: 227-238, 1992.

CHAPTER 7

PROTEIN KINASE C AND PLATINUM SENSITIVITY

Isonishi, S.[§], Howell, S. B.* and Terashima, Y.
Department of Obstetrics/Gynecology Jikei University School of Medicine, 3-25-8 Nishi-shinbashi, Minato-ku, Tokyo 105, Japan, *Department of Medicine and the Cancer Center, University of California, San Diego, La Jolla, California 92093, U.S.A.; [§] Corresponding author.

Key words: protein kinase C, platinum drugs

ABSTRACT

In our 2008 human ovarian carcinoma cells, activation of a number of different pathways induced 2 to 4-fold sensitivity to platinum compounds. One of these signaling pathways is that activated by protein kinase C. Enhanced sensitivity to chemotherapeutic agents is presumed to be mediated by phosphorylation of target proteins. With the growing understanding of how signaling events relate to platinum sensitivity, new and potentially useful stratagies for modulating platinum sensitivity are involved.

TEXT

Protein kinase C (PKC) plays a crucial role in signal transduction for variety of biologically active substances which activate cellular functions (1). PKC is transiently activated by diacylglycerol which is produced in the membrane during the signal induced turnover of inositol phospholipids. Activation of PKC results in serine or threonine phosphorylation on target molecules and induces many cellular functions, including cellular differentiation, proliferation, and the cellular program of gene expression (1). PKC may play a role in the in vitro transformation process caused by the oncogenes such as ras, cis (2), fms, and fes (3).

Isolation and analysis of cDNA clones have revealed the existence of a family of PKC genes (4). PKC family now can be classified into conventional (cPKC; α, β, γ) and novel PKCs (nPKC;ε, δ, ξ, η) based on their requirement or lack of requirement of Ca^{2+} for activity. The isoenzymes display cell-type-specific expression (5), may have different substrate specificities, and may perform different specilized functions.

PKC is a target for phorbol esters such as 12-O-tetradecanoylphorbol-13-acetate (TPA), as the tumor promoters directly activate this enzyme and there is a correlation between the ability of individual phorbol esters to promote tumors and to activate the enzyme (6, 7). Kinetic analysis indicates that TPA, which has a diacylglycerole-like structure, is able to substitute for diacylglycerole at extremely low concentrations. Like diacylglycerole, TPA dramatically increases the affinity of the enzyme for Ca^{2+}, resulting in its full activation without detectable cellular mobilization of Ca^{2+} (7). Thus the effect of TPA appear to be largely mediated through stimulation of PKC and the subsequent phosphorylation of a variety of protein substrate.

Recently, we have shown that α- and ζ-isotype PKC were the dominant forms present in both human ovarian carcinoma 2008 cells and its 10-fold cisplatin-resistant variant 2008/C13*5.25 cells, whereas none of the other isoforms could be identified in these cells (8). Thus PKCα is the only enzyme that is able to be responsive to TPA in those cells. This is indicating that both 2008 and 2008/C13*5.25 cells have a very simple PKC-signal transduction pathway and therefore good model to elucidate the PKC-associated cellular mechanism of platinum sensitivity.

Activation of PKC has been shown to regulate the sensitivity of cancer cells to chemotherapeutic agents (9-11). We have shown that TPA enhanced the sensitivity of 2008 cells to cisplatin by a factor of 2.5 fold. A similar degree of sensitization was produced in 2008/C13*5.25 cells (10). The synergistic interaction between TPA and cisplatin was completely inhibited by pretreatment with staurosporine, a potent inhibitor of PKC. These findings indicate that PKC regulates the sensitivity to cisplatin by phosphorylation of a substrate of PKC in both cisplatin sensitive and resistant cells. Furthermore activation of PKC by TPA was found to enhance the sensitivity of 2008 cells to cisplatin analogues such as carboplatin and (Glycolato-o, o')diammineplatinum(II) (254-S) (12). TPA sensitized the cells to carboplatin and 254-S by factors of 2.8 and 2.4 respectively. Including cisplatin all these three are platinum(II) compounds, but each has a different leaving ligand. In the cytosol, aquation displaces the two

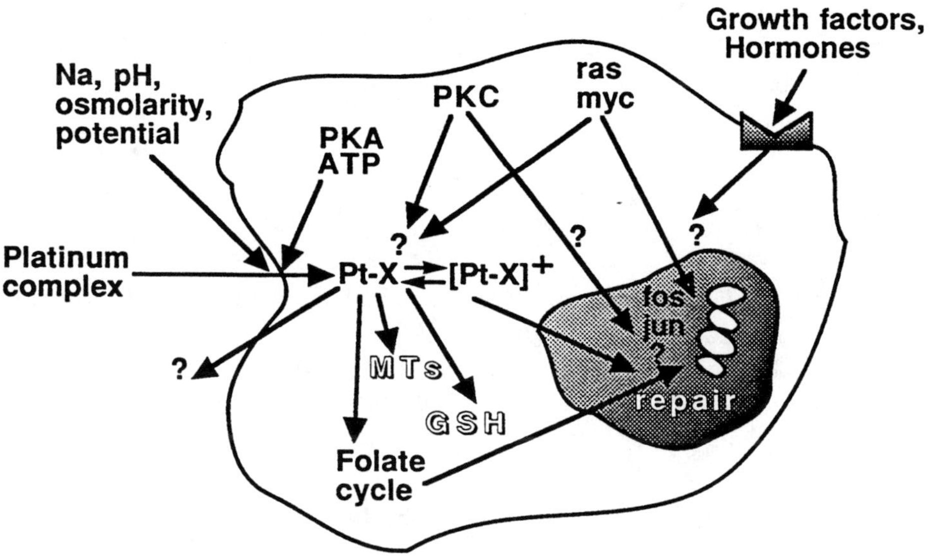

chlorides from cisplatin, the cyclobutane dicarboxylate from carboplatin, and glycolato group from 254-S. All three drugs generate the same $Pt(NH_3)_2(H_2O)_2^{++}$ reactive species, and produce the same types of DNA-adducts. The fact that TPA was able to sensitize cells to all three agents, and by approximately equivalent degrees, indicates that the effect was not specific to any one type of leaving ligand. TPA was also able to enhance the sensitivity of the cisplatin-resistant 2008/C13*5.25 subline to each of the three drugs to the same extent as for the 2008 cells. TPA sensitized the 2008/C13*5.25 cells by a factor of 3.2 for carboplatin and 2.5 for 254-S. TPA was as effective at sensitizing the resistant cells as it was at sensitizing the sensitive 2008 cells, and therefore the mechanism must be independent of those factors that render the 2008/C13*5.25 cells resistant.

The mechanisms by which TPA enhances platinum cytotoxicity to tumor cells are currently not understood (12) (Fig. 1). TPA produced no significant change in the cellular accumulation of platinum, and did not alter the cellular content of glutathione or activity of glutathione-S-transferase. Activation of PKC induced, rather than suppressed metallothionein IIa mRNA levels in 2008 cells. Increased metallothionein levels would be expected to result in resistance to cisplatin rather than increased sensitivity. Hence, alteration of metallothionein levels cannot accout for the observed chemosensitization following activation of PKC. TPA did increase the formation of intrastrand cross-links by a factor of 1.5-fold. The effect was relatively small in magnitude, and it is currently not known to what extent small changes in the intrastrand adducts are biologically relevant. The mechanism by which activation of PKC modulates platinum sensitivity is not understood at this point of time.

REFERENCES

1. Nishizuka, Y. The role of protein kinase C in cell surface signal transduction and tumor promotion. Nature 308, 693-698, 1984.
2. Preiss, J., Loomis, C., Bishop, W., Stein, R., Niedel, J., and Bell, R. M. Quantitative measurement of sn-1, 2-diacylglycerols present in platelets, hepatocytes and ras- and cis-transformed normal rat kidney cells. J. Biol. Chem. 261, 8597-87600, 1986.
3. Jakowski, S., Rettenmier, C. w., Sherr, C. J., and Rock, C. O. A guanine-nucleotide-dependent phosphotidalinositol-4, 5-diphosphate phospholipase C in cells transformed by the v-fms and v-fes oncogenes. J. Biol. Chem. 261, 4978-4985, 1986.
4. Housey, G. M., O'Brian, C. A., Johnson, M. D., Kirschmeier, P., and Weinstein, I. B. Isolation of cDNA clones encoding protein kinase C: evidence for a protein kinase C-related gene family. Proc. Natl. Acad. Sci. USA 84, 1065-1069, 1987.
5. Brandt, S. J., Niedel, J. E., Bell, R. M., and Young, W. S., III. Distinct patterns of expression of different protein kinase C mRNAs in rat tissues. Cell 49, 57-63, 1987.
6. Castagna, M., Takai, Y., Kaibuchi, K., Sano, K., Kikkawa, U., and Nishizuka, Y. Direct activation of calcium-activated, phospholipid-dependent protein kinase by tumor-promoting phorbol esters. Biol. Chem. 257, 7847-7851, 1982.
7. Yamanishi, J., Takai, Y., Kaibuchi, K., Sano, K., Castagna, M., and Nishizuka, Y. Synergistic functions of phorbol ester and calcium in serotonin release from human platelets. Biochem. Biophys. Res. Commun. 112, 778-786, 1983.
8. Isonishi, S., Ochiai, K., Yasuda, M., Ohkawa, K., and Terashima, Y. Mechanism-related circumvention of cisplatin resistance in human ovarian carcinoma cells by (-) - ® -2 - aminomethylpyrrolidine (1, 1 - cyclobutane-

dicarboxylato)-platinum(II) monohydrate and modulation of its sensitivity by 12-O-tetradecanoylphorbol-13-acetate. Int. J. Oncolo. (in press).

9. Fine R. L., Patel, J., Chabner, B. A. Phorbol esters induce multidrug resistance in human breast cancer cells. Proc. Natl. Acad. Sci. USA 85, 582-586, 1988.
10. Isonishi, S., Andrews, P. A., and Howell, S. B. Increased sensitivity to cis-Diamminedichloroplatinum(II) in humanovarian carcinoma cells in response to treatment with 12-O-tetradecanoylphorbol-13-acetate. J. Biol. Chem., 265, 3623-3627, 1990.
11. Basu, A., Teicher, B. A., and Lazo, J. S. Involvement of protein kinase C in phorbor ester-induced sensitization of Hela cells to cis-Diamminedichloroplatinum(II). J. Biol. Chem., 265, 8451-8457, 1990.
12. Isonishi, S., Hom, D. K., Eastman, A. and Howell, S. B. Enhancement of sensitivity to platinum(II)-containing drugs by 12-O-tetradecanoyl-phobol-13-acetate in a human ovarian carcinoma cell line. Br. J. Cancer. 69, 217-221, 1994.
13. Huang, K. P., Nakabayashi, H., and Huang, F. L. Isozymic forms of rat brain Ca^{2+}-activated and phospholipid-dependent protein kinase. Proc. Natl. Acad. Sci. USA 83, 8535-8539, 1986.

CHAPTER 8

SENSITIZATION OF HUMAN OVARIAN CARCINOMA CELLS TO PLATINUM ANTICANCER DRUGS BY AMPHOTERICIN B

Fumitaka Kikkawa*, Osamu Maeda, Koji Tamakoshi, Hidenori Oguchi and Yutaka Tomoda

Department of Obstetrics and Gynecology, Nagoya University School of Medicine, Tsurumai-Cho 65, Showa-Ku, Nagoya 466, Japan

ABSTRACT

The ability of amphotericin B (AMB), an antifungal drug, to modulate the cytotoxicity of 5 platinum anticancer drugs was investigated in human ovarian carcinoma cell lines sensitive (NOS2), or with experimentally induced resistance (NOS2CR) to, cis-diamminedichloroplatinum (II) (CDDP). NOS2CR cells had 7.4-fold resistance to CDDP and were partially cross-resistant to 4 CDDP analogues. In NOS2CR cells, intracellular platinum accumulation was significantly lower than in NOS2 cells at each concentration and exposure time tested. The percentage platinum accumulation level of 5 platinum anticancer drugs in NOS2CR cells compared to NOS2 cells was inversely correlated with resistance factors, suggesting that resistance to 5 platinum anticancer drugs was due, in part, to reduced intracellular drug levels. Treatment with AMB enhanced the cytotoxicity of 5 platinum anticancer drugs in both types of cells. In particular, the CDDP IC_{50} value was reduced 4.2-fold in NOS2 cells and 7.2-fold in NOS2CR cells. Intracellular platinum accumulation of CDDP was remarkably increased by the treatment with AMB in both of these cells. In NOS2 cells, AMB a caused marked increase in the intracellular platinum

* Correspondence to Fumitaka Kikkawa, Department of Obstetrics and Gynecology, Nagoya University School of Medicine, Tsurumai-cho 65, Showa-ku, Nagoya 466, Japan Tel No. Japan 52-741-2111 Ext. 2245, Fax No. Japan 52-731-6136

accumulation of platinum anticancer drugs except for one drug, while in NOS2CR cells a remarkable increase was observed only in the combination treatment with CDDP and AMB. These results indicate that AMB can enhance the cytotoxicity of CDDP most among 5 platinum anticancer drugs at a low concentration in both NOS2 and NOS2CR cells, mainly due to the increasing intracellular platinum anticancer drugs.

INTRODUCTION

Although combination chemotherapy including CDDP has dramatically improved survival of patients with ovarian carcinoma, the long-term prognosis is still poor (1), presumably due to the intrinsic and acquired resistance to CDDP. It is important to clarify the mechanism of CDDP resistance in order to further improve survival. Several mechanisms possibly contributing to the resistance to CDDP have been proposed including increased removal of DNA-bound CDDP, increased intracellular glutathione (GSH) levels and enhanced activity of glutathione S-transferase (GST), which are thought to play a key role in intracellular detoxification (2,3). Using a better understanding of the possible resistance mechanism, several approaches have been followed to overcome resistance, such as inhibition of poly-ADP ribose synthesis by 3-aminobenzamide (3AB), reduction of intracellular GSH by D,L-buthionine-sulfoximine (BSO), and inhibition of α polymerase by aphidicolin (4,5).

A variety of cell lines with acquired resistance to CDDP exhibit reduced intracellular platinum accumulation of CDDP as part of their resistant phenotype (6,7). It has been assumed for many years that CDDP enters cells by a passive diffusion process, but the exact mechanisms involved have not been completely defined and may differ between functionally different cell types.

Cis-diammine (1,1-cyclobutanedicarboxylato) platinum (II) (CBDCA) is the first clinically available analogue with lower emetic potential and nephrotoxicity, but it causes severe thrombocytopenia. Further, most CDDP resistant cell lines, as well as NOS2CR, have a cross resistance to CBDCA. Indeed, treatment with CBDCA has often failed in patients with CDDP-resistant ovarian carcinoma. Several CDDP analogues were developed in Japan and phase II or III trials are now under way. Their cytotoxic effects *in vivo* are almost the same as those of CDDP, and they cause lower side effects.

Enhancing intracellular platinum accumulation is possible to sensitize sensitive cells as well as resistant cells. AMB can potentiate the cytotoxicity of anticancer drugs, such as adriamycin (ADM) and

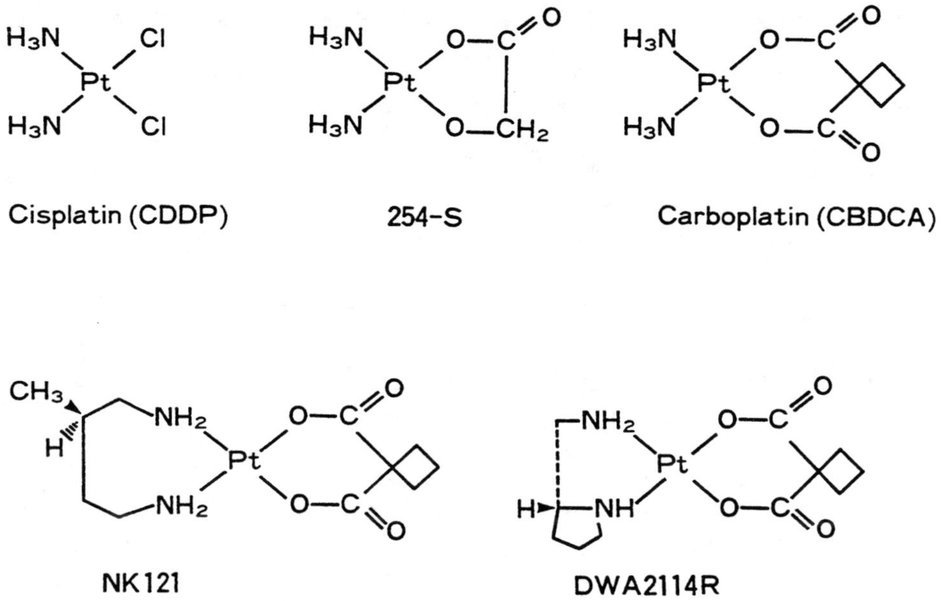

Figure 1. Chemical structure of platinum anticancer drugs.

mitomycin C (MMC) by enhancing intracellular drug levels (8,9). In this article, we evaluated the capacity of AMB to enhance the intracellular drug accumulation and the cytotoxicity of 5 platinum anticancer drugs in human ovarian carcinoma cell lines sensitive, or with experimentally induced resistance to, CDDP.

SENSITIVITY TO PLATINUM ANTICANCER DRUGS

As shown in figure 1, CBDCA and 254-S are modified at the chloric residues with the dioxylato group, while NK121 and DWA2114R have the CBDCA structure, which is further modified at the amine residues with the unsymmetrical diammine group.

NOS2 cells, established from a patient with serous cystadenocarcinoma of the ovary, were used in these studies. By continuous exposure to CDDP while slowly escalating the concentration for 18 months, these cells acquired CDDP resistance, and were then designated NOS2CR. Sensitivity to drugs was measured by MTT assay as described in our previous report (10). IC_{50} was used as the measure of relative cytotoxicity. The resistance factor (RF) was considered to be the

Table 1. Sensitivity of the NOS2 and NOS2CR cells to platinum anticancer drugs.

	IC_{50} (μM)		
	NOS2	NOS2CR	Resistance Factor
CDDP	3.73	27.5	7.4
254-S	11.7	50.1	4.3
CBDCA	75.4	223	3.0
NK121	48.7	111	2.3
DWA2114R	50.5	80.8	1.6

ratio of the IC_{50} of the NOS2CR cells to the IC_{50} of the NOS2 cells. The IC_{50} and the RF to 5 platinum anticancer drugs were summarized in table 1. The results indicated that NOS2CR cells, while particularly resistant to CDDP, were cross-resistant to the 4 CDDP analogues tested, although the RF was lower for the analogues. A modest level of cross-resistance to CBDCA has been observed in several CDDP-resistant cell lines (11,12,13,14). Katabami et al. reported that a human lung squamous-carcinoma cell line, 11.4-fold resistant to CDDP, is cross-resistant to CBDCA and 254-S (7). NOS2CR cells also showed a modest level of cross-resistance to CBDCA and 254-S, and the RF of 254-S was larger than that of CBDCA. This might be due to the structural similarity to CBDCA. A low level of cross-resistance to NK121 and DWA2114R, further modified at the amine residues of CBDCA, was observed. The mechanism underlying cross-resistance to CDDP analogues is not clear, but it is possible that the same mechanism operating in CDDP might be responsible.

INTRACELLULAR PLATINUM ACCUMULATION

Exponentially growing cells were incubated in freshly changed RPMI1640 medium containing 10% fetal bovine serum and each platinum drugs at various concentrations for 2 hours except as indicated. After washing with phosphate-buffered saline, analysis for intracellular platinum accumulation was performed by a modified method of Pera and Harder (15). Figure 2 shows that platinum accumulation in the NOS2 and the NOS2CR cells was a linear function of cisplatin concentration up to at least 300 μM. The accumulation of CDDP was also linear over a 3-hour incubation time. At each exposure concentration and exposure time,

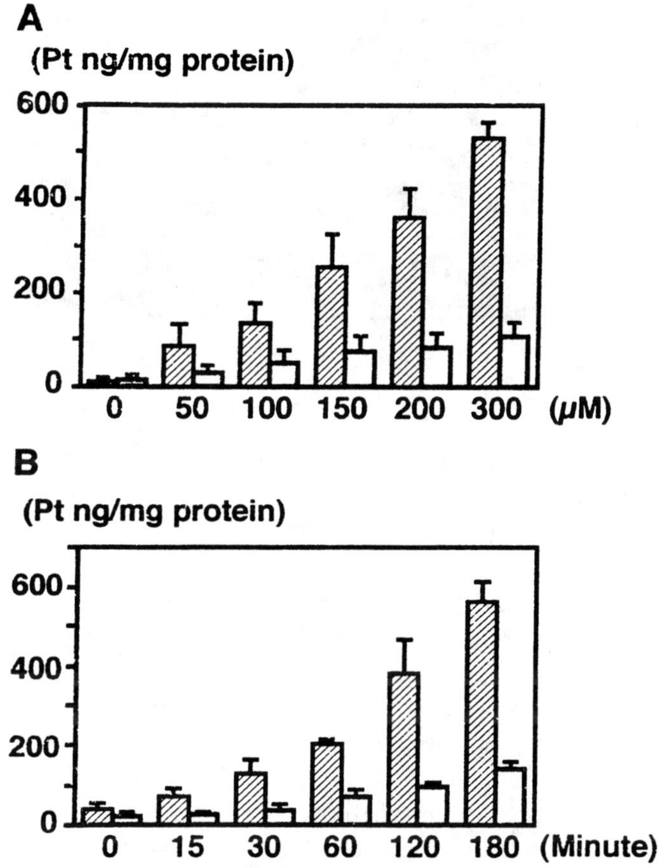

Figure 2. Intracellular platinum accumulation of CDDP in NOS2 ( ) and NOS2CR cells ( ) as measured by atomic absorption. A, Intracellular platinum accumulation of CDDP after 2 h exposure of CDDP with various concentrations. B, Intracellular platinum accumulation of CDDP after exposure of 200 μM CDDP for various times. Points are the mean values for 4 independent experiments and bars indicate the S.D.

platinum levels were reduced significantly in the NOS2CR cells compared to the NOS2 cells. These results suggested that the reduced sensitivity to CDDP in NOS2CR cells was predominantly due to reduced intracellular CDDP levels, although various other mechanisms have been proposed. Further, we investigated intracellular platinum accumulation of CDDP

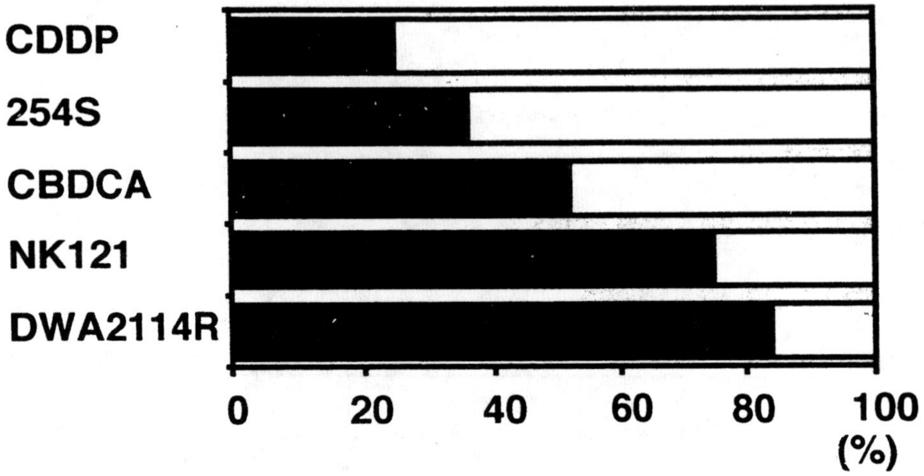

Figure 3. Intracellular platinum accumulation of each platinum anticancer drug in the NOS2CR cells was expressed as a percentage of that in the NOS2 cells.

analogues following 2-hour exposure of the respective drugs. As shown in figure 3, NOS2CR cells accumulated 25% and 16% less platinum than NOS2 cells following exposure to NK121 and DWA2114R, respectively, whereas accumulation of 254-S and CBDCA was only 36 and 52% of that in NOS2 cells, respectively. The platinum level in NOS2CR cells, as a percentage of that in NOS2 cells, was inversely correlated with RF, suggesting that reduced intracellular platinum levels were involved in resistance to platinum anticancer drugs.

MODULATION OF ANTICANCER DRUGS BY AMPHOTERICIN B

The polyene antibiotic, AMB, has a unique mechanism of action related to its affinity for sterol in the cell membrane (16). Studies have shown that AMB binds to cholesterol and causes 0.4 to 1.0 nm pores in the cell membrane, increasing permeability and facilitating uptake of various molecules (17,18). Medoff et al. reported that AMB in combination with actinomycin D resulted in a significant decrease in the number of variable cells and increase in the cellular uptake of actinomycin D incorporated in HeLa cells resistant to actinomycin D up to 6-fold (8).

Since AMB had little effect on cell survival at concentrations below 10 mg/ml in the NOS2 and the NOS2CR cells, we investigated the enhancing effect of 5 and 10 mg/ml of AMB on the intracellular drug

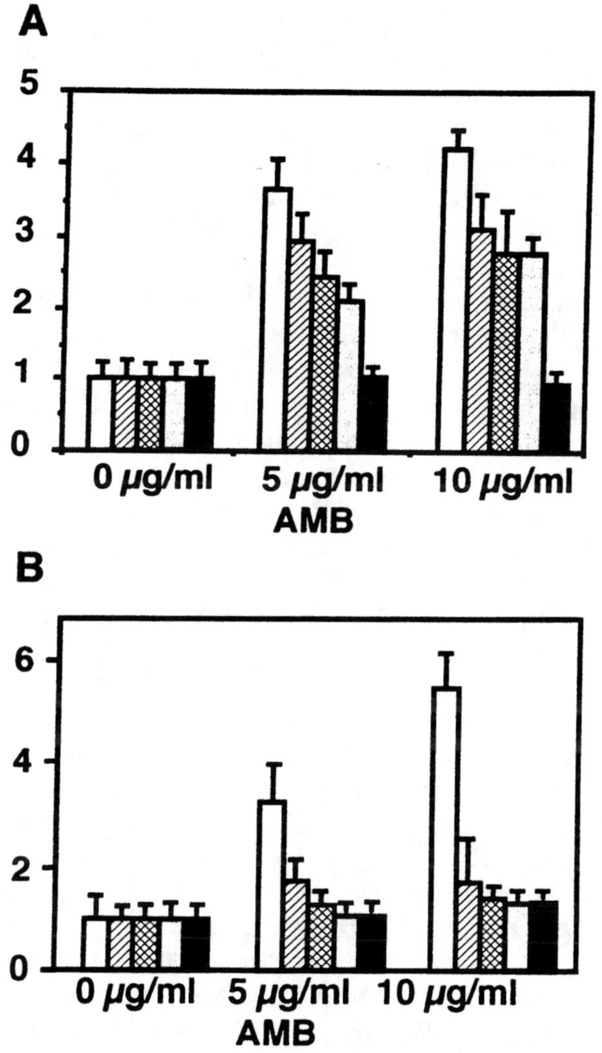

Figure 4. Intracellular platinum accumulation of CDDP ( ), 254-S ( ), CBDCA ( ), NK121 ( ), and DWA2114R ( ) in combination with or without AMB in the NOS2 (A) and the NOS2CR cells (B). Each bar indicates a ratio of the value for anticancer drug without AMB to that with AMB.

levels and the cytotoxicity of platinum anticancer drugs. Figure 4 shows the intracellular platinum levels in combination with AMB expressed relative to the values for each anticancer drug alone. In the NOS2 cells 5 mg/ml AMB enhanced significantly intracellular platinum except for

DWA2114R, and a further increase was observed in combination with 10 ug/ml. In the NOS2CR cells, intracellular platinum accumulation of 4 CDDP analogues increased only slightly even in the combination with 10 μM AMB, although that of CDDP increased remarkably in a dose-dependent manner. Only a few drugs are known to increase the intracellular CDDP level. Jekunen et al. reported that intracellular CDDP level increased markedly by the treatment with 20 μM dipyridamole, at which concentration it caused minimal inhibition of cell survival in 2008 cells (19). However, dipyridamole had little effect on CDDP cytotoxicity in the NOS2 and the NOS2CR cells (data not shown). Randolph et al. reported that forskolin and 3-isobutyl-1-methylxanthine (IBMX) enhanced intracellular CDDP accumulation as well as the CDDP cytotoxicity in CDDP-sensitive cells. In resistant cells, however, neither effect was observed. AMB enhanced markedly the CDDP cytotoxicity in both the NOS2 and the NOS2CR cells. The potency of the enhancing effect of AMB was expressed by dose modification factor (DMF), which is ratio of IC_{50} in the treatment with anticancer drug alone to IC_{50} in the combination treatment with AMB (Table 2). The order of DMFs was in accordance with the order of RFs of the NOS2CR cells to the NOS2 cells, suggesting that the mechanism of the potentiating effect of AMB was associated with the mechanisms of CDDP resistance. Several authors proposed that the effect of AMB at the cellular level is more complex than simply producing micropores in the cell membrane (18,20).

CDDP is one of the most important drugs utilized in ovarian carcinoma despite its severe side effects. Recurrent tumors often acquire resistance to this drug, limiting its clinical usefulness. Thus, CDDP analogues have been developed. Our results demonstrated that DWA2114R was the most effective platinum anticancer drug in the NOS2CR cells, an effect that may be due to the lower reduction of drug levels. However, AMB enhanced the cytotoxicity of this drug lower than 2-fold and the intracellular drug level increased little in both types of cells, while the CDDP cytotoxicity and the intracellular level were markedly enhanced. Various approaches have been employed in an attempt to overcome CDDP resistance (21,22). These attempts have met with limited success, since the modifying drug proved to be too toxic to be applied in vivo. AMB is a widely used antifungal drug, but its administration in large amounts causes renal failure. Thus, it is necessary to study how to administer AMB in vivo. The present findings suggest that combination therapy with CDDP and AMB may be useful in patients with CDDP-resistant ovarian carcinoma.

Table 2.
Dose modification factor in combination with AMB

	NOS2 (DMF)		NOS2CR (DMF)	
	AMB 5 μM	10 μM	AMB 5 μM	10 μM
CDDP	2.5	4.2	3.9	7.2
254-S	2.1	3.2	2.3	4.2
CBDCA	1.9	3.2	2.1	4.0
NK121	1.5	1.8	1.5	1.7
DWA2114R	1.2	1.5	1.5	1.7

REFERENCES

1. Omura G., Blessing J.A., Ehrlich C.E., Miller A., Yordan E., Creasman W.T., Homesley H.D. A randomized trial of cyclophosphamide and doxorubicin with or without cisplatin in advanced ovarian carcinoma. Cancer. 57: 1725-1730, 1986.
2. Fram R.J., Wonda B.A., Wilson J.M., Robichaud N. Characterization of acquired resistance to cis-diamminedichloroplatinum (II) in BE human colon carcinoma cells. Cancer Res. 50: 72-77, 1990.
3. Masuda H., Tanaka T., Matsuda H., Kusaba I. Increased removal of DNA-bound platinum in a human ovarian cancer cell line resistant to cis-diamminedichloroplatinum (II). Cancer Res. 50: 1863-1866, 1990.
4. Chen G., Zeller W.J. Enhancement of cisplatin (DDP) antitumor activity by 3-aminobenzamide in rat ovarian tumors sensitive and resistant to DDP in vivo. Cancer Chemother. Pharmacol. 26: 37-41, 1990.
5. Hrubisky M., McGown A.T., Fox B.W. The role of metallothionein, glutathione S-transferases and DNA repair in resistance to platinum drugs in a series of L1210 cell lines made resistant to anticancer platinum agents. Biochem. Pharmacol. 45: 253-256, 1993.
6. Katabami M., Fujita H., Haneda H., Akita H., Kuzumaki N., Miyamoto H., Kawakami Y. Reduced drug accumulation in a newly established human lung aquamous-carcinoma cell line resistant to cis-diamminedichloroplatinum (II). Biochem. Pharmacol. 44: 394-397, 1992.
7. Kelland L.R., Mistry P., Abel G., Loh S.Y., O'Neill C.F., Murrer B.A., Harrap K.R. Mechanism-related circumvention of acquired cis-diamminedichloroplatinum (II) resistance using pairs of human ovarian carcinoma cell lines by ammine/amine platinum (IV) dicarboxylates. Cancer Res. 52: 3857-3864, 1992.

8. Medoff J., Medoff G., Goldstein M.N., Schlesinger D., Kobayashi G.S. Amphotericin B-induced sensitivity to actinomycin D in drug-resistant HeLa cells. Cancer Res. 35: 2548-2552, 1975.
9. Krishan A., Sauerteig A., Gordon K. Effect of amphotericin B on adriamycin transport in P388 cells. Cancer Res. 45: 4097-4102, 1985.
10. Mizuno K., Furuhashi Y., Maeda O., Iwata M., Misawa T., Kawai M., Kano T., Tomoda Y. Mitomycin C cross-resistance induced by adriamycin in human ovarian cancer cells in vitro. Cancer Chemother. Pharmacol. 26: 333-339, 1990.
11. Twentyman P.R., Wright K.A., Mistry P., Kelland L.R., Murrer B.A. Sensitivity to novel platinum compounds of panels of human lung cancer cell lines with acquired and inherent resistance to cisplatin. Cancer Res. 52: 5647-5680, 1992.
12. Hill B.T., Shellard S.A., Hosking L.K., Dempke W.C., Fichtinger-Schepman A.M., Tone T., Scanlon K.J., Whelan R.D. Characterization of a cisplatin-resistant human ovarian carcinoma cell line expressing cross-resistance to 5-fluorouracil but collateral sensitivity to methotrexate. Cancer Res. 52: 3110-3118, 1992.
13. Fram R.J., Wonda B.A., Wilson J.M., Robichaud N. Characteriza- tion of acquired resistance to cis-diamminedichloroplatinum (II) in BE human colon carcinom cells. Cancer Res. 50: 1963-1866, 1990.
14. Kraker A.J., Moore C.W. Accumulation of cis-diamminedichloro-platinum (II) and platinum analogues by platinum-resistant murine leukemia cells in vitro. Cancer Res. 48: 9-13, 1988.
15. Pera M.F.Jr., Harder H.C. Analysis for platinum in biological material by flameless atomic absorption spectrometry. Clin. Chem. 23: 1245-1249, 1977.
16. Hamilton-Miller J.M.T. Chemistry and biology of the polyene macrolide antibiotics. Bacteriol. Rev. 73: 166-196, 1973.
17. Zygmunt W.A. Intracellular loss of potassium in candida albicans after exposure to polyene antifungal antibiotics. Appl. Microbiol. 14: 953-956, 1966.
18. Presant C.A., Valeriote F., Proffitt R., Metter G. Amphotericin B-interactions with nitrosoureas and other antineoplastic agents. In: Prestayko A.W., Cooke S.T., Baker L.H., Carter S.K., Schein P.S. eds. Nitrosoureas: Current status and new developments, New York: Academic Press, Inc. 343-360, 1981.
19. Jekunen A., Vick J., Thomas R., Chan C.R., Howell S.B. Synergism between dipyridamole and cisplatin in human ovarian carcinoma cells in vitro. Cancer Res. 52: 3566-3571, 1992.
20. Medoff G., Valeriote F., Dieckman J. Potentiation of anticancer agents by amphotericin B. J. Natl. Cancer Inst. 67: 131-135, 1981.

21. Chen G., Zeller W.J. Enhancement of cisplatin (CDDP) antitumor activity by 3-aminobenzamide in rat ovarian tumors sensitive and resistant to DDP in vivo. Cancer Chemother. Pharmacol. 26: 37-41, 1990.
22. Ikeda H., Nakano G., Nagashima K., Sakamoto K., Hasegawa N., Kitamura T., Nakamura T. Verapamil enhancement of antitumor effect of cis-diamminedichloroplatinum (II) in nude mouse-grown human neuroblastoma. Cancer Res. 47: 231-236, 1987.

CHAPTER 9

MODE OF ACTION OF MICROTUBULE INHIBITORS (PACLITAXEL/TAXOTERE) IN CDDP-SENSITIVE AND -RESISTANT OVARIAN CANCER CELL LINES.*

Kazuo Imamura, M.D., Yasuhiko Kiyozuka, M.D., Ph.D., Michiaki Yakushiji, M.D., Ph.D.

Department of Obstetrics and Gynecology, Kurume University, School of Medicine.

Key words : Paclitaxel, Taxotere, CDDP-resistant cell line, Ovarian cancer

SUMMARY

We studied the cytotoxicity of paclitaxel and taxotere against cisplatin (CDDP)-sensitive (MN-1, EC) and -resistant cell lines (SHIN-3, KEN-3). To establish an optimal schedule for clinical administration in combination with CDDP, the cytotoxicity of paclitaxel or taxotere alone and in sequential combination with CDDP were also investigated in vitro using the MTT assay.

Dose- and schedule-dependency were significant at lower concentrations of paclitaxel and taxotere, while only schedule-dependency was observed at higher concentrations of taxotere. No cross-resistance to CDDP was observed. Increasing the area under the curve (AUC) by dose escalation seemed to confer no advantageous effects on the cytotoxicity. The cytotoxicity of taxotere was approximately 0.71- to 129-fold that of paclitaxel, when the IC_{50s} of both agents were compared. The most

* Address for reprints and correspondence to: Kazuo Imamura, M.D. Department of Obstetrics and Gynecology, Kurume University School of Medicine, 67-Asahi-machi, Kurume 830, Fukuoka, Japan. Tel:0942-35-3311

prominent G2/M phase arrest was observed in response to 0.5 μM paclitaxel treatment.

In a combination with CDDP, treatment with these drugs over 48 hours followed by CDDP administration (CDDP>10 μg/ml)demonstrated the most effective "relative inhibition rate".

INTRODUCTION

Paclitaxel (taxol) is a natural plant product extracted from the bark of the Western Yew, *Taxus brevifolia*, which grows in the Pacific Northwest region of the United States.[1] This agent has a unique mechanism of action and a broad spectrum of antineoplastic activity. Paclitaxel promotes the assembly of microtubules as well as stabilize their formation by preventing depolymerization.[2, 3] In contrast, other antimicrotubule agents such as colchicine or vincristine induce the disassembly of microtubules.[4] Paclitaxel is also known to be a potent inhibitor of cell proliferation, blocking the cell cycle in the late G2 or M phase.[1] This agent has also been reported to significantly improve the response rate of platinum- treated refractory ovarian neoplasms and to be superior to conventional salvage therapy.[5, 6] However, because of problems of supply, its usage have been limited.

Taxotere (N-debenzoyl-N-tert-butoxycarbonyl-10-deacetyl taxol; RP 56976; NSC 628503) is a semisynthetic analog of paclitaxel. Taxotere is prepared from a noncytotoxic precursor extracted from the needles of the European Yew, *Taxus baccata*, which is then esterified with the synthetic side-chain.[7, 8] It has been reported that taxotere is more active against cancer cell lines in vitro than paclitaxel, [9] and also no cross-resistance has been reported to this class agent with topoisomerase I and II-related multidrug resistance phenotypes.[10]

In the present study, we investigated the cytotoxicity of paclitaxel and taxotere against established ovarian cancer cell lines (cisplatin(CDDP)-sensitive and -resistant). In addition, to establish a clinically optimal administration schedule for combination with CDDP, the cytotoxicity of paclitaxel or taxotere alone and in sequential combination with CDDP were investigated in vitro using the 3-(4, 5-dimethylthiazol-2-yl)-2, 5-diphenyl tetrazolium bromide (MTT) assay.[11, 12]

MATERIALS AND METHODS

CELL LINES

We studied the effects of these agents on four established cell lines: SHIN-3, ovarian serous cystadenocarcinoma cells obtained from a patient who became resistant to CDDP13); KEN-3, an ovarian fibrosarcoma cell line resistant to CDDP [14]; EC, a cell line derived from a mixed germ cell tumor which was sensitive to CDDP [15]; and MN-1, a cell line developed from a patient with mucinous cyst- adenocarcinoma who responded to CDDP-based chemotherapy.[16] These established cell lines were incubated in Dulbecco's minimum essential medium (DMEM) supplemented with 10% FCS (Gibco, Grand Island, N.Y.), and grown at 37°C in a humidified atmosphere of 5% CO_2 in air.

To assay cytotoxicity, single cell suspensions in medium in the presence or absence of drugs were plated in 96-well multiplates. A total of 10^4 cells per 50 µl of culture medium were plated and incubated for 24 hours before drug administration.

DRUG PREPARATION

Paclitaxel (Bristol-Myers Oncology Division, Bristol Laboratories, Evansville, IN) and taxotere (Rhône-Poulenc Rorer, Vitry-sur-Seine, France) were reconstituted in sterile dimethylsulfoxide (DMSO) at a concentration of 1000 µM and diluted to the final concentration immediately before use. The final concentration of DMSO in the culture medium was adjusted to less than 1.0% (V/V) which was found to have no antiproliferative effect on any cell line used.

MTT ASSAY

The number of cells plated in each of the 96-wells was deter- mined from the results of preliminary studies of cell growth using the MTT assay (data not shown) so that the untreated cells were in the exponential growth phase during the experiment. An equal number of cells (10^4 cells/well) were inoculated into each well in 50 µl of culture medium. Then, 150µl of 4/3 fold concentration of drug diluted in medium was added. We studied 10 concent- rations of paclitaxel and taxotere, covering a 4-log range of concentrations chosen to span the 50% inhibitory concentration (IC_{50}) as determined by preliminary assays (data not shown). Following culture, 13 µl (5 mg/ml) of 3-[4, 5-

dimethylthiazol-2-yl]-2, 5- diphenyl tetrazolium bromide (MTT:Sigma Chemical Co., St.Louis, Mo) diluted with phosphate buffered saline (PBS, pH 7.6) was added to each well, and then incubated at 37°C for an additional 4 hours. The medium was then aspirated from each well by an auto- matic plate washer (Eimax 601, Fujirebio Inc., Japan). Dimethyl-sulfoxide (DMSO:Dojin chem. Res. Co.Ltd, Kumamoto, Japan) (150 μl) was added to each well using a multichannel pipetter and the plates were placed on a plate shaker (Timer Mixer MB-1, Torika Corp., Japan) for 2 minutes. Plates were read immediately at 540 nm on a scanning multiwell spectrophotometer (Eimax A-4, Fujirebio Inc., Japan).

Data points represent the mean of 8 wells. The percentage of control absorbance represented the surviving cell fraction. Additional controls consisted of culture medium alone. The IC_{50} value was determined as the concentration of drug that produced a 50% reduction in absorbance at 540 nm.

DRUG EXPOSURE

Paclitaxel or taxotere were added to each cell line at concent- rations between 0.1 nM and 10 μM, or 0.469 nM and 24.8 μM, respectively. The percentages of surviving cells exposed to paclitaxel or taxotere were determined by MTT assay after incubation for 21 to 71 hours, or 11 to 76 hours, respectively. Survival of fractional absorbances were expressed as percentages of control absorbance values; that is, the absorbances of the drug- treated cells were corrected by the untreated control absorbance values, from which we defined the schedule- and dose-dependent growth inhibition curves. The area under the curve (AUC) values for the assay, expressed as μM•hours, was calculated as concentration of drug × the duration of continuous exposure. A relationship between the inhibition of growth produced by paclitaxel or taxotere and the assay AUC was indicated.

FLOW CYTOMETRY

Single-cell suspensions of 5×10^5 cells of SHIN-3 or EC cells were inoculated into 75 cm^2 culture flasks. After preincubation for 24 hours, paclitaxel was added at concentrations of 0.5, 3.0 and 10.0 μM. Samples of the control and paclitaxel-treated cells were obtained by trypsinization following culture for 24 hours. Cells were filtered through a 60 μm metal mesh, then stained with propidium iodine (50 μg/ml). The amount of nuclear DNA in the stained samples was measured by flow cytometry

(Spectrum-III, Ortho Diagnostic System, Mass., U.S.A.) using the CELLFIT program.

INTRACELLULAR UPTAKE OF PACLITAXEL

An equal number of 5×10^5 SHIN-3 cells or EC cells were inoculated into 75 cm^2 culture flasks in 20 ml of medium. After preincubation for 24 hours, paclitaxel was added at concentrations of 0.5, 3.0 and 10.0 μM for another 24 hours. Trypsinized cells were washed hree times in cold PBS and stored in PBS until the next procedure. Intracellular uptake of paclitaxel was analyzed by high performance liquid chromatography (HPLC). The samples were injected onto an Inertsil 5-150 column(4.6×150 mm, GL science). Drugs were eluted from the column using 2mM H3PO4-acetonytrile (55:45) at a flow rate of 1.5 ml/min at 40°C. Compounds were detected at 227 nm using a spectrophotometer. Intracellular protein concentrations of same samples were measured by BCA (Bicin- choninic acid) protein assay. Data represent intracellular uptake of paclitaxel per protein, which were the mean of two samples at each level.

COMBINATION WITH CDDP

SHIN-3 (CDDP-resistant) cells were evaluated for an optimal administration schedule for combined treatment with paclitaxel or taxotere plus CDDP. An equal number of cells (10^3 cells/well) were exposed to 0.6 or 6 ng/ml (almost compatible with IC20 for 48 hour exposure) of paclitaxel or taxotere continuously for 6 days. CDDP wasadded during this period on the first day (group I'), the second day (group II'), the third day (group III') or the fourth day (group IV') for 24 hours. Groups I, II, III and IV represented the use of CDDP alone following the same schedule as groups I' to IV' (Fig. 1). The number of cells in each group was determined by MTT assay as the absorbance relative to that of the untreated group. The effectiveness of combined treatment according to the different schedules of CDDP administration (relative inhibition rate) was determined for each group as follows:

Relative inhibition rate (%) = [(% inhibition in the group treated with cisplatin alone to untreated control - % inhibition in combination therapy group to untreated control) ÷ % inhibition of the group treated with cisplatin alone to untreated control] ×100

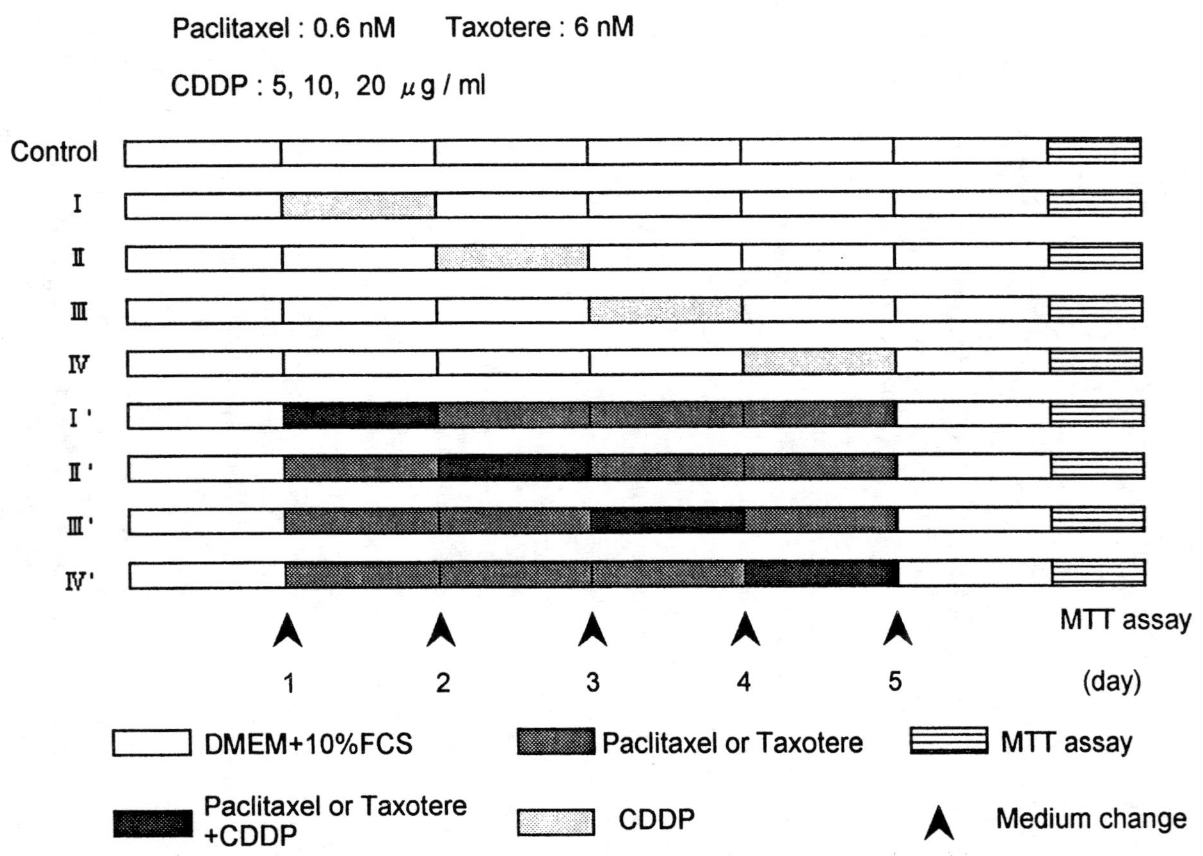

Figure 1 : In vitro administration schedule of a combination of paclitaxel or taxotere and CDDP in SHIN-3 and MN-1 cell lines.

The medium in the wells of all groups was exchanged at the same time, to ensure an equal background in each group. CDDP was added at concentrations of 5, 10 or 20μg/ml.

STATISTICAL METHODS

Statistical significance was determined by trend analysis for proportion for the experiment of "relative inhibition rate". P values < 0.05 were considered significant.

RESULTS

CYTOTOXIC EFFECTS OF PACLITAXEL AND TAXOTERE

Dose- and schedule- dependencies were observed in both SHIN-3 cells (CDDP-resistant) and MN-1 cells (CDDP-sensitive) at lower concentrations of paclitaxel (0.1 to 3 nM). At concentrations over 3 nM, schedule-dependency was significant. The effects of exposure for periods longer than 48 hours exceeded those with 24 hour exposure. The dose-dependency of the effects of paclitaxel on KEN- 3 cells (CDDP-resistant) and EC cells (CDDP-sensitive) was significant at concentrations over 3 μM, while the growth of EC cells was stimulated at concentrations below 3 μM (Fig. 2). The degree of resistance of SHIN-3 cells to CDDP was 13-fold that of MN-1, while cross-resistance to paclitaxel was 2.4-fold higher in SHIN-3 cells than MN-1 cells when comparing IC_{50s} of paclitaxel in for 20 to 72 hours continuous exposure. The tolerance of KEN-3 and EC cells to CDDP were approximately 556-fold and 2.4-fold, respectively, that of MN-1 cells. In contrast, the paclitaxel tolerance of KEN-3 and EC cells were approximately 1330-fold and 3900-fold, respectively, that of MN-1 cells (data not shown).

Both dose- and schedule-dependency of taxotere were observed at concentrations between 0.469 nM and 240 nM in all four cell lines. The percent inhibition of taxotere relative to control in KEN-3 and EC cells were lower than those of paclitaxel (Fig. 3). At higher concentrations of taxotere (0.049 to 24.8 μM), only schedule- dependency was observed (data not shown).

The antitumor effect of paclitaxel in CDDP-resistant SHIN-3 cells was AUC-dependent at AUC less than 0.1μM•hours, and was saturated at AUC over this level. Taxotere showed the same trend, although AUC-

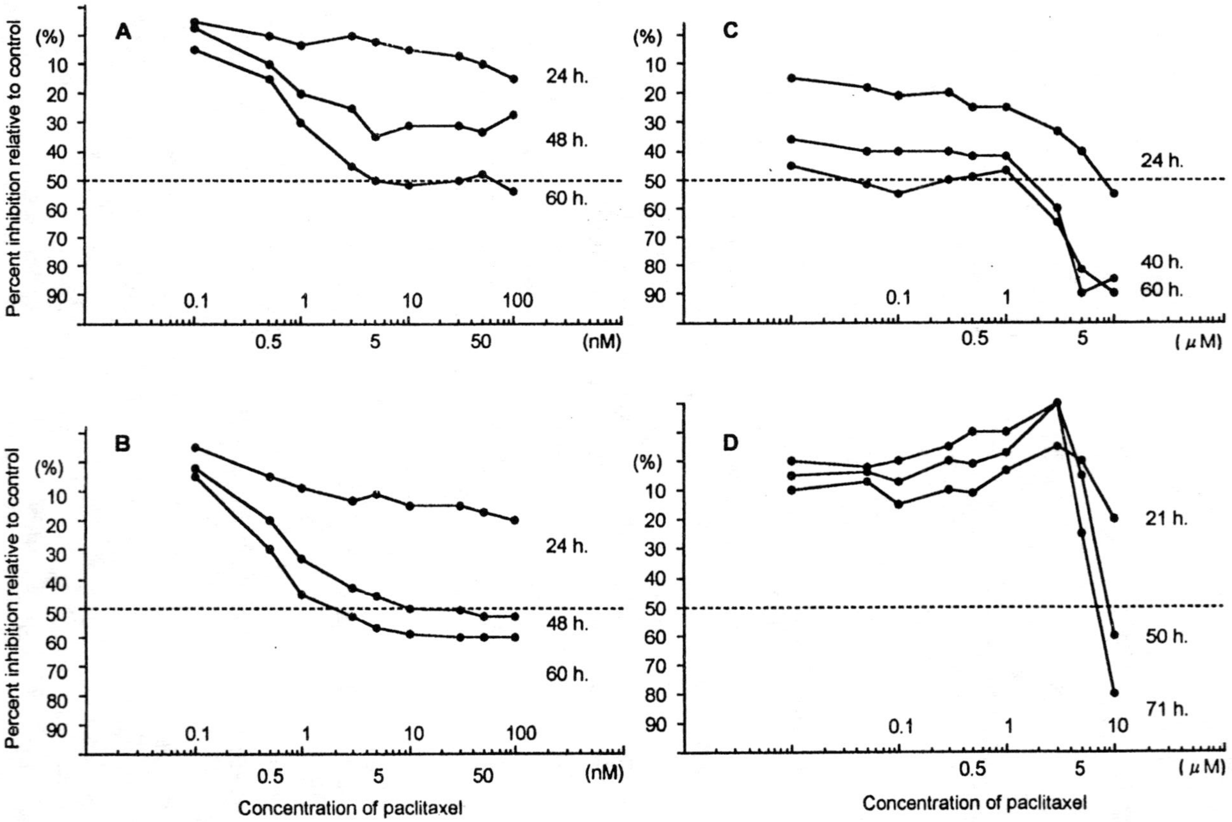

Figure 2 : Dose- and schedule-response curves of paclitaxel against established cell lines. Percent inhibition relative to untreated controls are indicated.

A : SHIN-3 (CDDP-resistant) C : KEN-3 (CDDP-resistant) B : MN-1 (CDDP-sensitive) D : EC (CDDP-sensitive)

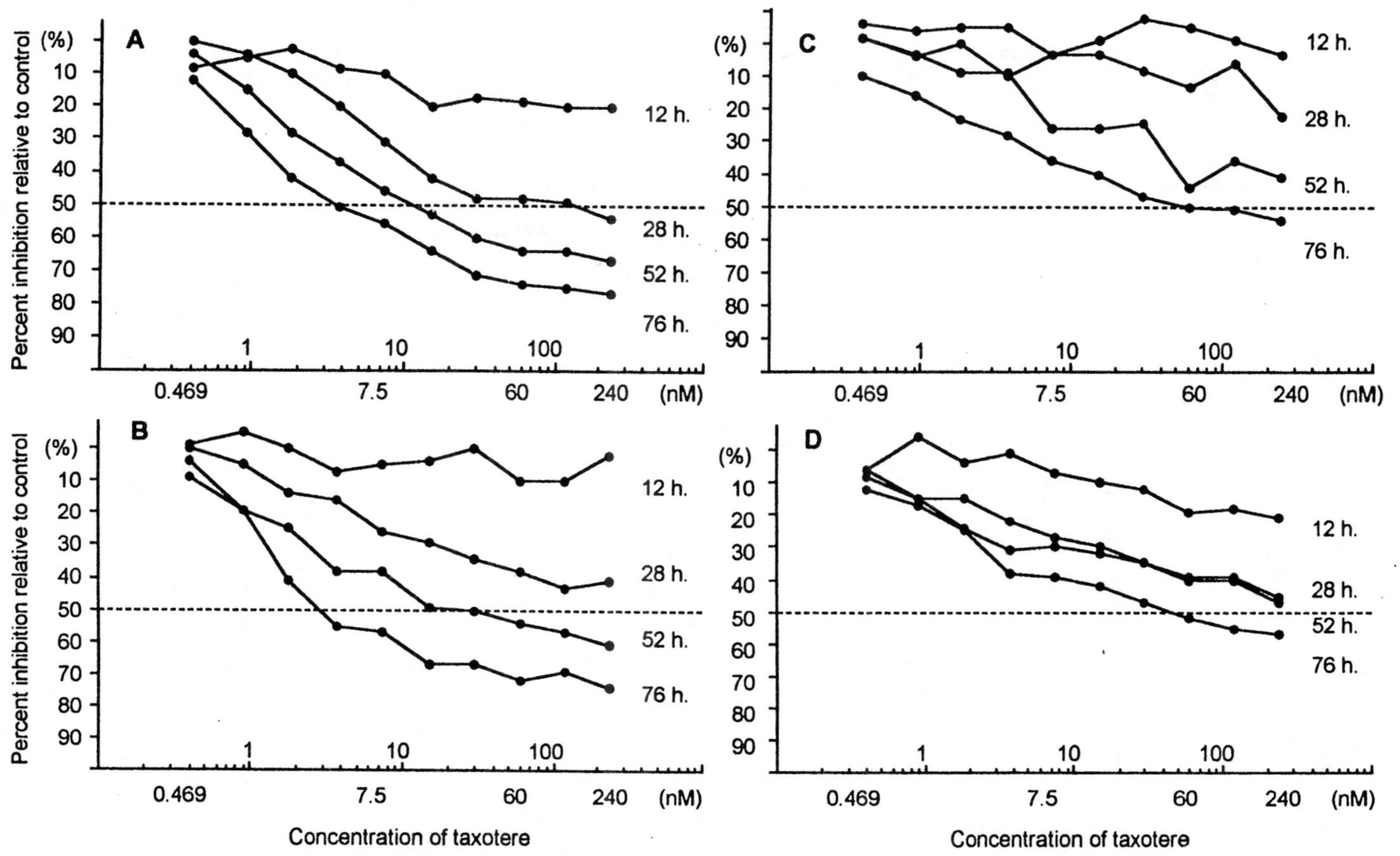

Figure 3 : Dose- and schedule-response curves of taxotere against established cell lines at lower concentrations. Percent inhibition relative to untreated controls are indicated.

A : SHIN-3 (CDDP-resistant) C : KEN-3 (CDDP-resistant)

B : MN-1 (CDDP-sensitive) D : EC (CDDP-sensitive)

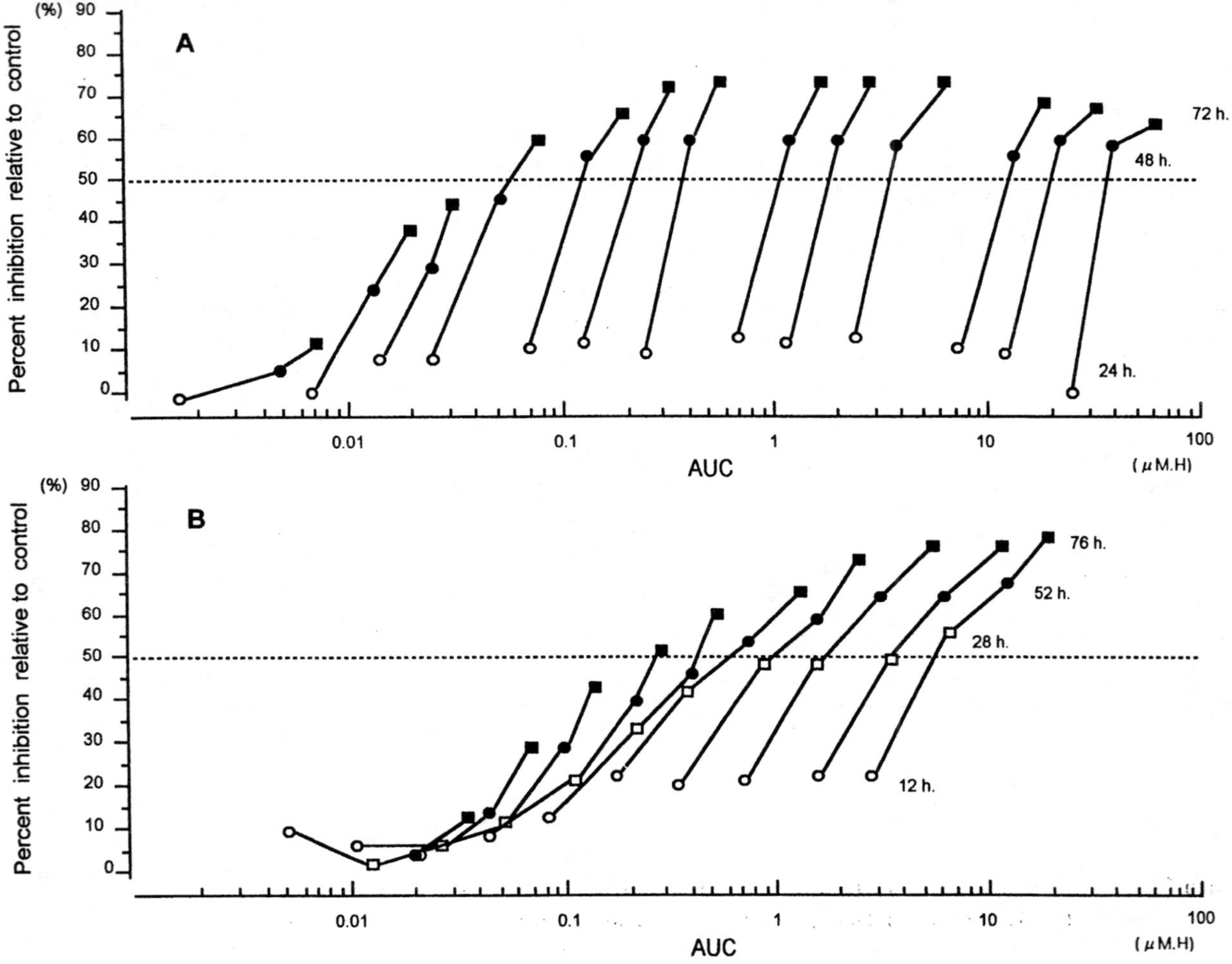

Figure 4 : Association between growth inhibition and assay AUC induced by continuous exposure of SHIN-3 cells to each drug. Response curves represents results obtained with each concentration of each drugs.
A: paclitaxel B:taxotere

dependency was observed at AUC less than 1.0 μM•hours. Greater growth inhibition was observed by paclitaxel with continuous exposure for over 48 hours compared with 24 hours exposure (Fig. 4).

IC_{50s} of paclitaxel for 60 hours exposure and of taxotere for 76 hours exposure are shown in Table I. The tolerance against paclitaxel and taxotere in order of potency were SHIN-3, KEN-3, EC and MN-1. Approximately 0.71- to 129-fold higher concentrations of paclitaxel were required for equivalence to the effects of taxotere.

FLOW CYTOMETRIC ANALYSIS

In the control specimens, the majority of cells (72.3%) occupied the G0/G1 phase fraction, while 21.3% were in the S phase, and 6.4% were in the G2/M phase. After exposure to paclitaxel, 0.5 μM for 24 hours, the S phase fraction comprised 64.4% of the population, the G2/M phase 19.0%, while the G0/G1 phase fraction decreased markedly to 16.1%. At concentrations of paclitaxel of 3.0 μM and 10.0 μM, the same was true for the G2/M phase fraction with proportions of 17.1% and 9.9%, respectively. In contrast, the number of cells in G0/G1 phase rose to the control level, being 27.6% and 66.9%, respectively. The highest number of cells in the G2/M phase was obtained with exposure to 0.5 μM of paclitaxel for 24 hours. The proportions of phase fractions of EC cells were similar to those of SHIN-3 cells (Table II).

INTRACELLULAR UPTAKE OF PACLITAXEL

The highest intracellular uptake of paclitaxel was obtained with exposure to 3.0 μM paclitaxel for 24 hours in both SHIN-3 and EC cells. Intracellular uptake of paclitaxel in SHIN-3 and EC cells were 8.689 and 10.220 μg/ ml. mg protein, respectively (Table III).

COMBINATION WITH CDDP

In combination with CDDP and paclitaxel, the "relative inhibition rate" rose as the time for preincubation with paclitaxel increased ($P<0.005$) at 5, 10 and 20 μg/ ml of CDDP. The same trend was seen with exposure to CDDP and taxotere in combination ($P<0.005$). The significantly higher "relative inhibition rate" was observed with continuous exposure to paclitaxel or taxotere over 24 hours prior to CDDP administration in comparison with that observed for shorter

	paclitaxel IC_{50} (μM)	taxotere IC_{50} (μM)	paclitaxel IC_{50} / taxotere IC_{50}
MN-1	0.002	0.0028	0.71
SHIN-3	0.005	0.0032	1.6
KEN-3	1.2	0.06	20
EC	8.0	0.062	129

Table I. Comparison of IC_{50s} between paclitaxel and taxotere on ovarian cancer cell lines

SHIN-3 (CDDP-resistant)	Control	0.5 μM	3 μM	10 μM
G0/G1 PHASE	73.40	16.15	28.55	66.90
S PHASE	22.35	64.40	54.30	23.10
G2/M PHASE	4.25	19.50	17.15	9.95

EC (CDDP-sensitive)	Control	0.5 μM	3 μM	10 μM
G0/G1 PHASE	69.50	29.25	32.95	56.55
S PHASE	24.80	42.65	35.05	26.00
G2/M PHASE	5.75	28.1	32.00	17.50

Table II. Change of cell cycle phase fraction after continuous exposure to paclitaxel for 24 hours. The population in each phase fraction is indicated as a percentage.

Concentration of paclitaxel (μM)	SHIN-3 (μg/ ml. mg protein) (μM)	EC (μg / ml. mg protein) (μM)
0.5	0.411 (0.048)	0.506 (0.059)
3.0	8.689 (1.017)	10.220 (1.197)
10.0	2.296 (0.269)	6.481 (0.759)

Table III. Intracellular uptake of paclitaxel determined by HPLC following 24 hours continuous exposure. Values are given as the concentation per mg. of protein.

duration of exposure at 5 μg/ml of CDDP, which was considered to be a clinically relevant concentration. However, continuous exposure to paclitaxel for over 48 hours prior to CDDP administration was necessary for an increase in "relative inhibition rate" at concentrations over 10 μg/ml of CDDP (Table IV).

DISCUSSION

In the present study, we investigated the cytotoxicity of paclitaxel and taxotere, and attempted to establish an optimal administration schedule for combined treatment with paclitaxel or taxotere and CDDP in an in vitro chemosensitivity test.

Paclitaxel shows significant clinical activity in advanced ovarian cancer. Subsequent trials confirmed the activity noted in patients with CDDP-refractory disease, as well as those with drug-sensitive relapse.[5, 6, 17] However, it was not clear whether paclitaxel or taxotere show dose and/or schedule dependency. McGuire et al. reported that no dose-response relationship was observed in a phase II trial.[18] However, Riou et al. reported that these drugs showed dose-dependent cytotoxic effects on proliferating cells which were considerably decreased on non-proliferating cells.[10] Kelland and Abel demonstrated that paclitaxel and taxotere showed pronounced schedule-dependency in vitro, while taxotere showed no such effect in a test against syngeneic transplantable tumors in

Cisplatin dose	Groups I - I'	Groups II - II'	Groups III - III'	Groups IV-IV'
5 μg/ml *	32.0	80.2	87.1	91.7
10 μg/ml *	23.4	31.8	70.9	85.0
20 μg/ml *	1.7	18.1	44.4	73.0

Cisplatin dose	Groups I - I'	Groups II - II'	Groups III - III'	Groups IV-IV'
5 μg/ml *	30.4	87.7	90.5	92.2
10 μg/ml *	41.8	82.3	91.5	92.9
20 μg/ml *	42.9	57.4	82.5	90.7

Table IV. Comparison of "relative inhibition rate" (%) achieved by administration of combinations of paclitaxel (above) or taxotere (below) with CDDP and CDDP alone to SHIN-3 cells.
Chi-square test for linear trend: *P<0.005

mice representing a variety of tissue types and chemosensitivity patterns.[19, 20] In the present study, dose- and schedule- dependency were observed at lower concentrations of paclitaxel and taxotere. Only schedule dependency was observed in higher concentrations of taxotere. Further investigation is required to determine whether paclitaxel and taxotere show significant dose- and/or schedule-dependency.

Increasing AUC by dose escalation seemed to confer no advantages regarding cytotoxicity in the present study. However, it was shown previously that paclitaxel dose intensification in a study of combinatorial administration with granulocyte colony stimulating factor (G-CSF), was associated with an enhanced rate of response.[21] A comparison of continuous (96-h.) and brief (2-h.) drug exposure also indicated that the cytotoxicity of paclitaxel and taxotere were highly AUC-dependent as compared with that of CDDP.[20] A phase I trial with a 5-day schedule of taxotere administration demonstrated a relationship between AUC on day 1 and percent decrease in absolute granulocyte counts.[22]

By comparison of IC_{50s}, higher concentrations of paclitaxel and taxotere were required as the resistance to microtubule inhibitor increased, and the ratio of IC_{50s} suggested that taxotere was more potent than paclitaxel. The mechanism of action of taxotere has been shown to be correlated with that of paclitaxel, [10] and Ringel and Horwitz reported that of these two agents taxotere was slightly more active as a promoter of tubulin polymerization.[9] Without grossly affecting DNA, RNA or protein synthesis, paclitaxel and taxotere inhibited cell proliferation.[3, 9] Antiproliferative activity of paclitaxel and taxotere was also observed against freshly explanted human tumor specimens in a soft agar cloning system.[23] Ringel and Horwitz reported that taxotere was 2.5-fold more potent in J774.2 and P388 cells than paclitaxel, [9] and Riou et al. also demonstrated that taxotere was 1.3-12 fold more active than paclitaxel.[10] Taxotere was also more cytotoxic than paclitaxel following both continuous (96-h.) and brief (2-h.) exposure.[21] Bissery et al. reported that taxotere was active against both CDDP-sensitive and CDDP-refractory tumors. However, they also reported taxotere was inactive on a CDDP-sensitive tumor (M5076) and on a tumor with acquired resistance to CDDP (L1210/CDDP).[19]

A previous study by Kelland and Abel showed that three pairs of cell lines made resistant to platinum exhibited no cross-resistance to paclitaxel and taxotere, and these two drugs virtually abolished the large (71-fold) range of CDDP sensitivity.[20] Our previous experiment [24] and the present study demonstrated that a CDDP-resistant cell line (i.e. SHIN-3) showed little cross-resistance to paclitaxel and taxotere, suggesting that these agents may be effective as second-line chemotherapy against CDDP-refractory disease. In addition, our results suggested that low-dose and long- term exposure schedules might be efficacious in administration as a single agent. However, there were also tumor types such as the EC cell line (CDDP-sensitive, paclitaxel-resistant) in clinical, and thus it was necessary to consider combination of paclitaxel or taxotere and CDDP as first-line chemotherapy.

The greater potency of taxotere compared with that of paclitaxel for paclitaxel-resistant cell line might be related, in part, to the increased aqueous solubility of the analogue.[9] Investigations using paclitaxel have shown two major mechanisms to be responsible for paclitaxel resistance, namely, transport-related and tubulin-related processes. Resistance to paclitaxel is associated with amplification of the 170-kDa membrane P-glycoprotein which is encoded by the multidrug resistance gene in man. A second major mechanism of resistance to paclitaxel appears to involve alterations in α- and β-tubulin, resulting in impaired microtubule assembly.[25] Robert et al. reported that development of polyploidization was observed in a paclitaxel-resistant K562 cells.[26] This observation suggested that the resistance of a cancer to antitubulin agents may be predictable by this polyploidization.

Manfredi and Horwitz reported that paclitaxel causes accumulation of cells in G2/M and prolongs interphase in a dose- dependent manner.[27] Steren also reported that low doses of paclitaxel may serve to synchronize the population cell cycle, allowing more cells to accumulate in G2/M, thus making the cell line more radiosensitive.[28] In the present study, flow cytometric analysis showed that the number of cells in each phase of the cell cycle changed according to the concentration of paclitaxel. As the most prominent G2/M arrest was observed with 0.5 μM paclitaxel treatment, the effect of paclitaxel on the cell cycle was different at each concentration. Further investigations should be performed to clarify this effect in details.

The intracellular uptake of paclitaxel was independent of the administered concentration. Intracellular uptake of paclitaxel in EC (CDDP-sensitive) cells at various concentrations was only 1.2- to 3- fold higher than those in SHIN-3 (CDDP-resistant) cells. This result suggested that the intracellular uptake was not correlated with the degree of resistance to paclitaxel.

CDDP, cytotoxicity in vitro was increased by pretreatment with paclitaxel or taxotere, suggesting that sequential administration of paclitaxel prior to CDDP might be the most clinically effective administration schedule. This observation was consistent with the report of Citardi et al. that the paclitaxel-CDDP sequence was more active than the CDDP-paclitaxel sequence in L1210 cells.[32] McGuire reported that the toxicities observed in a phase II trial of paclitaxel overlapped little with those of CDDP, making paclitaxel an excellent agent for combinatorial administration with CDDP.[18] Since the doses of paclitaxel that could be safely administered with CDDP in a previous phase I study of this combination were only 50% of that recommended as a single agent from phase I studies, Forastiere et al. evaluated the combination of CDDP, paclitaxel, and G-CSF.[33] Finally, the dose of paclitaxel that could be safely administered was shown to be increased relative to original estimations from 135 to 250 mg/m^2. A phase III randomized trial in patients with suboptimally debulked stage III and stage IV ovarian cancer comparing combined administration of CDDP and paclitaxel or CDDP and cytoxan is currently in progress by the GOG group.

ACKNOWLEDGMENT

We thank Bristol-Myers Oncology Division and Rhône-Poulenc Rorer for providing paclitaxel and taxotere. We also thank Professor Yoshiteru Terashima and Dr.Yoshihiro Kikuchi for this opportunity to describe.

REFERENCES

1. Wani, M.C., Taylor, H.L., Wall, M.E., Coggan, P., and McPhail, A.T. Plant antitumor agents VI. The isolation and structure of taxol, a novel antileukemic and antitumor agent from taxus brevifolia, *J.Am.Chem.Soc.* 93, 2325-2327 (1971).
2. Kumar, N. Taxol-induced polymerization of purified tubulin:mechanism of action, J.Biol.Chem. 256, 10435-10441(1981)
3. Shiff, P.B., Fant, J., and Horwitz, S.B. Promotion of microtubule assembly in vitro by taxol, *Nature* 22, 665-667(1979)
4. Tucker, R.W., Owellen, R.J., and Harris, S.B. Correlation of cytotoxicity and mitotic spindle dissolution by vinblastine in mammalian cells, *Cancer Res.* 37, 4346-4351(1977)
5. Tigpen, T., Blessing, J., and Ball, H. Phase II trial of taxol as second-line therapy for ovarian carcinoma:A gynecologic oncology group study, *Proc.* ASCO 9, 604(1990)
6. McGuire, W., P. Taxol: A new drug with significant activity as a salvage therapy in advanced epithelial ovarian carcinoma, Gynecol.Oncol., 51, 78-85(1993)
7. Dennis, J.N., Greene, A.E., Guénard, D., Voegelein, G.F., Mangatal, L., and Potier, P. A highly efficient, practical approach to natural taxol, *J.Am.Chem.Soc.* 110, 5917-5919(1988)
8. Mangatal, L., Adeline, M.T., Guénard, D., Voegelein, G.F., and Potier, P Application of the vicinal oxyamination reaction with asymmetric induction to the hemisynthesis of taxol and analogues, *Tetrahedron* 45, 4177-4190(1989)
9. Ringel, I., Horwitz, S.B. Studies with RP56976 (Taxotere):A semisynthetic analogue of taxol, *J. Natl .Cancer Inst.* 83, 288-291(1991)
10. Riou, J.F., Naudin, A., and Lavelle. F. Effects of taxotere on murine and human tumor cell lines, *Biochem. Biophy. Res. Comm.* 187, 164-170(1992)
11. Mossman, T. Rapid colorimetric assay for cellular growth and survival: Application to proliferation and cytotoxic assays, *J. Immunol. Methods* 65, 55-63(1983)
12. Twentyman, P.R. and Luscombe, M. A study of some variables in a tetrazolium dye (MTT) based assay for cell growth and chemosensitivity. *Br. J. Cancer*, 56, 279-285 (1987).
13. Kiyozuka, Y. Establishment of human ovarian carcinoma cell line: Characterization and tumor marker expression in vitro, *J. Nara. Med. Association* 38, 459-479(1987) (in Japanese)
14. Kiyozuka, Y., Nishimura, H., Iwanaga, S., Yakushiji, M., Ito, K., Nakano, S., Tamori, N., Adachi, S. Establishment and

characterization of human ovarian fibrosarcoma cell line and its sensitivity to anticancer agents, *Acta Obst. Gynaec. Jpn.* 44, 461-468(1992)(in Japanese)

15. Imamura, K., Kiyozuka, Y., Nishimura, H., Yakushiji, M. Novel germ cell tumor cell line established from a testicular feminization syndrome. (Contributed to *International Journal of Oncology*)
16. Yosida, M., Kiyozuka, Y., Noda, T., Imai, S., and Ichijo, M. Establishment and characterization of human cell line derived from mucinous cystadenocarcinoma of ovary, *J. Jpn. Soc. Clin. Cytol* 32, 1- 8(1993) (in Japanese)
17. Einzig, A.I., Wiernik, P.H., Sasloff, J., Runowicz, C.D., and Goldgerg, G.L. Phase II study and long-term follow-up of patients treated with taxol for advanced ovarian adenocarcinoma, *J. Clin. Oncol.* 10, 1748-1753(1992)
18. McGuire, W.P., Rowinsky, E.K., Rosenshein, N.B., Grumbine, F.C., Ettinger, D.S., Armstrong, D.K., and Donehower, R.C. Taxol:A unique antineoplastic agent with significant activity in ovarian epithelial neoplasms, *Ann.Int.Med.* 111, 273-279(1989)
19. Bissery, M.C., Guénard, D., Voegelein, G.F., and Lavelle, F. Experimental anti-tumor activity of taxotere (RP 56976, NSC 628503), a taxol analogue, Cancer Res. 51, 4845-4852(1991)
20. Kelland, L.R., and Abel, G. Comparative in vitro cytotoxicity of taxol and taxotere against cisplatin-sensitive and -resistant human ovarian carcinoma cell lines, *Cancer Chemother. Pharmacol* 30, 444-450(1992)
21. Sarosy, G., Kohn, E., Stone, D.A., Rothenberg. M., Jacob, J., Adamo, D.O., Ognibene, F. P., Cunnion, R.E., and Reed, E. Phase I study of taxol and granulocyte colony- stimulating factor in patients with refractory ovarian cancer, *J. Clin. Oncol.* 10, 1165-1170(1992)
22. Pazdur, R., Newman, R.A., Newman, B.M. , Fuentes, A., Benvenuto, J., Bready, B., Moore, D., Jaiyesimi, J.I., Vreeland, F., Bayssas, M.M.G., Raber, M.N. Phase I trial of taxotere: Five-day schedule, *J.Natl.Cancer Ins.* 84, 1781-1788(1992)
23. Hanauske, A.R., Degen, D., Hilsenbeck, S.G., Bissery, M.C., and Von Hoff, D.D. Effects of taxotere and taxol on in vitro colony formation of freshly explanted human tumor cells, *Anti-Cancer Drugs* 3, 121- 124(1992)
24. Murakami, F., Kiyozuka, Y., and Nishimura, H. Etoposide/cisplatin (CDDP) combined chemotherapy for ovarian cancer:Evaluation of optimum schedule for CDDP administration in chronic continuous exposure of low-dose etoposide to ovarian cancer cells, in vitro, *Acta. Obst. Gynaec .Jpn.* 45, 42-50(1993)(in Japanese)

25. Rowinsky, E.K., Cazenave, L.A., and Donehower, R.C. Taxol:A novel investi-gational antimicrotubule agent, *J.Natl.Cancer Ins.* 82, 1247-1259(1990)
26. Roberts, J.R., Allison., D.C., Donehower, R.C., and Rowinsky, E.K. Development of polyploidization in taxol-resistant human leukemia cells in vitro, *Cancer Res.* 50, 710-716(1990)
27. Manfredi, J.J., and Horwitz, S.B. Taxol:An antimitotic agent with a new mechanism of action, *Pharmacol. Ther.* 25, 83-125(1984)
28. Steren, A., Sevin, B., Perras, J., Angioli, R., Nguyen, H., Guerra, L., Koechli, O., and Averette, H.E. Taxol sensitizes human ovarian cancer cells to radiation, *Gyneol.Oncol.* 48, 252-258(1993)
29. Terashima, T. and Tolmach, L.J. Change in X-ray sensitivity of HeLa cells during the division cycle, *Nature* 190, 1210-1211(1961)
30. Terashima, T. and Tolmach, L.J. Growth and nucleic acid synthesis in synchronously dividing population of HeLa cells, *Exp.Cell Res.* 30, 344-362(1963)
31. Robbins, E. and Marcus, P.I. Mitotically synchronized mammalian cells:A simple method for obtaining large populations, *Science* 144, 1152-1153(1964)
32. Citardi, M.J., Rowinsky, E.K., Schaefer, K.L., and Donehower, R.C. Sequence-dependent cytotoxicity between cisplatin and the antimicrotubule agents taxol and vincristine, *Proc.Am.Assoc.Cancer Res.* 31, 2431(1990)
33. Forastiere, A.A., Rowinsky, E., Chaudry, V., Sartorius, S., Lubejko, B., Ettinger, D., Growchow, L., and Donehower, R.C. Phase I trial of taxol and cisplatin + G-CSF in solid tumors, *Proc.Am.Soc.Clin.Oncol.* 11, 289(1992)

CHAPTER 10

THE MECHANISMS OF CISPLATIN-RESISTANCE AND THE POSSIBILITY OF CIRCUMVENTION OF THE RESISTANCE BY PACLITAXEL

Akira Yoshizaki[1], Noboru Yoshizumi[2], Jun Fujiwara[3], Tatsuya Honda[1], Ikuyo Takamura[1], Toshikazu Izutsu[1] and Iwao Nishiya[1]

[1]Department of Obstetrics and Gynecology, Iwate Medical University, Morioka, Iwate, [2]Department of Obstetrics and Gynecology, Iwate Prefectural Takada Hospital, Rikuzentakada, Iwate, and [3]Department of Obstetrics and Gynecology, Morioka Red Cross Hospital, Morioka, Iwate, Japan.

SUMMARY

We have demonstrated the several mechanisms on cis-diammine-dichloroplatinum(II) (CDDP) resistance in human ovarian cancer cell lines (KF_1, KFr and KFrb) by means of flow cytometry. These cell lines were derived from the same tumor and the CDDP resistant cell lines (KFr and KFrb) showed about 2-fold higher resistance to CDDP, compared to the original cell line (KF_1). The possible mechanisms of CDDP resistance are shown in Table 1. In the present study, the mechanisms of CDDP resistance of KFr and KFrb seemed to be involved in DNA repair and CDDP influx, namely increased DNA repair and decreased CDDP uptake. We also observed the cross-resistance of KFr and KFrb cells to CDDP analogues (DWA2114R and CBDCA) and adriamycin (ADM). The cross-resistance to these platinum (Pt) derivatives was found to be resulted by increased DNA repair and by decreased influx of Pt derivatives, while that to ADM seemed to be due to decreased uptake of ADM but not increased DNA repair. Moreover, paclitaxel showed the possibility to overcome the CDDP resistance. Although the mechanisms of paclitaxel to overcome the CDDP resistance is still unclear, the induction of polypoid cells observed in this study may be the cue to solve this question. The implication of apoptosis, the expression of MDR-1 genes and the glutathione synthetase level are considered as the other possibilities to explain the mechanisms of CDDP resistance. Regarding the apoptosis, our preliminary study showed that 24 hr exposure to 10^{-6}M paclitaxel had the most marked effect for induction of apoptosis in KFr cells and these apoptotic cells were mainly found in the floating cells. The effect of paclitaxel on the expression of Fas antigen and bcl-2 remained to be elucidated. P53-related genes and the gene products have also been pointed out to be involved in CDDP-resistance.

We expect that the CDDP-resistance mechanism is elucidated and the new strategy to overcome the CDDP-resistance will be developed in near future.

INTRODUCTION

Introduction of platinum (Pt) derivatives, especially cis-diamminedichloroplatinum(II) (CDDP) for ovarian cancer treatment had improved the outcome of patients dramatically. At least, the short term survival rate (less than 5 year) has turned better by CDDP. On the other hand, when the cases acquired resistance to CDDP during chemotherapy or at relapse, we have to suffer deep frustration because there is no superior combination chemotherapy to substitute for CDDP-based combination chemotherapy. Therefore, better understanding of the mechanisms of CDDP-resistance is necessary and essential to improve chemotherapeutic efficacy especially for relapse or recurrent cases. Several possibilities have been reported to explain the mechanisms of CDDP resistance. As shown in Table 1, the cancer cells seem to have a complex mechanism of CDDP resistance [1]. Complexity in the resistance mechanisms is observed against other anticancer drugs, such as anthracyclines, alkylating agents and antimetabolic agents [2]. We have studied to reveal the mechanisms of CDDP resistance using human ovarian cancer cell lines and also to demonstrate the cross-resistance to drugs which are widely used to combine with CDDP.

The KF cell lines used in this study were established by Dr. Kikuchi in 1984 from patients with serous cystadenocarcinoma of the ovary [3, 4]. A human ovarian cancer cell line, KF_1 is the original cell line which is sensitive to CDDP. KFr and KFrb are CDDP resistant cell lines developed by continuous exposure of KF_1 cells to CDDP. The IC_{50} of KFr to CDDP was 0.8 μg/ml and that of KF_1 was 0.4 μg/ml. To elucidate the mechanisms of CDDP resistance in KFr cells, effects of CDDP on DNA damage, DNA repair and CDDP uptake in the KFr cells were examined in addition to the cross-resistance of Pt derivatives, doxorubicine (adriamycin; ADM) and paclitaxel to CDDP. Thus, we now report several data to be involved in the mechanisms of CDDP resistance.

Material and Methods

Cells lines.

Human ovarian cancer cell lines, KF_1 and CDDP-resistant KFr and KFrb derived from KF_1 were kindly provided by Dr. Kikuchi [5]. These cell lines were grown at 37 in the presence of 5% CO_2 in RPMI 1640 medium (Nissui Pharmacol. Co., Ltd., Tokyo, Japan), supplemented with 10% fetal bovine serum (Mitsubishi Kasei, Co., Ltd., Tokyo, Japan), 100 units penicillin/ml and 100 μg/ml streptomycin (Cosmo Bio Co., Ltd., Tokyo, Japan).

Anticancer drugs.

CDDP, cis-diammine (1,1-cyclobutane-dicarboxylato)platinum(II) (CBDCA) and paclitaxel were kindly supplied by Bristol-Myers Squibb K.K., Tokyo, Japan. (-)- (R)-2-aminomethyl-pyrolidine (1,1-cyclobutanedicarboxylato) platinum(II) monohydrate (DWA2114R) was kindly provided by Chugai Pharmaceutical Co., Ltd., Tokyo, Japan. ADM was purchased by Kyowa Hakkou Co., Ltd., Tokyo, Japan.

Cell cycle analysis.

For cell cycle analysis, cells were fixed in 70% ethanol and stored at 4 until the analysis. Fixed cells were washed several times with cold phosphate buffered saline (PBS) and stained by 5 μg/ml of propidium iodide (PI) after treatment with RNase for non-base specific total DNA, mithramycin for G-C base DNA and Hoechst 33342 for A-T base DNA. DNA histograms were obtained by Cytofluorograhic 50H and 2150 computer (Ortho Instrument, Westwood, MA, USA) using 488 nm argon laser for excitation, 630 nm for emission for PI, 457 nm argon ion laser for excitation, 515 nm for emission for mithramycin, 351 nm UV laser for excitation and 460 nm for emission for Hoechst 33342. Analysis by paclitaxel was performed by FACScan Flow Cytometer (Becton-Dickinson, Mountain View, CA, USA). Cells were excited with a single 488 nm argon laser. Linear fluorescence red (FL2) and forward-angle scatter (FCS) were collected for 10,000 to 30,000 events in the list mode files. The data were analyzed on Cell Fit software (Becton-Dickinson, Mountain View, CA, USA). For DNA repair study, BrdU monoclonal antibody was used to distinguish the growth fraction of cells during and after drug exposure.

INTRACELLULAR PLATINUM CONTENTS.

KF_1 and KFrb cells at exponential growth phase were exposed to 1.0 or 2.0 μ/ml CDDP, 15 or 30 μg/ml CBDCA and 10 or 20 μg/ml DWA2114R for 4 hr. The cells were divided into two cellular fractions, cytosol and nuclear fractions. The preparation of cellular fractions was performed as follows; Cells were harvested, washed twice with cold PBS, transferred to Politrone Homogenizer (PT-10, Kinematic, Switzerland), homogenized for a few seconds and centrifuged at 800 x g for 10 min. The resultant supernatants were centrifuged at 10,000 x g for 60 min using a ultracentrifuge (Hitachi 75P-72, Tokyo, Japan). The supernatants were collected as the cytosol fraction and the sediments after washing with cold PBS were used as the nuclear fraction. The Pt contents in both cytosol and nuclear fractions were measured using atomic absorption method by Nac, Co., Ltd., Takasaki, Japan. The number of cells were counted and adjusted before the preparation of the cell fractions, and the Pt concentrations of each cell fractions were presented as μg Pt/10^7 cells.

TO EXAMINE EFFECTS OF PACLITAXEL ON CELL PROLIFERATION.

Cells were allowed to attach to culture flasks (Nunc, Denmark) for 72 hr and then incubated for 3, 6, 12 and 24 hr with concentrations of paclitaxel indicated.

At each time point, cells were harvested with trypsin (GIBCO, Grand Island, New York, USA) and EDTA (Kanto Pharmaceutical Co., Ltd., Tokyo, Japan). Drug concentrations used for this experiment were 10^{-8}M, 10^{-7}M and 10^{-6}M which are clinically equivalent doses. The cells were counted with a Coulter counter (Hialeath, New York, USA). Viable cells were counted with a hematocytometer using nigrosin (Sigma Co., St. Louis, MO, USA).

MEASUREMENT OF CELLULAR DNA.

To determine cellular DNA, 10^6 cells at preconfluent state were harvested with trypsin, washed with PBS and suspended in 500 µl Triton X. The suspension was passed through 40 µm nylon mesh after treatment with 500 µl PNase and stained by 50 µl of 1 mg/ml PI for 15 min in the dark.

RESULTS AND DISCUSSION

EFFECTS OF CDDP AND ADM ON DNA DAMAGE IN KF1 AND KFR CELLS BY BASE SPECIFIC ANALYSIS [5]

PI intensity, mithramycin intensity and Hoechst 33342 intensity are presumed to show the non-base specific total DNA content, the G-C base DNA content and the A-T base DNA content, respectively. The non-base specific total DNA and the A-T base DNA analyses revealed significant G_2 + M phase cell accumulations and a decrease of G_{0+1} phase cells after exposure of both KF_1 and KFr cells to 0.5 and 1.0 µg/ml CDDP for 48 to 72 hr. On the other hand, the G-C base DNA content in KFr showed a significant decrease of accumulation in G_2 + M phase cells and an increase of S phase fraction only after 24 hr of 1.0 µg/ml CDDP exposure. One of the mechanisms of CDDP to damage DNA is believed to be due to intrastrand cross-link to guanine base. These results suggest that the G-C base DNA in KFr was less affected by CDDP than that of KF_1 or the content of the G-C base pair of KFr was less than that of KF_1.

The base specific DNA, A-T base DNA and G-C base DNA in KF_1 and KFr showed no significant difference by ADM exposure. Cell growth inhibition by

ADM was almost the same degree in both KF_1 and KFr. These results suggest that KFr cells had the cross-resistance to ADM.

STUDIES ON DNA REPAIR OF KF_1 AND KFR AFTER CDDP EXPOSURE [5]

The effect of CDDP on DNA synthesis of KFr cells was observed by BrdU labeling rate before CDDP exposure and after 2, 4, 6, 8, 10, 12 and 24 hr of CDDP exposure. After 24 hr of drug exposure, the medium was changed to the drug-free medium. Further observations were performed at 2, 4, 6, 8, 10, 12 and 24 hr. Figs. 1 and 2 show the changes in BrdU labeled S phase fractions of KF_1 and KFr without CDDP exposure (control). The cell cycle times (Tcs) of KF_1 and KFr were 15.3 and 16.4 hr, respectively. The DNA synthesis times (Tds) were 5.0 and 6.0 hr, respectively according to this figure.

When KF_1 and KFr cells were exposed to 0.5 and 1.0 μg/ml CDDP, both Tcs and Tds of KF_1 and KFr cells were elongated by CDDP in a dose-dependent fashion. Twenty 4 hr after CDDP exposure, the late S phase fractions of KF_1 and KFr cells were remarkably increased than those of control. Exposure to 1.0 μg/ml CDDP resulted in a decrease of mid S and early S phase fractions of KF_1 and KFr, compared to the drug free control. These results show the delay of cell cycle progression to G_1 and S phase. However, no clear difference in the delay of cell cycle progression was observed between KF_1 and KFr cells. The changes in BrdU labeled S phase fractions after CDDP removal (after 27 hr and more) were also shown in Figs. 1 and 2. Unless cells were exposed to CDDP, BrdU labeled S phase fractions, Tcs and Tds of each KF_1 and KFr cells were not changed after 27 hr and more. On the other hand, the Tcs and Tds were prolonged if KF1 and KFr were exposed to 0.5 and 1.0 μg/ml CDDP. Remarkable late S phase accumulations were observed by exposure of KF_1 and KFr to 1.0 μg/ml CDDP for 33 hr. This late S phase accumulation in KF_1 was maintained for 36 hr after removal of CDDP and the cell cycle seemed to be almost stopped (Fig. 1). The late S phase cell fraction in KFr decreased and the early S phase cell fraction increased gradually (Fig. 2). These phenomena suggest strongly that even if the cell cycle of KFr had been affected and elongated by CDDP, KFr cells had still the possibility to recover from the late S accumulation and to recruit to the other cell cycle.

CROSS-RESISTANCE OF KFR TO PT ANALOGUES [6]

Cross-resistance of DWA2114R and CBDCA to CDDP was examined using KF_1 and KFr cells. Growth inhibition curves by CDDP, DWA2114R and CBDCA in KF_1 and KFr cells are shown in Fig. 3. The IC_{50} values were 0.42 μg/ml for CDDP, 2.4 μg/ml for DWA2114R and 6.8 μg/ml for CBDCA in KF_1 cells, while those in KFr cells were 0.8 μg/ml for CDDP, 6.2 μg/ml for DWA2114R and 11.5 μg/ml for CBDCA. These results suggest that DWA2114R and CBDCA had cross-resistance to CDDP as shown in KFr cells. The cell cycle analysis revealed that 1 μg/ml (3.3 μM) CDDP, 15 μg/ml (40.4 μM) CBDCA and 10 μg/ml (22.0 μM) DWA2114R showed similar G_2 + M cell accumulation.

PT UPTAKES BY KF1 AND KFR CELLS [7]

As shown in Table 2, when KF_1 cells were exposed to 1 μg/ml CDDP, 15 μg/ml CBDCA and 10 μg/ml DWA2114R for 4 hr, the nuclear Pt content was 10.4, 7.3 and 12.9 μg/10^7 cells, respectively. When KFr cells were exposed to the same concentrations of CDDP and CBDCA, the nuclear content was not detectable. When KFr cells were incubated with 2 μg/ml CDDP, 30 μg/ml CBDCA and 20 μg/ml DWA2114R, the nuclear Pt content was 15.7, 8.5 and 7.8 μg/10^7 cells, respectively. Pt content in the cytosol fraction of KF_1 cells was 9.0, 32.5 and 57.5 μg/10^7 cells by exposure with 1 μg/ml CDDP, 15 μg/ml CBDCA and 10 μg/ml DWA2114R, respectively. That of KFr cells was not detectable by exposure with CDDP and CBDCA but showed 47.3 μg/10^7 cells level by exposure with DWA2114R. Even if KFr cells were exposed to 2-fold higher concentration of CDDP, the Pt content in the cytosol fraction was not detectable, while that was 65.3 μg/10^7 cells by CBDCA and 82.1 μg/10^7 cells by DWA2114R. These results suggest that KFr cells may have some mechanisms to

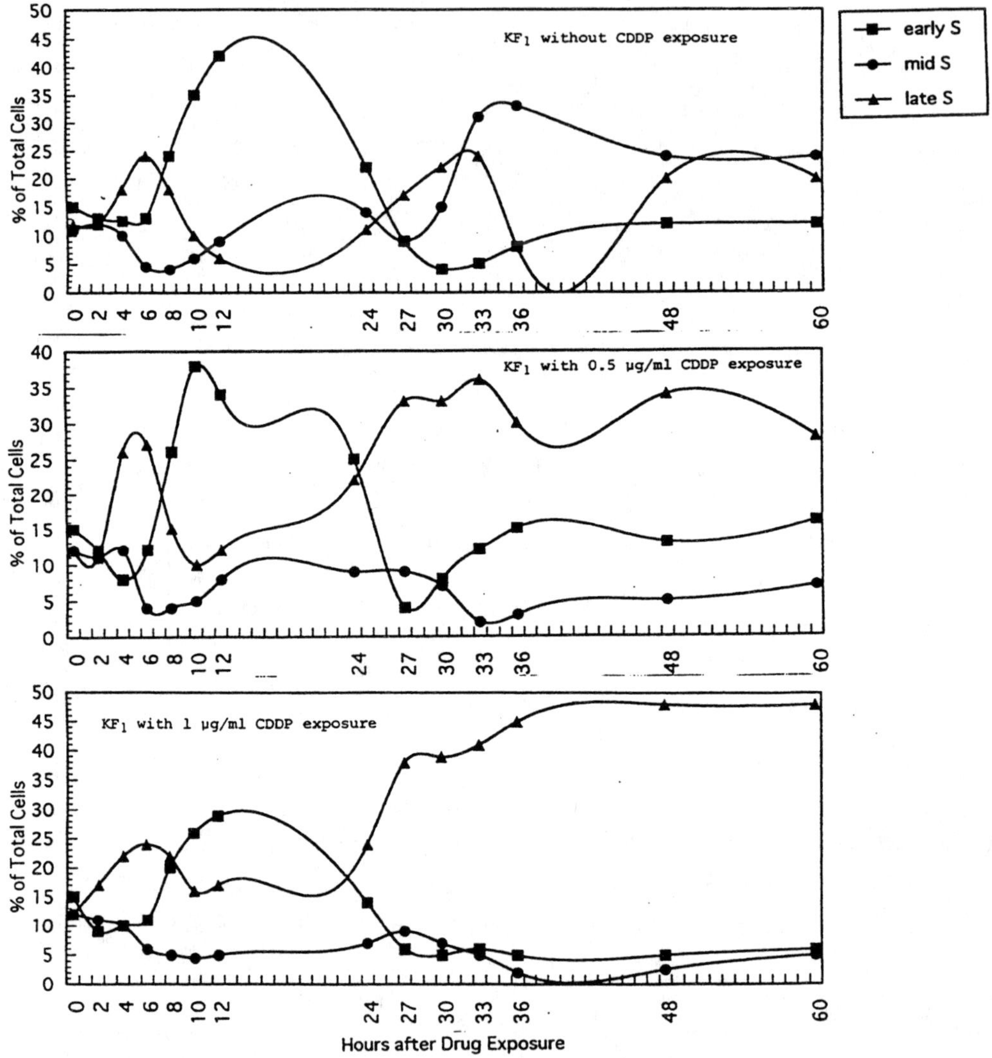

Fig. 1. Changes in the S phase fractions of KF_1 cells after CDDP exposure.

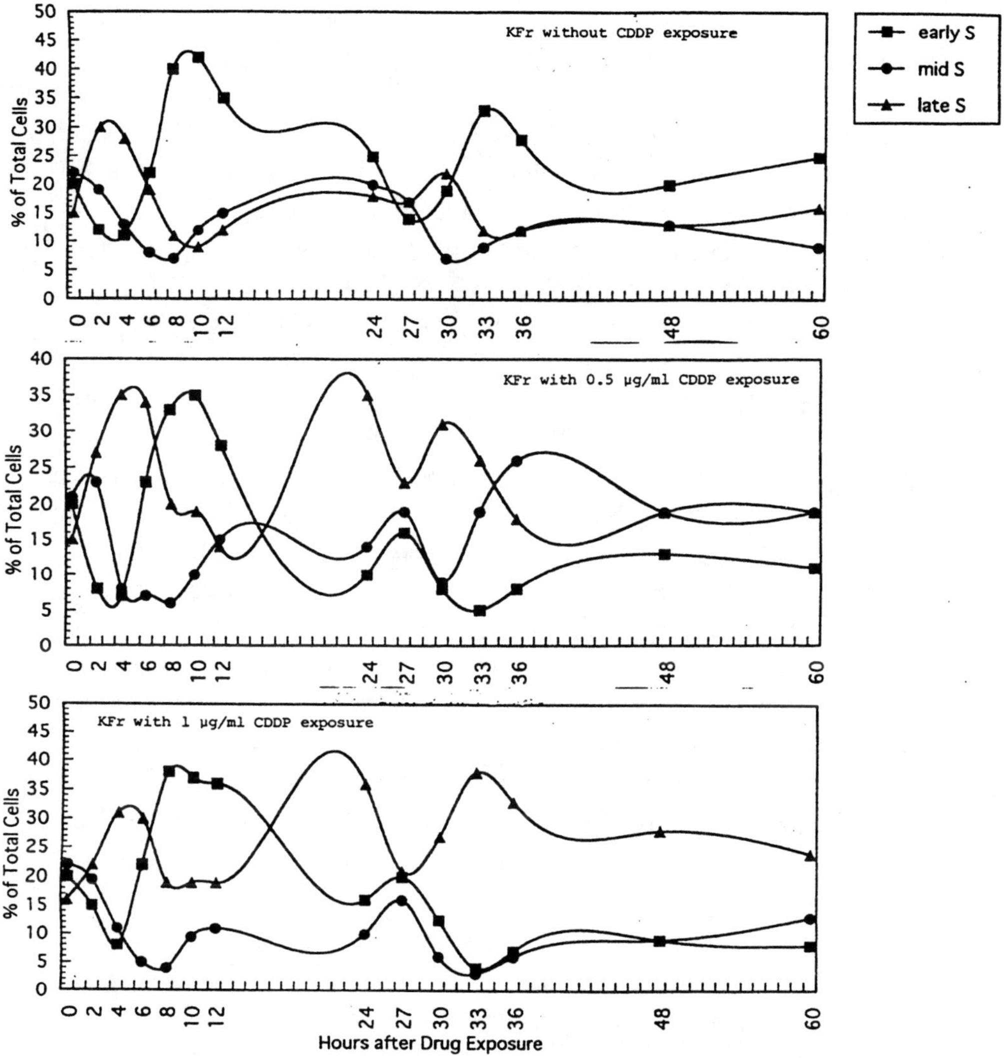

Fig. 2. Changes in the S phase fractions of KFr cells after CDDP exposure.

the nucleus, because Pt in KFr cells was not detected after CDDP and CBDCA exposure.

EFFECTS OF PACLITAXEL ON THE PROLIFERATION KF1 AND KFR CELLS

Recently, paclitaxel has been expected to substitute for CDDP especially in refractory ovarian cancer. Therefore, we attempted to clarify the effect of paclitaxel on cell growths and cell cycle changes of KF_1 and KFr. When KF_1 and KFrb cells were incubated in the presence of 10^{-7}M and 10^{-6}M paclitaxel for 24 hr, the cell proliferations were significantly ($P<0.05$) inhibited. KF_1 cells with exposure to 10^{-6}M paclitaxel for 24 hr showed 41.9 ± 9.8% survival while KFrb cells with the same exposure showed 65.7 ± 26.7% survival (Fig. 4).

Remarkable G_2 + M phase accumulation and a decrease in proportion of G_{0+1} phase cells were observed in KF_1 and KFrb cells after 12 and 24 hr of exposure to 10^{-7}M and 10^{-6}M paclitaxel (Fig. 5). These changes began 6 hr after exposure to paclitaxel, and after 12 hr of exposure to 10^{-6} and 10^{-7}M paclitaxel the proportions of G_{0+1} phase cells were significantly ($P<0.05$) lower than those without exposure to paclitaxel. On the other hand, when cells were exposed to 10^{-6} and 10^{-7}M paclitaxel for 12 hr, G_2 + M cell proportions in KF_1 and KFrb cells were significantly ($P<0.05$) increased, compared to those when cells were not exposed to paclitaxel (Fig. 5). After 24 hr of drug exposure, further decreases in the proportions of G_{0+1} phase cells and further increases in the proportions of G_2 + M phase cells were observed in both KF_1 and KFrb cells. These findings suggest that paclitaxel induces polypoid cells in both KF_1 and KFrb cells.

Table 1. Changes found in A2780 human ovarian carcinoma cells after in vitro CDDP resistance induction

Changes found in resistant cells	A possible role for
Reduced accumulation potential	Membrane Na^+/K^+ adenosine triphosphate
Increased detoxification	Glutathione Metallothionein
Increased DNA repair	DNA synthesis DNA polymerase Thymidine triphosphate synthetase Folate metabolism

Modified from Timmer-Bosscha et al., [1].

Table 2. Nuclear Pt contents in KF_1 and KFr cells

Pt derivatives	KF_1 cells	KFr cells
CDDP (1.0 μg/ml)[a]	10.4[b]	undetectable
(2.0 μg/ml)	nd	15.7
CBDCA (15.0 μg/ml)	7.3	undetectable
(30.0 μg/ml)	nd	8.5
DWA2114R (10.0 μg/ml)	12.9	10.5
(20.0 μg/ml)	nd	7.8

[a]Cells were exposed to concentrations of each drug shown in parenthesis.
[b]Pt contents; $\mu g/10^7$ cells.
nd, not done.

Table 3. Cytosol Pt contents in KF_1 and KFrb cells

Pt derivatives	KF_1 cells	KFrb cells
CDDP (1.0 μg/ml)[a]	9.0[b]	undetectable
(2.0 μg/ml)	nd	undetectable
CBDCA (15.0 μg/ml)	32.5	undetectable
(30.0 μg/ml)	nd	65.3
DWA2114R (10.0 μg/ml)	57.5	47.3
(20.0 μg/ml)	nd	82.1

[a]Cells were exposed to concentrations of each drug in parenthesis.
[b]Pt contents; $\mu g/10^7$ cells.
nd, not done.

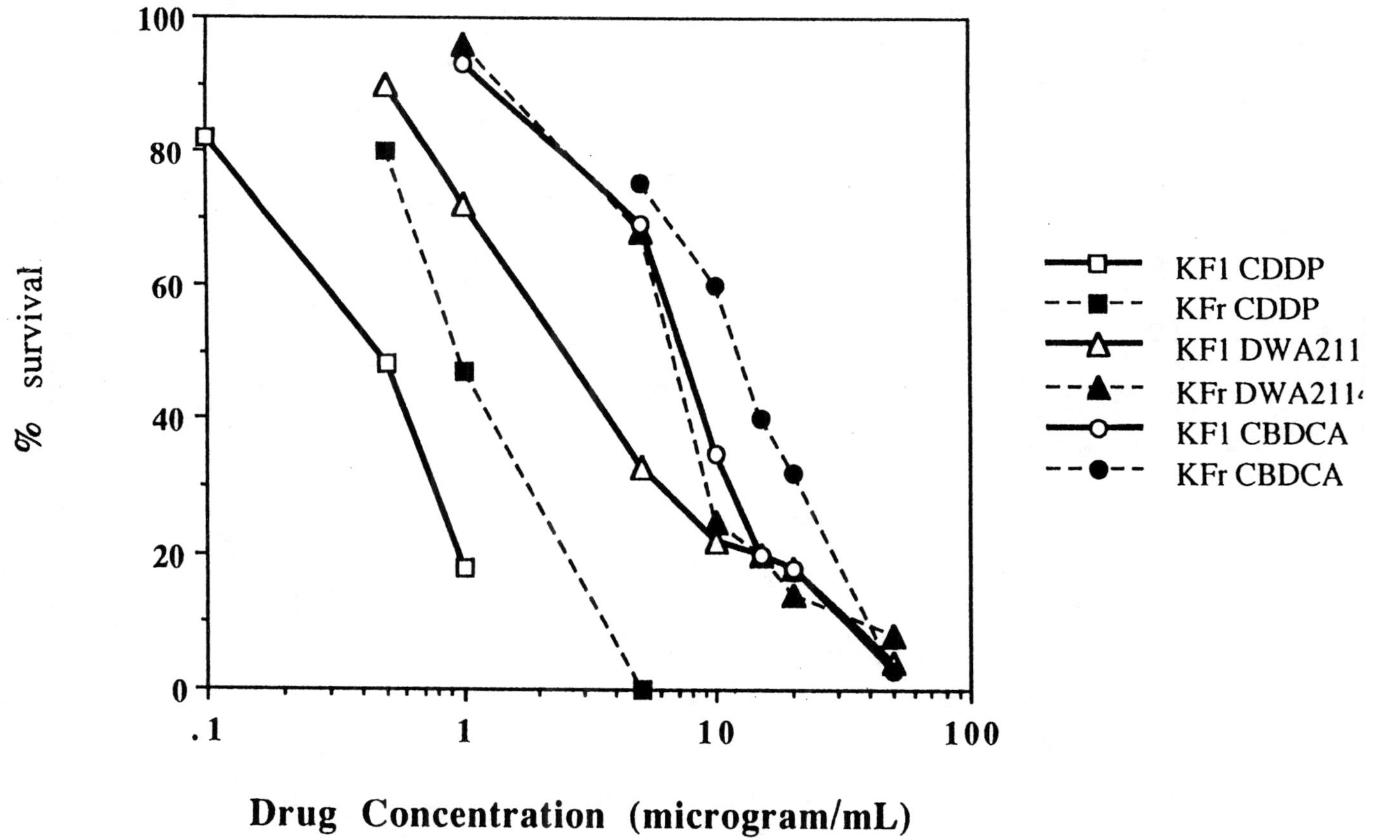

Fig. 3. Effects of CDDP and its analogues on the cell growth in vitro.

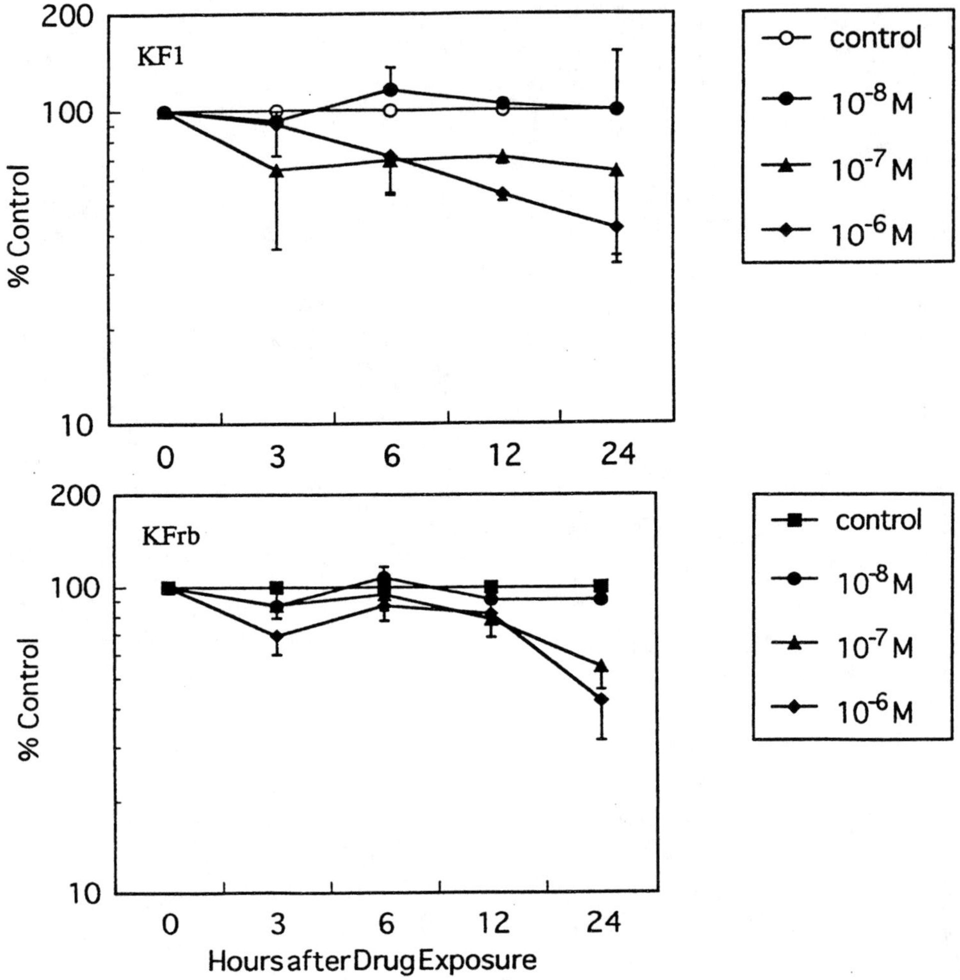

Fig. 4. Effects of paclitaxel on the cell growth of KF_1 and KFrb.

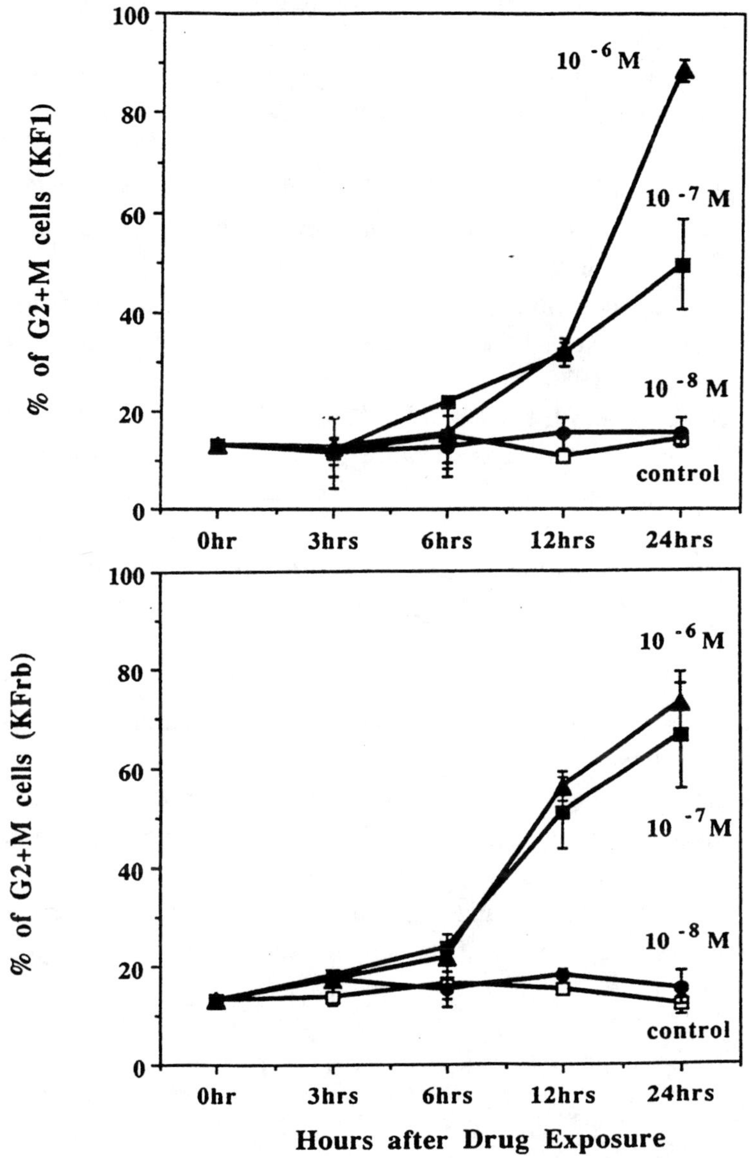

Fig. 5. Changes in the G_2 + M fractions of KF_1 and KFrb cells after exposure to paclitaxel.

REFERENCES

1. Timmer-Bosscha H, Mulder NH and de Vries EGF: Modulation of cis-diamminedichloroplatinum(II) resistanc: a review. *Br J Cancer* 66:227-238, 1992.
2. van der Zee AGT, Hollema HH, Brujin HWA, Willemse PHB, Boostra H, Mulder NH, Aalders JG and de Vries EGE: Cell biological markers of drug resistance in ovarian carcinoma. *Gynecol Oncol* 58:165-178, 1995.
3. Kikuchi Y, Miyauchi M, Kizawa I, Oomori K and Kato K: Establishment of a cisplatin-resistant human ovarian cancer cell line. *J Natl Cancer Inst* 77:1181-1185, 1986.
4. Kikuchi Y, Iwano I, Miyauchi M, Kita T, Sugita M, Tenjin Y and Nagata I: Possible mechanisms of resistance to cis-diamminedichloroplatinum(II) of human ovarian cancer cells. Jpn J Cancer Res 81:701-706, 1990.
5. Nishiya I, Yoshizumi N, Fujiwara J and Kagabu K: Drug resistant mechanisms of platinum derivatives in a human cisplatin resistant ovarian cancer cell line. *Gan To Kagaku Ryouhou* 15:2871-2881, 1988 (in Japanese).
6. Fujiwara J, Yoshizumi N, Hirama T and Nishiya I: The cytokinetic effects and cross-resistance of platinum derivatives on human ovarian cancer cells in vitro. *J Iwate Med Assoc* 42:823-836, 1990.
7. Yoshizaki A, Fujiwara J, Fukushima A, Yoshizumi N and Nishiya I: Mechanism of cross resistance of platinum derivatives. *Proc Jpn Cancer Assoc*, 49th Annual Meeting:1954, 1990.
8. Yoshizaki A, Izutsu T and Nishiya I: The effects of paclitaxel on CDDP-sensitive and CDDP-resistant human ovarian cancer cell lines. *J Jpn Soc Cancer Ther* 30:730-739, 1995 (in Japanese).

CHAPTER 11

INHIBITORY EFFECT OF GINSENOSIDE RH_2 ON THE GROWTH OF OVARIAN CANCER CELLS AND ITS ADJUVANT EFFECT TO CISPLATIN

Takehiko Tode, Yoshihiro Kikuchi, Junko Hirata, Tunekazu Kita and Ichiro Nagata

Department of Obstetrics and Gynecology, National Defense Medical College, Namiki 3-2, Tokorozawa, Saitama 359, Japan

I. INTRODUCTION

Multiple drug chemotherapy containing cisdiammine-dichloroplatinum(II) (cisplatin) has been used for the treatment of advanced ovarian carcinoma. Consequently, the response rate of patients with advanced ovarian carcinoma has been significantly improved. However, most patients who respond to such chemotherapy relapsed and become resistant to cisplatin (CDDP). So that it is very important to develop ways to enhance the antitumor effect of CDDP and/or to find out new agents which reveal antitumor activity as well. In Asian countries, especially in Korea, Japan, and China, Panax ginseng CA Meyer (so called red ginseng) has been used commonly by oral administration as a tonic medicine or elixir of life for more than 2000 years. Red ginseng contains many useful components such as ginseng saponin (ginsenoside) showing antineoplastic, antithrombotic, and antiatherogenic actions.

In 1979, Odashima et al have reported the direct effect of crude ginseng saponin on Morris hepatoma cells (1). They concluded that crude ginseng saponin induces reverse transformation or redifferentiation of Morris hepatoma cells. Since then, they isolated new components designated ginsenoside Rh_1 (Rh_1) and ginsenoside Rh_2 (Rh_2) from the ethanol extract of

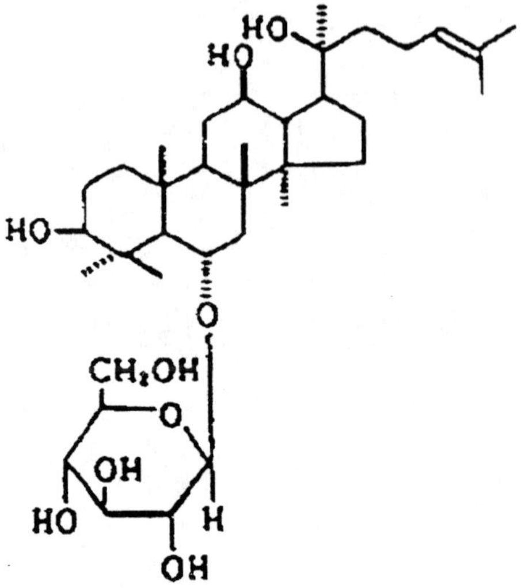

ginsenoside Rh_1

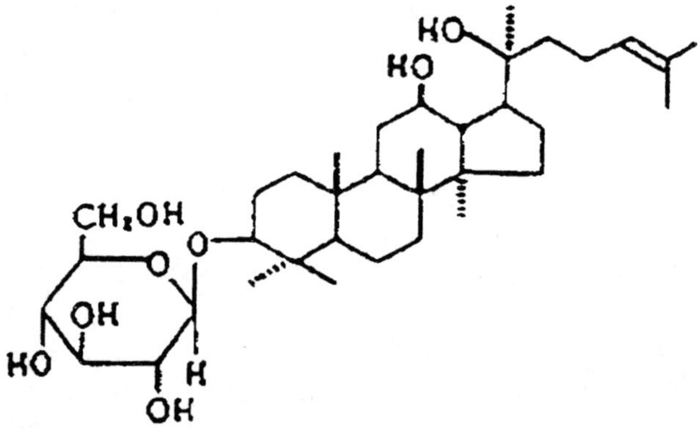

ginsenoside Rh_2

Fig. 1 Chemical structures of ginsenoside Rh_1 and ginsenoside Rh_2

the processed root of Panax ginseng CA Meyer. As shown in Fig.1, Rh_1 and Rh_2 are plant glycoside with a dammarane skelton resembling steroid skelton as an aglycon. Rh_1 has a glucose molecule at C-6, while Rh_2 possesses a same molecule at C-3. Despite their similarity in the chemical structure, the actions on cancer cells are very different. Rh_1 enhances melanogenesis in B16 melanoma cells but neither stimulates nor inhibits their growth, while Rh_2 remarkably inhibits the cell proliferation in addition to induction of melanogenesis of B16 melanoma cells(2). Rh_2 inhibits the B16 melanoma cell in a dose dependent manner and results in a complete inhibition at more than 15 μM. In addition, red ginseng has been reported to contain other antineoplastic substances (3). Thus, we examined the effects of Rh_2 on the growth of human ovarian cancer cell line (HRA) (4) in vitro and its adjuvant effect to CDDP in nude mice bearing HRA cell tumor.

II. EFFECTS OF RH_2 ON THE HRA CELL PROLIFERATION IN VITRO

Purified ginsenoside Rh_2 was supplied by Korean Ginseng and Tobaco Research Institute, Korea and Seikansho Co. Ltd., Japan. Rh_2 was dissolved in ethanol and diluted by distilled water to desired concentrations. HRA cell line was established from ascites of a patients with serous cystadenocarcinoma of the ovary. The cells were cultured in RPMI1640 medium, supplemented with 10% fetal bovine serum, penicillin and streptomycin (100 mU/ml and 100 mg/ml, respectively; Grand Island Biological Co.) in 5% CO2 at 37°C. Effects of Rh_2 on HRA cell proliferation and uptake of radiolabeled precursors by tumor cell were examined in vitro. To determine the effect of Rh_2 on HRA cell proliferation, 10^4 viable HRA cells were seeded into 24 well Nunce-multidishes and incubated in a humidified atmosphere of 5% CO_2 at 37°C. After 24 h of culture, various concentrations of Rh_2 were added to the medium. After additional 4 days' culture, cells in each well were harvested and counted with a hematocytometer. The cell numbers in wells containing fresh medium alone were used as controls. As shown in Fig. 2, Rh_2 inhibited the HRA cell proliferation in a dose dependent manner between 10 and 100 μM. Concentration of Rh_2 required for 50% inhibition of cell proliferation (IC50) was about 30 μM (5). To elucidate the mechanism of action of Rh_2, the effect of Rh_2 on synthesis of DNA, RNA and protein by HRA cells were examined. HRA cells (10^4/ml) were seeded into 24 well Nunc-multidishes. After 24 h of culture, various concentrations of Rh_2 were added into each well. The DNA, RNA or protein synthesis by HRA cells was assayed by adding 37 kBq of ^{3}H-thymidine, ^{3}H-uridine, or ^{3}H-valine to each well during

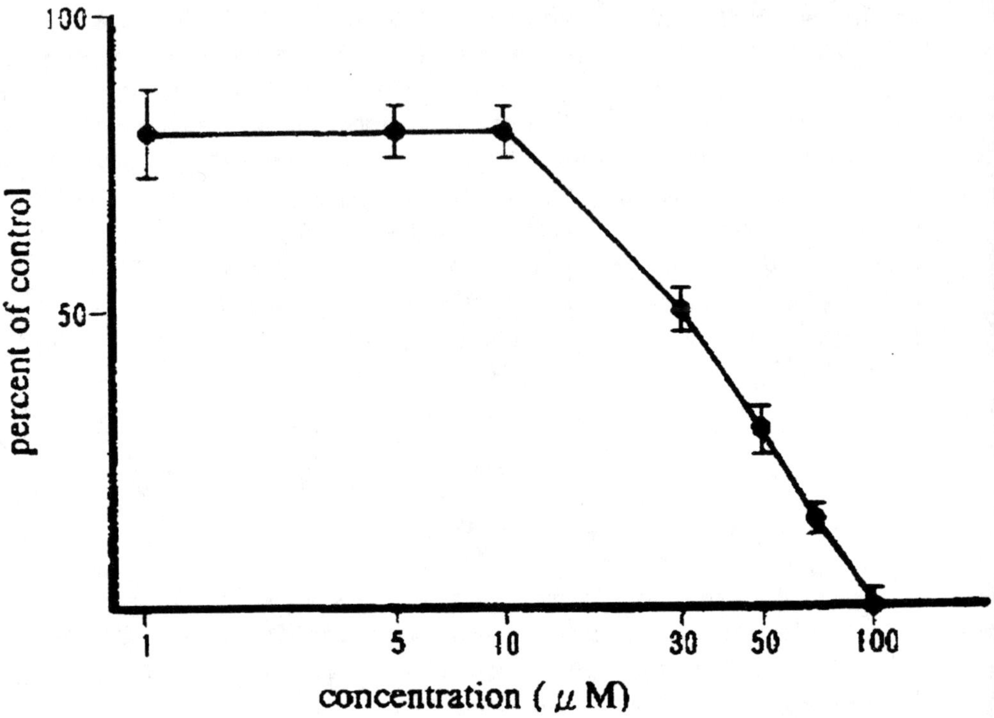

Fig. 2 Effect of Rh_2 on the HRA cell proliferation in vitro. The 10^4 viable cells were seeded into 24 well Nunc multidishes. After 24h of culture, various concentrations of Rh_2 were added to the medium. After 48h of additional culture, cells in each well were harvested and counted. Vertical bars show the mean ± SD.

the last 4 h of the 48 h incubation period. The collected cells were precipitated with 15% trichloroacetic acid (TCA) and the amount of radioactivity in the TCA insoluble material solubilized by 8% sodium dodecyl sulfate was determined by a liquid scintillation counter. As shown in Table 1, 60 μM Rh_2 reduced the uptakes of ^{3}H-thymidine and ^{3}H-uridine to about 50% of that by 30 μM Rh_2. Uptake of ^{3}H-valine was decreased by 60 μM Rh_2 to about one-fifth of that by 30 μM Rh_2. The uptakes of radiolabeled precursors were completely inhibited by 100 μM Rh_2.

Table 1. Inhibitory effects of Rh_2 on uptakes of radiolabeled precursors by HRA cells

Rh_2 Concentrations (μM)	Radiolabeled precursors (cpm)		
	^{3}H-thymidine	^{3}H-uridine	^{3}H-valine
0	6481	5091	43834
15	4628	4181	56892
30	4844	3849	50591
60	2426	1897	9513
100	111	21	64

60 μM Rh_2 reduces the uptakes of ^{3}H-thymidine and ^{3}H-uridine to about 50% of that by 30 μM Rh_2. Uptake of ^{3}H-valine is decreased by 60 μM Rh_2 to about one-fifth of that of 30 μM of Rh_2.

III. EFFECTS OF RH_2 ON THE TUMOR GROWTH IN NUDE MICE

We attempted to determine whether such direct inhibition of the HRA cell proliferation by Rh_2 can bring about the adjuvant effect to cisplatin on the growth of HRA tumor in nude mice. 9 x 10^5 HRA cells were inoculated s.c into the right flank of nude mice. After 7 days of tumor inoculation, 2 mg/kg CDDP was administered i.p every week for 5 weeks. Various concentrations of Rh2 were administered i.p or orally with or without CDDP. In the first experiment, Rh_2 was administered i.p every week for 5 weeks with or without CDDP. The mice were divided into the following groups. 1; 10 mice treated with 0.1 ml medium alone containing 0.1% ethanol (control group), 2; 10 mice treated with 2 mg/kg CDDP alone, 3; 10 mice treated with 0.1 ml of 1 μM Rh_2 alone, 4; 10 mice treated with 2 mg/kg CDDP and 0.1 ml of 1 μM Rh_2 , 5; 10 mice treated with 0.1 ml of 10 μM Rh_2 alone, 6; 10 mice treated with 2 mg/kg CDDP and 0.1 ml of 10 μM Rh_2, 7; 10 mice treated with 0.1 ml of 100 μM Rh_2 alone, 8; 10 mice treated with 2 mg/kg CDDP and 0.1 ml of 100 μM Rh_2. Tumor volume (cm^3) was calculated according to the following formula, $4\pi/3(r1+r2)^3/8$, where r1 is the longitudinal radius and r2 is the transverse radius. Results were presented as the mean ± SD and analysed statistically by non-parametric method. As shown in Fig. 3 i.p treatment with Rh_2 alone had no significant inhibitory effect on the tumor growth. On the other hand, when 10 μM Rh_2 (not 1 μM or 10 μM) was combined with CDDP, a significant inhibition ($p < 0.05$) of the tumor growth was observed at 31 days after tumor inoculation compared to that of the control group. Consequently, the survival of nude mice treated with 2 mg/kg CDDP and 10 μM Rh_2 was significantly ($p < 0.05$) prolonged, compared to that not only of the control group but also the group treated with CDDP or Rh_2 alone.

In the second experiment, we attempted to determine the effect of oral administration of Rh_2 on the HRA cell tumor growth in nude mice, because red ginseng containing Rh_2 has been commonly used by oral administration as a traditional medicine. HRA cells were inoculated into nude mice in the same way as in the first experiment. CDDP (2 mg/kg) was administered i.p every week after 7 days of tumor inoculation for 5 weeks, while Rh_2 was administered orally every day using a cannula for 90 days after the next day of tumor inoculation. The volume of Rh_2 solution administered to each mouse was 0.4 ml and the final concentration of ethanol was less than 0.4 %. The experimental groups were divided as follows: 1; 10 mice were treated orally with distilled water containing 0.4% ethanol alone (control group), 2; 10 mice were treated i.p with 2 mg/kg CDDP alone, 3; 10 mice were treated orally with 1 μM Rh_2 solution, 4; 10 mice were treated orally with 15 μM Rh_2 solution, 5; 10 mice were treated orally with 120 μM Rh_2 solution. As shown in Table 2, the tumor volumes of nude mice treated with only 1 μM Rh_2 were significantly ($p< 0.05$) smaller than those of CDDP treated mice as well as those of control group at 56 and 77 days after tumor inoculation. Oral administration of 15 μM or 120 μM Rh_2 remarkably inhibited the tumor growth during the experimental period and the tumor volumes were about 1/4 and 1/3 of those in a control group and a CDDP treated group, respectively on day 91. Consequently, the survival time in nude mice treated with 15 μM or 120 μM Rh_2 (not 1 μM Rh_2) were significantly prolonged, compared to that of a control group or a CDDP treated group (data not shown). During the experimental period no adverse effects were seen both in the first and second experiment as confirmed by monitoring body weight and hematocrit (6).

IV. DISCUSSION

Rh_2 is a new antineoplastic agent isolated from ethanol extract of Panax ginseng CA Meyer so called red ginseng. We have demonstrated that Rh_2

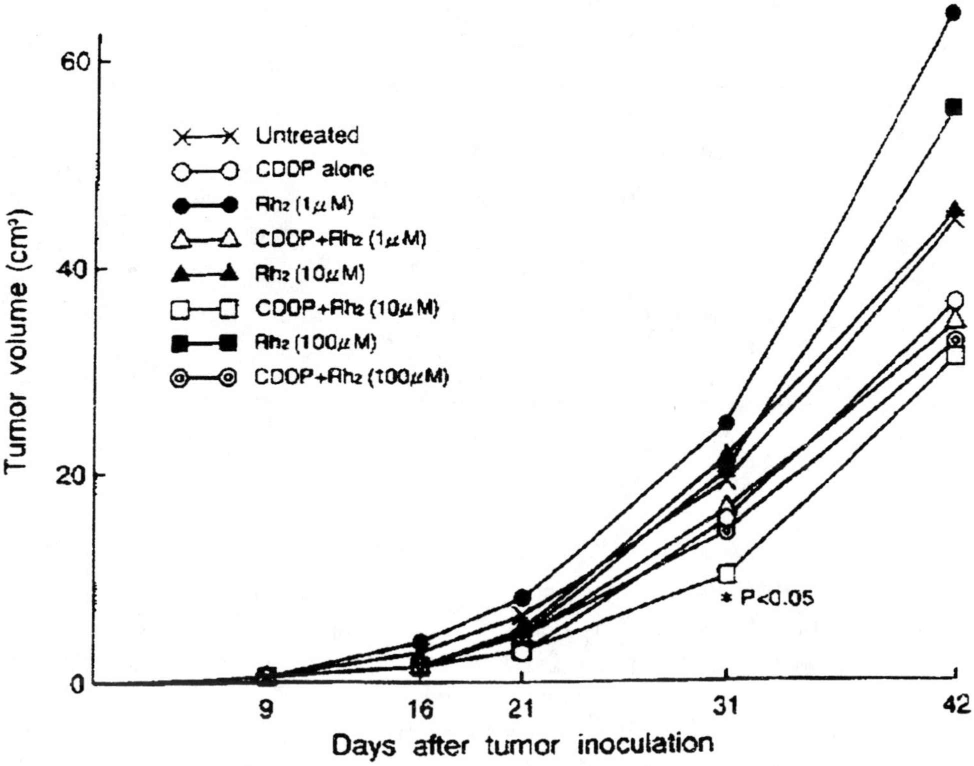

Fig. 3 Effects of Rh_2 alone or combinations of Rh_2 and CDDP on growth of the HRA tumor inoculated in nude mice. The $9x10^5$ HRA cells were inoculated s.c into the right flank of nude mice. After 7 days of tumor inoculation, CDDP (2mg/kg) alone or 0.1ml of Rh_2 (1, 10, 100 μM) solution was administered i.p once a week for 5 weeks. *$p<0.05$, compared to the control group.

Table 2. Effects of Rh_2 on tumor growth in nude mice bearing HRA cells

Days	Control	CDDP	1μM Rh_2	15μM Rh_2	120μM Rh_2
35	4.43±1.74	[a] 2.08±0.60	2.32±1.34	1.46±0.57	0.84±0.24*
42	6.44±1.74	3.36±1.01	2.69±0.94	1.36±0.38*	0.70±0.19*
49	9.57±6.12	5.49±1.90	3.84±2.00	2.97±0.49*	1.22±0.37*
56	10.37±5.37	6.28±1.67	3.69±1.21*	2.61±0.53*	1.36±0.39*
63	13.43±5.49	8.22±2.85	4.94±1.62	3.99±0.76*	2.25±0.92*
70	15.37±4.58	11.85±4.22	7.13±3.56	4.42±1.58*	3.45±2.10*
77	17.22±5.78	13.55±3.94	7.51±3.17*	5.17±1.76*	3.56±1.76*
84	21.12±8.87	14.26±5.43	9.05±3.99	5.53±2.37*	5.33±3.08*
91	21.44±9.31	14.67±8.17	8.61±5.10	5.20±2.23*	5.23±3.15*

[a] Tumor volume (cm^3), Mean ± SD, μM $p<0.05$, compared to control and CDDP treated group.

inhibited HRA cell proliferation in vitro in a dose dependent manner between 10 and 100 μM. When Rh_2 was administered i.p with CDDP to nude mice bearing HRA cell tumor, marked retardation of tumor growth and prolongation of survival time was revealed, suggesting that Rh_2 has adjuvant effects to CDDP. Red ginseng containing Rh_2 is a useful traditional medical agent which has been used widely in Asian countries, especially Korea, Japan, and China. This agent has been exclusively administered orally. Thus, antitumor effects of oral administration of Rh_2 were examined in nude mice bearing HRA cell tumor. We have demonstrated that oral but not i.p administration of Rh_2 alone had a remarkable antitumor effect. The precise mechanism of action of Rh_2 were still unknown. The inhibitory effect of Rh_2 on the DNA, RNA and protein synthesis by HRA cells was elucidated in this study. In addition, we suggested that Rh_2 has the capacity to inhibit growth by arresting HRA cells in the G1 phase of the cell cycle (data not shown). Moreover, Rh_2 has been demonstrated to increase cell adhesiveness to plastic surfaces and cell agglutinability (7). Thus, it is conceivable that Rh_2 may affect functions of cell surface and membrane, which are involved in the regulation of phenotypic expression of the cells. Recently, Ota et al (8) reported that protopanaxadiol (PPD), which is an aglycon of Rh_2, is formed from Rh_2 as a result of it's deglycosylation by the cells and the inhibitory effect of PPD on the cancer cell growth was stronger than that of Rh_2. Therefore, PPD converted from Rh_2 in the tumor cells may inhibit the tumor growth mainly rather than Rh_2 itself. Red ginseng has been used as a tonic medicine, which may be act as a biological response modifier. In our study (data not shown), Rh_2. significantly enhanced natural killer (NK) activity of spleen cells in nude mice bearing HRA cells. Further investigation will be necessary to elucidate the precise mechanism of action of Rh_2.

REFERENCES

1. Odashima, S., Nakayama, Y., Honjyo, N., Abe, H., and Arichi, S.: Induction of phenotypic reverse transformation by ginsenosides in cultured Morris hepatoma cells. *Eur. J. Cancer*, 15: 885-892, 1979.
2. Odashima, S., Ota, T., Kohno, H., Matsuda, T., Kitagawa, I., Abe, H., and Arichi, S.: Control of phenotypic expression of cultured B16 melanoma cells by plant glycosides. *Cancer Res.*, 45: 2781-2784, 1985.
3. Matsunaga, H., Katano, M., Yamamoto, H., Mori, M., and Takata, K.: Determination of panaxytriol, a new type of tumor growth inhibitor from Panax ginseng, by capillary gas chromatography. *J. Chromatograph*, 483: 368-372, 1989.
4. Kikuchi, Y., Kizawa, I., Oomori, K., Miyauchi, M., Kita, T., Tenjin, Y., and Kato, K. : Establishment of a human ovarian cancer cell line capable of forming ascites in nude mice and effects of tranexamic acid on cell proliferation and ascites formation. *Cancer Res.*, 47: 592-596, 1987.
5. Kikuchi, Y., Sasa, H., Kita, T., Hirata, J., Tode, T., and Nagata, I.: Inhibition of human ovarian cancer cell proliferation in vitro by ginsenoside Rh2 and adjuvant effects to cisplatin in vivo. *Anti-Cancer Drugs,* 2: 63-67, 1991.
6. Tode, T., Kikuchi, Y., Kita, T., Hirata, J., Imaizumi, E., and Nagata, I.: Inhibitory effects by oral administration of ginsenoside Rh_2 on the growth of human ovarian cancer cells in nude mice. *J. Cancer Res. Clin. Oncol.*, 120: 24-26, 1993.
7. Ota, T., Fujikawa-Yamamoto, F., Zhi-Ping Zong, ZP., Yamazaki, M., Odashima, S., Kitagawa, I., Abe, H., and Arichi, S.: Plant-glycoside modulation of cell surface related to control of differentiation in cultured B16 melanoma cells. *Cancer Res.*, 47: 38633-3867, 1987.
8. Ota, T., Maeda, M., and Odashima, S.: Mechanism of action of ginsenoside Rh2; Uptake and metabolism of ginsenoside Rh_2 by cultured B16 melanoma cells. *J. Pharm. Sci.*, 80: 1141-1147, 1991.

CHAPTER 12

CHEMOSENSITIVITY OF OVARIAN CLEAR CELL CARCINOMA REVEALED BY DISEASE ORIENTED SCREENING SYSTEM[1]

Masato Nishida*, Hajime Tsunoda, Sadahiko Shigemitsu, Keiko Kohno, Ken Nishide, Yuko Arisawa and Takeshi Kubo

Department of Obstetrics and Gynecology, Institute of Clinical Medicine, Tsukuba University, Tsukuba City, Ibaraki-Ken, Japan

ABSTRACT

This study was undertaken to examine the chemosensitivity of ovarian clear cell carcinoma cells in vitro by MTT assay. Using four established human ovarian clear cell carcinoma cell lines (HAC-2, OVAS-21, RMG-I and KK), their sensitivity to 23 antitumor agents was investigated. The antitumor effects of each drug were evaluated based on the surviving fraction curves. The four cell lines showed strong resistance to most of the drugs tested. Especially, RMG-I cells were resistant to all the drugs investigated. The other cell lines showed similar drug sensitivity and the most eligible drugs for chemotherapy against ovarian clear cell carcinoma seemed to be actinomycin-D, mitomycin-C, CDDP and 254-S. From these results, a more effective combination therapy for this tumor may be a combination of actinomycin-D, mitomycin C, and CDDP or 254-S or of all these 4 drugs.

[1] This work was supported by Grants-in-Aid for Scientific Research from the Ministry of Education, Science and Culture (No63570767) and from the University of Tsukuba Project Research.

* Masato Nishida MD., Department of Obstetrics and Gynecology, Institute of Clinical Medicine, Tsukuba University, 1-1-1, Tennoudai, Tsukuba-shi, 305 Ibaraki-ken, Japan, Telephone number: 0298-53-3210, Fax number: 0298-53-3039,

Key Words: Chemosensitivity, Ovarian cancer, Clear cell carcinoma, Cell line, Disease oriented screening system.

INTRODUCTION

Owing to rapid progress in chemotherapy, the prognosis for various tumor diseases, which used to be very poor, has greatly been improved in recent years. In the field of obstetrics and gynecology, for example, the prognosis for chorionic tumors has been improved with development of a combination chemotherapy containing methotrexate, actinomycin-D and etoposide (1,2). In addition, the prognosis of germ cell tumors has also been improved by PVB therapy (3), i.e., the combination of CDDP, vinblastine and bleomycin. Surprisingly, these both tumors show a consistent sensitivity to the corresponding chemotherapeutic regimen with high response rate. These findings suggest that histologically identical tumors show a consistent response to the same drug.

At present, CAP therapy, i.e., the combination of cyclophosphamide, adriamycin and cisplatin, is most commonly administered to patients with epithelial ovarian cancer (4-7). However, ovarian clear cell carcinoma, which has tendency to increase in recent years, is resistant to this chemotherapeutic regimen and its prognosis is very poor (8).

Thus, in the present study, we attempted to determine which drugs are more effective against ovarian clear cell carcinoma using the MTT assay (9-12).

MATERIALS AND METHODS

CELL LINES.

Four cell lines, HAC-2, OVAS-21, RMG-1 and KK, established from human ovarian clear cell carcinoma were used. HAC-2 cells (13) were established in our laboratory. OVAS-21 cells (14) were kindly provided by Dr. T. Morisawa of Kitasato University, RMG-1 cells (15) by Dr. S. Nozawa of Keio University and KK cells (16) by Dr. Y. Kikuchi of the National Defense Medical College. All cell lines showed stable growth and were maintained under conditions recommended by the suppliers.

CHEMICALS.

Pirarubicin (THP-ADM), peplomycin sulfate (PEP), bleomycin hydrochloride (BLM), cisplatin (CDDP) and etoposide (ETP) were supplied by Nippon Kayaku Co., Ltd. (Tokyo, Japan). Doxorubicin hydrochloride (ADM), epirubicin hydrochloride (EPI), L-asparaginase (L-ASP), mitomycin C (MMC) and 5-fluorouracil (5-FU) were supplied by Kyowa Hakko Co., Ltd. (Tokyo, Japan). Vincristine sulfate (VCR), vinblastine sulfate (VLB), vindesine sulfate (VDS), 4-hydroperoxy cyclophosphamide, the active metabolite of cyclophosphamide (CPM) and glycolate-o,o' diammineplatinum (254-S) were supplied by Shionogi Seiyaku Co., Ltd., Tokyo, Japan. Aclarubicin hydrochloride (ACR) and neocarzinostatin (NCS) were supplied by Yamanouchi Seiyaku Co., Ltd., Tokyo, Japan. Actinomycin-D (Act-D), ranimustine (MCNU), daunorubicin hydrochloride (DM), cytarabine (Ara-C), methorexate (MTX) and carboplatin (CBDCA)was supplied by Banyu Seiyaku Co., Ltd., Tokyo, Japan, by Tokyo Tanabe Seiyaku Co., Ltd., Tokyo, Japan, by Meiji Seika Co., Ltd., Tokyo, Japan, by Nippon Shinyaku Co., Ltd., Tokyo, Japan, by Takeda Yakuhinkogyo Co., Ltd., Tokyo, Japan and by Bristol-Myers Squibb Co., Ltd., Tokyo, Japan, respectively. MTT-cell growth assay kit was purchased from Chemicon International Co., Ltd., CA, USA.

DRUG CONCENTRATIONS.

Drugs concentrations (0.01, 0.05, 0.1, 0.2, 0.5, 1, 2, 5 and 10 mg/ml) were selected because the peak plasma concentrations reported in humans for the drugs used in the present study were around this range. Drugs with the IC50 (more than 10 mg/ml) were tested at higher concentrations. L-asparaginase was used at concentrations equivalent to 0.005-5 IU/ml.

EXPOSURE TIME.

Cells were exposed to the drugs for 1, 3, 6, 12, 24, 48 or 72 hrs. These exposure times seemed to be necessary to reflect the in vivo effect of each drug.

CYTOTOXICITY ASSAY.

The effect of chemotherapeutic agents on cell growth was determined by the MTT assay(1). Briefly, HAC-2, OVAS-21 and KK cells were seeded at a density of 1 x 10^4 cells/well in 96-well microplates (Falcon Labware, CA, USA). RMG-I cells were seeded at a density of 3 x 10^4 cells/well. After incubation of cells for 72 h, the media were changed for media containing various agents at different concentrations. After cells were incubated at 37°C for 1, 3, 6, 12, 24, 48 and 72 h , they were rinsed 3 times with phosphate buffered saline (PBS, pH7.4) to eliminate the drugs. After additional 3 days' incubation with drug free growth media, MTT assay was performed as previously described. (12, 17, 18). Briefly, 3-(4,5-dimethylthiazol-2-yl)-2,5-diphenyl tetrazolium bromide (MTT) (5 mg/ml: 10 ml/well) was added to each well and incubated at 37°C for 4 h. The medium was aspirated from the wells without disturbing the formazan crystals and cells on the plastic surface. 100 ml of dimethyl sulfoxide (DMSO) was added to each well to solubilize the formazan crystals and the absorbance at 570 nm of these formazan solutions was measured using a microplate assay reader (MPR A4, Toyo-soda, Tokyo, Japan). Cells cultured in drug free media and rinsed three times with PBS were served as the control. Percentage of control absorbance was considered to be the surviving fraction of the cells. The IC_{50} value of each drug was obtained based on the surviving fraction curves at each exposure time, and the effect of drugs was evaluated. Results were shown as the mean (± SD) from quadruplicate experiments.

RESULTS

CHARACTERISTICS OF SURVIVING FRACTION CURVES OF THE CHEMOTHERAPEUTIC AGENTS.

Anthracycline anticancer drugs (ADM) inhibited the growth of the HAC-2 cells in both time- and concentration- dependent fashion (Fig.1). Anticancer antibiotic agents (Act-D) also showed time- and concentration- dependent inhibitory effects on the HAC-2 cell growth (Fig.2), but BLM had no inhibitory effects on the HAC-2 cell growth. (Fig. 3). VCR showed inhibitory effects (although weak) on the KK cell growth in both time- and dose- dependent manner (Fig. 4), while VCR had no inhibitory effects on the cell growth of the other clear cell carcinoma lines (data not shown). Metabolic antagonist (5-FU.) showed no inhibitory effects on the KK cell growth and the IC50 value could not be obtained ever after exposure for 72 h at 10 mg/ml (Fig. 5). More than 5 mg/ml cyclophosphamide showed time- and concentration- dependent inhibitory effects on the KK cell growth(Fig. 6), but the IC50 could not be obtained for OVAS-21 and RMG-I (data not shown). Cisplatin (CDDP) resulted in time- and concentration- dependent inhibition of the HAC-2 at more than 0.1 mg/ml concentrations (Fig. 7). Although data was not shown, MCNU was ineffective to any cell line used in this study. Although l-asparaginase showed a tendency to inhibit the HAC-2 cell growth after exposure for 72 h, it could not decrease the surviving fraction to less than 50% (data not shown). ETP showed a tendency to inhibit the HAC-2 cell growth without obtaining the IC_{50} (Fig. 8).

CHARACTERISTICS OF CHEMOSENSITIVITY TO THE FOUR CLEAR CELL CARCINOMA LINES USED.

Tables 1, 2, 3 and 4 show the IC_{50} values to various drugs for each cell line at different exposure times, in addition to the peak plasma concentration of each drug in human. Based upon these results, the four cell lines were classified into relatively sensitive cell line to various drugs (HAC-2, OVAS-21 and KK cells) and a cell line (RMG-I cell) resistant to almost all drugs tested. These three sensitive cell lines could obtain the IC50 values to several drugs at less than 72 h exposure time. However, 21 of 23 anti-cancer drugs tested at concentration of 10 mg/ml for 72 h failed to result in 50% inhibition of the RMG-I cell growth. These three sensitive cell lines seemed to have a similar sensitivity to each drug.

DRUG EFFICACY EVALUATION.

Since none of the drugs tested seemed inhibitory effects on the RMG-I cell growth, the efficacy of drugs was evaluated only regarding the other three cell lines. The drugs were considered effective when their values were lower than the reported peak plasma concentrations at 1 h exposure time, and eligible when their IC_{50} values were lower than the reported peak plasma concentration at 72 h exposure time for these three cell lines. ADM, THP-ADM, DM, BLM, PEP, NCS, VDS, Ara-C, 5-FU, MCNU, MTX, L-ASP and ETP did not meet these criteria and thus were regarded as ineffective. The drugs which resulted in 50% inhibition of cell growth at 1 h exposure time were Act-D and 254-S for HAC-2 cells. Since the IC_{50} values to Act-D and 254-S of OVAS-21 and KK cells were higher than the reported peak plasma concentrations at 1 h exposure time, these drugs were considered ineffective on ovarian clear cell carcinoma. However, EPI, Act-D, MMC, CDDP and 254-S were considered eligible for this tumor.

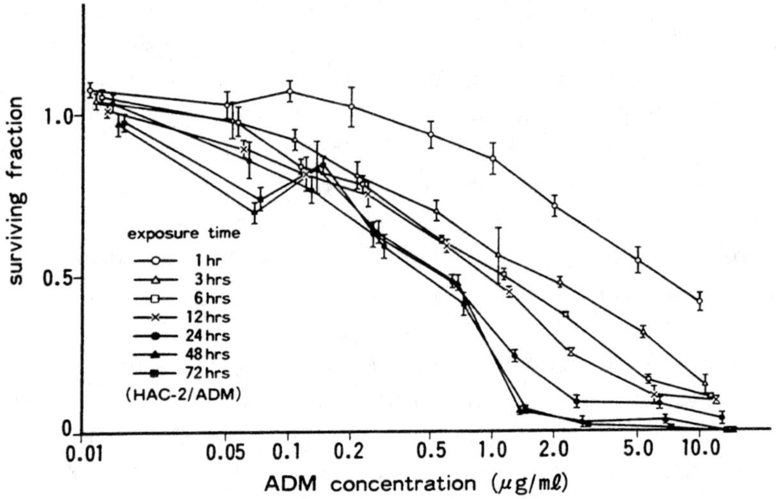

Fig. 1. Surviving fraction curves of ADM on HAC-2 cells. ADM inhibited the HAC-2 cell growth in both time- and concentration- dependent fashion. The IC_{50} value was 6 mg/ml after exposure for 1 h. Efficacy did not increase even if exposure was continued for more than 24 h. The IC_{50} value was about 0.5 mg/ml at 24 h and over. Vertical bars show the mean ± SD from quadruplicate experiments.

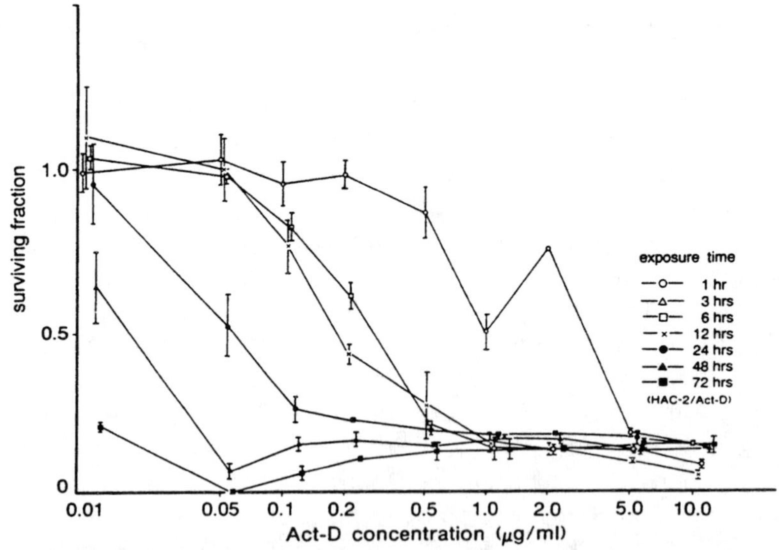

Fig. 2. Surviving fraction curves of Act-D on HAC-2 cells. Act-D showed time- and concentration- dependent inhibitory effects. The effects were particularly time-dependent, and IC_{50} values of 1.0, 0.27 and 0.18 mg/ml were obtained after exposure for 1, 6 and 12 h, respectively, and IC_{50} value of less than 0.1 mg/ml was obtained after exposure for 72 h. Vertical bars show the mean ± SD from quadruplicate experiments.

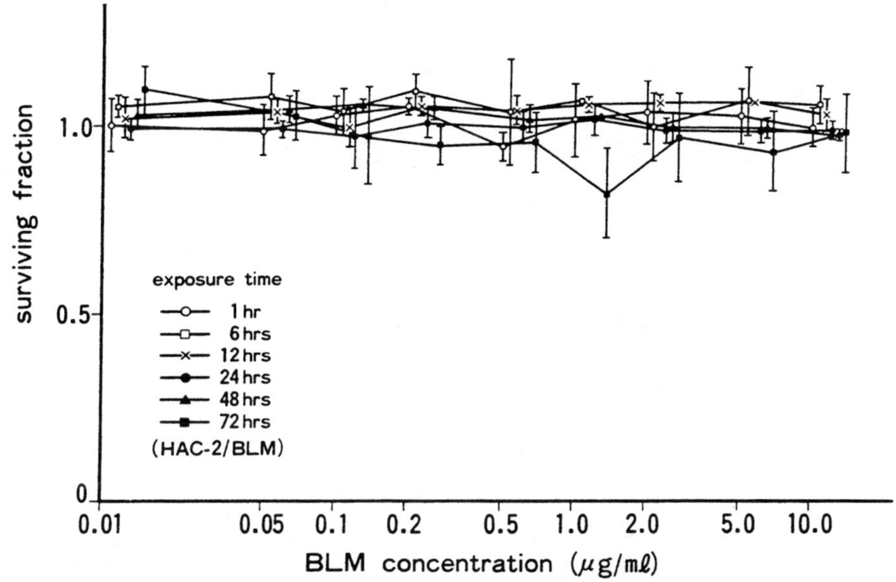

Fig. 3. Surviving fraction curves of BLM on HAC-2 cells. No inhibitory effects were observed even at 10 mg/ml after exposure for 72 h. Vertical bars show the mean ± SD from quadruplicate experiments.

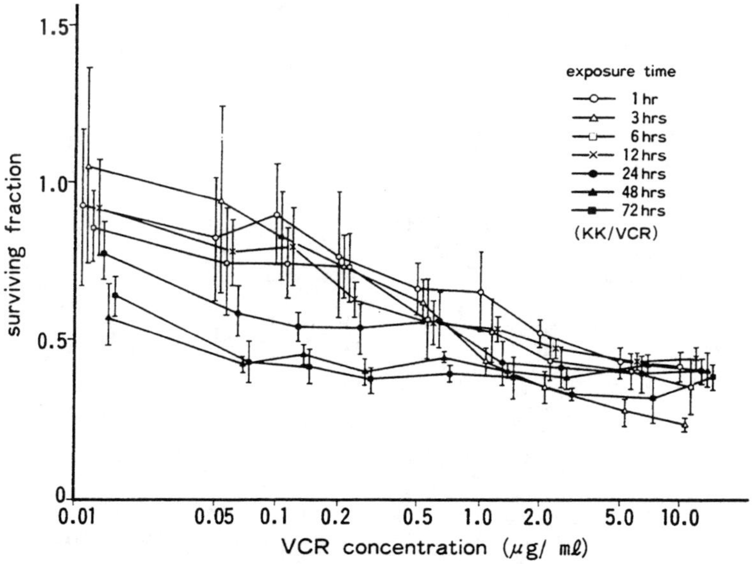

Fig. 4. Surviving fraction curves of VCR on KK cells. IC_{50} values to VCR of KK cells were 2.35, 0.77, 1.23, 1.4, 0.68, 0.02 and 0.03 mg/ml after exposure for 1, 3, 6, 12, 24, 48 and 72 h, respectively showing both time- and concentration- dependent inhibition. Efficacy was thus observed at lower concentration with longer exposure time. Vertical bars show the mean ± SD from quadruplicate experiments.

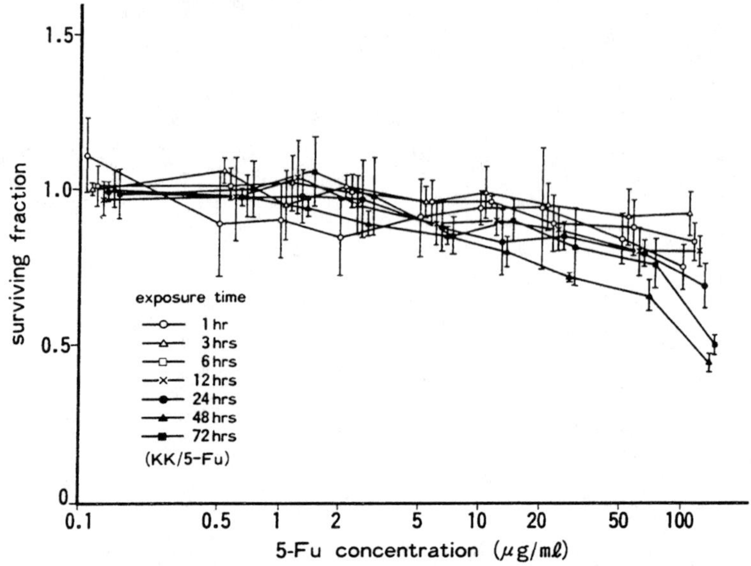

Fig. 5. Surviving fraction curves of 5-FU on KK cells. The IC50 value could not be obtained even at 100 mg/ml when exposure time was 24 h or less. The IC50 values of 84 and 100 mg/ml were obtained after exposure for 48 and 72 h, respectively. Vertical bars show the mean ± SD from quadruplicate experiments.

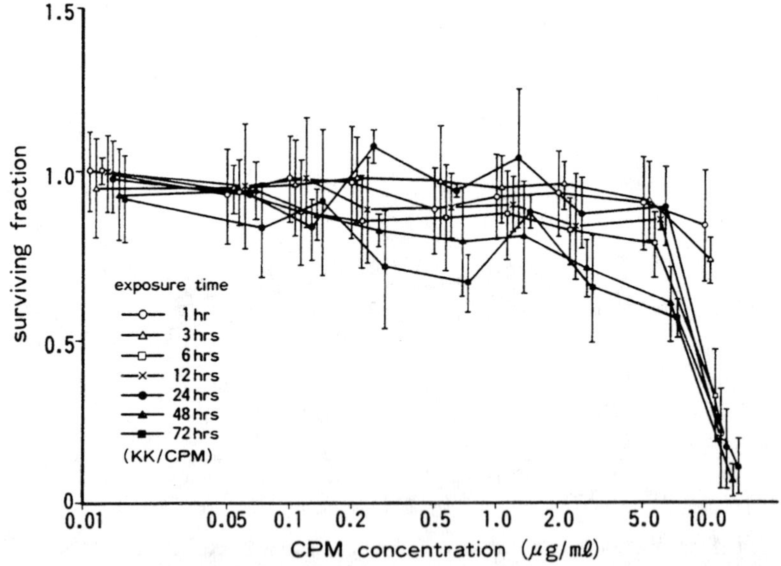

Fig. 6. Surviving fraction curves of CPM on KK cells. Inhibitory effects on KK cells increased with concentration and the IC_{50} values were 5 to 7 mg/ml when exposed for more than 6 h. Vertical bars show the mean ± SD from quadruplicate experiments.

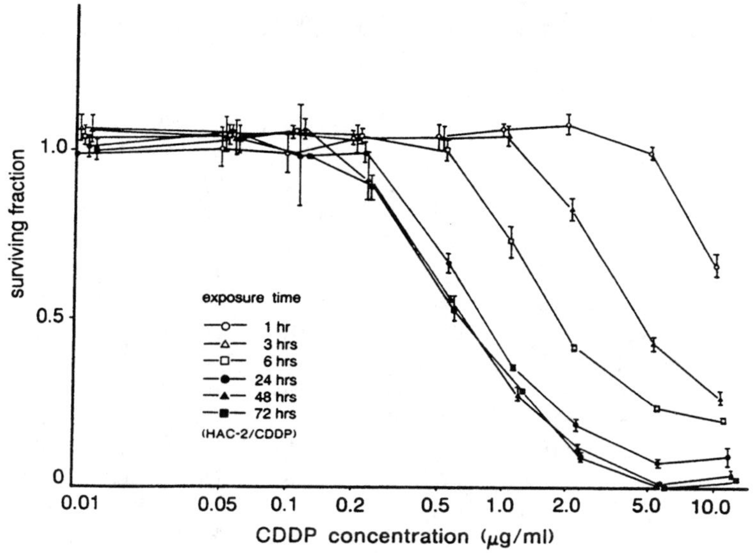

Fig. 7. Surviving fraction curves of CDDP on HAC-2 cells. CDDP showed both time- and concentration- dependent inhibitory effects on the HAC cell proliferation. The IC_{50} values were 4.4, 1.8, 0.8, 0.6 and 0.6 mg/ml after exposure for 3, 6, 24, 48 and 72 h, respectively. Vertical bars show the mean ± SD from quadruplicate experiments.

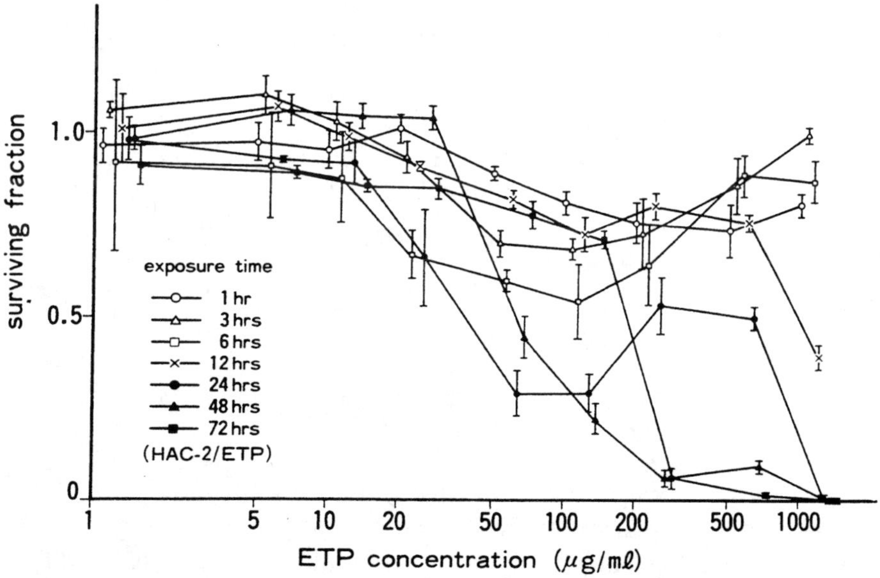

Fig. 8. Surviving fraction curves of ETP on HAC-2 cells. ETP showed both time- and concentration- dependent inhibitory effects on the HAC-2 cell growth. However, the IC_{50} value could not be obtained even at high dose of 10 mg/ml after exposure for 48 h or less. In repeat experiments conducted at higher concentrations, the IC_{50} value could not be obtained even at 1,000 mg/ml when exposure time was 6 h or less, indicating that inhibitory effects of ETP on the HAC-2 cell growth are time- dependent. The IC_{50} values of about 50 mg/ml were obtained after exposure for 48 and 72 h. Vertical bars show the mean ± SD from quadruplicate experiments.

Table 1. IC_{50} values (mg/ml) to each drug of RMG-I cells at different exposure times.

Drugs	PPC[1]	Exposure time (h)						
		1	3	6	12	24	48	72
ADM	0.17	10<	10<	10<	10<	10<	10<	10<
THP-ADM	0.1	10<	10<	10<	10<	10<	10<	10<
EPI	10	10<	10<	10<	10<	10<	10<	10<
ACR	0.2	10<	10<	10<	10<	10<	10<	10<
DM	0.1	10<	10<	10<	10<	10<	10<	10<
Act-D	1.6	10<	10<	10<	10<	10<	10<	10<
BLM	0.651	10<	10<	10<		10<	10<	10<
PEP	0.7	10<	10<	10<	10<	10<	10<	10<
NCS	0.3	10<	10<	10<	10<	10<	10<	10<
MMC	2.4	10<	10<	10<		10<	4.0	4.0
VLB	0.1	10<	10<	10<	10<	10<	10<	10<
VCR	0.7	10<	10<	10<	10<	10<	10<	10<
VDS	0.017	10<	10<	10<	10<	10<	10<	10<
Ara-C	5	10<	10<	10<	10<	10<	10<	10<
5-FU	15.3	100<	100<	100<	100<	100<	100<	100<
MTX	0.7	10<	10<	10<	10<	10<	10<	10<
CPM	8	10<	10<	9.8	9.9	9.6	10<	10<
CDDP	1.5	10<	10<	10<	10<	4.6	3.0	4.2
CBDCA	40	100<	100<	100<	100<	100<	100<	7.8
254-S	7	10<	10<	10<	10<	10<	10<	10<
MCNU	8	10<	10<	10<	10<	10<	10<	10<
L-ASP	5[2]	5<	5<	5<		5<	5<	5<
ETP	30	100<	100<	100<	100<	100<	100<	100<

[1]Peak plasma concentration (mg/ml).
[2]IU/ml.

DISCUSSION

The four ovarian clear cell carcinoma cell lines selected for the present study showed strong resistance to most of the drugs tested. In particular, RMG-I cells showed no sensitivity to any of them. Therefore, some types of ovarian clear cell carcinomas may have intrinsic resistance to the chemotherapeutic agents available at present, while other types of their tumors may be sensitive to certain drugs. Of the various drugs tested, Act-D appeared to be the most effective to these four clear cell carcinoma lines.

Table 2. IC$_{50}$ values (mg/ml) to each drug of HAC-2 cells at different exposure times.

Drugs	PPC[1]	Exposure time (h)						
		1	3	6	12	24	48	72
ADM	0.17	6.0	1.62	1.1	0.84	0.48	0.49	0.38
THP-ADM	0.1	2.0	0.96	0.66		0.32	0.26	0.28
EPI	10	10<	9.0	3.6		0.9	0.5	0.46
ACR	0.2	0.29	0.33	0.27	0.20	0.24	0.22	0.11
DM	0.1	3.2	1.9	1.4	0.7	0.5	0.48	0.4
Act-D	1.6	1.0		0.27	0.18	0.06	0.02	0.01>
BLM	0.65	10<	10<	10<	10<	10<	10<	10<
PEP	0.7	10<	10<	10<	10<	10<	10<	10<
NCS	0.3	4.0	1.5	1.6	1.4	1.9	1.6	1.9
MMC	2.4	4.6		0.55	0.23	0.10	0.06	0.06
VLB	0.1	10<	10<	10<	10<	10<	10<	10<
VCR	0.7	10<	10<	10<	10<	10<	10<	10<
VDS	0.017	10<	10<	10<	10<	10<	10<	10<
Ara-C	5	10<	10<	10<	10<	10<	10<	10<
5-FU	15.3	10000<	10000<	10000<	10000<	5600<	2200<	250<
MTX	0.7	10<	10<	10<	10<	10<	10<	10<
CPM	8	10<	10<	9.5	7.0	9.0	8.5	7.8
CDDP	1.5	10<	4.4	1.8		0.8	0.6	0.6
CBDCA	40100<	100<	78	56	16.5	9.2	52	
254-S	7	7.0	3.4	0.98		0.68	0.3	0.14
MCNU	8	10<	10<	10<	10<	10<	10<	10<
L-ASP	5[2]	5<	5<	5<	5<	5<	5<	5<
ETP	30	1000<	1000<	1000<	980<	30<	46<	120<

The values less than PPC are underlined.
[1]Peak plasma concentration (mg/ml).
[2]IU/ml.

It is noteworthy that Act-D is difficult to be metabolized in vivo, showing that half-life is about 36 h (19) and thus its plasma concentration can be maintained for long time. It has been clinically administered at 10-15 mg/kg for 5 consecutive days. This treatment regimen seems to be very rational for this drug, because its effects depend strongly on the time of exposure, as shown in the present study, especially at lower doses. Since Act-D has a long half-life, an effective concentrations is maintained over a long period of time and continuous administration contributes to the maintenance of high blood concentrations for a long time.

Table 3. IC_{50} values (mg/ml) to each drug of RMG-I cells at different exposure times.

Drugs	PPC[1]	Exposure time (h)						
		1	3	6	12	24	48	72
ADM	0.17	10<	10<	10.0	5.0	5.0	1.8	1.5
THP-ADM	0.1	0.68		0.48		0.32	0.28	0.20
EPI	10	10<		4.4		0.88	0.70	0.60
ACR	0.2	0.78	0.75	1.20	0.54	0.60	0.60	0.36
DM	0.1	4.4	10.0	3.2		3.6	0.58	0.8
Act-D	1.6	5.4	0.6	4.67	0.3	0.3	0.04	0.02
BLM	0.65	10<	10<	10<		10<	10<	10<
PEP	0.7	1000<	1000<	1000<	1000<	360	190	60
NCS	0.3	10<	10<	10<	10<	10<	9.0	6.2
MMC	2.4	10<	10<	7.0		2.4	1.0	1.2
VLB	0.1	340	320	250	200	95	100	70
VCR	0.7	10<	10<	10<	10<	10<	10<	10<
VDS	0.017	10<	10<	10<	10<	10<	10<	10<
Ara-C	5	10<	10<	10<	10<	10<	10<	10<
5-FU	15.3	100<	100<	100<	100<	100<	52	42
MTX	0.7	1000<	1000<	1000<	1000<	1000<	1000<	1000<
CPM	8	10<	10<	9.8	9.9	9.6	10<	10<
CDDP	1.5	10<	10<	5.0		1.8	0.95	0.88
CBDCA	40	100<	100<	100<	100<		16	14
254-S	7	10<	10<	10.0	3.8	2.4	1.1	0.9
MCNU	8	10<	10<	10<	10<	10<	10<	10<
L-ASP	5[2]	500<	500<	500<	500<	500<	500<	500<
ETP	30	1000<	1000<	1000<	500	220	550	120

The values less than PPC are underlined.
[1]Peak plasma concentration (mg/ml).
[2]IU/ml.

On the other hand, it is extremely difficult to assess the efficacy of any anthracycline anticancer drug in vitro, because of anthracycline anticancer drugs adhere to the cell surface in vitro, and especially ACR can not be removed by washing (17). Moreover, the peak plasma concentration of EPI is 100 times that of other anthracyclines (20), while the plasma concentration after 24 h does not differ from those of other anthracycline anticancer drugs. From results of the in vitro experiments, it is difficult to compare their treatment efficacy under the experimental conditions used in this study. Therefore, the results obtained in this study were presented only as a reference value.

Table 4. IC_{50} values (mg/ml) to each drug of KK cells at different exposure times.

Drugs	PPC[1]	Exposure time (h)						
		1	3	6	12	24	48	72
ADM	0.17	10<	5.0	1.9	1.05	0.66	0.43	0.33
THP-ADM	0.1	0.62	0.38	0.28	0.27	0.22	0	0.1
EPI	10	10<	5.8	2.8	1.6	1.13	0.7	0.37
ACR	0.2	0.46	0.64	0.68	0.4	0.22	0.17	0.15
DM	0.1	1.3	0.76	0.7	0.42	0.29	0.25	0.25
Act-D	1.6	1.65	0.26	0.12	0.03	0.03	0.01	0.01
BLM	0.65	10<	10<	10<	10<	10<	10<	10<
PEP	0.7	10<	10<	10<	10<	10<	10<	10<
NCS	0.3	10<	3.3	3.05	5.5	5.6	6.0	3.8
MMC	2.4	10<	10<	10<	3.9	2.45	1.2	1.4
VLB	0.1	0.19	0.12	0.18	10<	10<	0.34	10<
VCR	0.7	2.32	0.77	1.23	1.4	0.68	0.02	0.03
VDS	0.017	10<	10<	10<	10<	10<	10<	10<
Ara-C	5	10<	10<	10<	10<	10<	10<	5
5-FU	15.3	100<	100<	100<	100<	100<	84	100
MTX	0.7	10<	10<	10<	10<	10<	10<	1.0
CPM	8	10<	10<	7.8	7.4	7.4	5.8	5.5
CDDP	1.5	10<	4.0	2.1	1.0	0.8	0.58	0.68
CBDCA	40	100<	100<	100<	63	22	10.5	13
254-S	7	10<	10<	8.0	3.6	2.4	0.9	0.81
MCNU	8	10<	10<	10<	10<	10<	10<	10<
L-ASP	5[2]	5<	5<	5<	5<	5<	5<	5<
ETP	30	100<	100<	100<	100<	100<	100<	100<

The values less than PPC are undelined.
[1]Peak plasma concentration (mg/ml).
[2]IU/ml.

CDDP has been proved to be effective as treatment for ovarian cancer in clinical practice (7). Our results indicate that its effects are time- and concentration- dependent. At present, the CDDP based combination chemotherapy consisting of CPM, ADM and CDDP is usually performed for treatment of epithelial ovarian cancer including ovarian clear cell carcinoma. (4-7). These three drugs (CPM, ADM and CDDP) were also tested in the present study, but only CDDP was considered eligible for clear cell carcinoma cell lines used. In the treatment of ovarian clear cell carcinoma, therefore, monotherapy with high doses of CDDP may be more effective than CAP therapy. A more effective combination chemotherapy for this tumor may be a combination of Act-D, MMC and CDDP or 254-S, or a combination of all these 4 drugs. Since both CDDP and 254-S are platinum complexes, a combination of these two agents may result in a higher incidence of adverse side-effects. Although the dose limiting factor of CDDP is renal dysfunction, 254-S does not seem to have any significant adverse effects on renal function (21). The combination of these two agents which have similar mode of action, is expected to produce effects comparable to high dose intensity of CDDP and may be better of clinical use.

ACKNOWLEDGMENTS

We wish to thank Hideko Terashima for excellent technical assistance and Patricia Lopetegui de Venegas for preparation of this manuscript.

REFERENCES

1. Carter, S. K., Bakowski, M. T., Hellmann, K., *Chemotherapy of cancer*, New York: John Wiley & Sons, Inc, 1977; 152-5.
2. Newlands, E.S., Bagshawe, K. D., Anti-tumor activity of the epipodophyllin derivative VP16-213 (etoposide: NSG-141540) in gestational choriocarcinoma. *Eur. J. Cancer*, 16: 401-5, 1980.
3. Jacobs, A. J., Harris, M., Deppe, G., DasGupta, I., Cohen, C.J., Treatment of recurrent and persistent germ cell tumors with cisplatin, vinblastine, and bleomycin. *Obstet. Gycencol.* 59: 129-32, 1982.
4. Ehrlich, C. E., Einhorn, L., Williams, S.D., Morgan, J. Chemotherapy for stage III-IV epithelial ovarian cancer with cis-dichlorodiamiineplatinum (II), adriamycin, and cyclophosphamide; A preliminary report. *Cancer Treat. Rep.* 63: 281-288, 1979.
5. Conte, P.F., Bruzzone, M., Chiara, S., Sertoli, M. R., Daga, M. G., Rubagotti, A. et al. A randomized trial comparing cisplatin plus cyclophosphamide versus cisplatin, doxorubicin and cyclophosphamide in advanced ovarian cancer. *J. Clin. Oncol.* 4: 965-971, 1986.
6. Omura, G., Blessing, J. A., Ehrlich, C. E., Miller, A., Yordan, E., Creasman, W. T. et al. A randomized trial of cyclophosphamide and doxorubicin with or without cisplatin in advanced ovarian carcinoma. *Cancer* 57: 1725-1730, 1986.
7. Williams, C.J., Whitehouse JMA. Cisplatin combination chemotherapy versus chlorambucil for stage III and IV ovarian

cancer. Long term results of a randomized study. *Proc Am Soc. Clin. Oncology* 4: 116, 1985.
8. Pettersson, F. (Ed.) *Annual report on the result of treatment in gynecological cancer.* 20th vol., Stockholm: Panorama Press AB, 1988; 118-119.
9. Alley, M. C., Scudiero, D. A., Monks, A., Hursey, M. L., Czerwinski, M. J., Fine, D. L. et al. Feasibility of drug screening with panels of human tumor cell lines using a microculture tetrazolium assay, *Cancer Res.* 48: 589-601, 1988.
10. Park, J. G. , Kramer, B. S., Steinberg, S. M., Carmichael, J., Collins, J. M. , Minna, J.G. et al. Chemosensitivity testing of human colorectal carcinoma cell lines using a tetrazolium-based colorimetric assay, *Cancer Res.* 47: 5875-5879, 1987.
11. Mosman, T. Rapid colorimetric assay for cellular growth and survival: Application to proliferation and cytotoxicity assays. *J. Immunol. Methods* 65: 55-63. 1983.
12. Carmichael, J., DeGraff, W. G., Gazdar, A. F., Minna, J.M., Mitchell, J.B., Evaluation of a tetrazolium-based semiautomated colorimetric assay: Assessment of chemosensitivity testing. *Cancer Res.* 47: 936-942, 1987.
13. Nishida, M., Kuramoto, T., Jobo, T., Taguchi, A., Osanai, K., Hayashi, H. Characterization of human ovarian clear cell carcinoma in applying a cultured cell-line. *Acta Obstet Gynaec Jpn.* 29: 1840-1841, 1977. (in Japanese)
14. Morisawa, T., Kuramoto, H., Shimoda, M., Kato, Y., Hata, H. Establishment and characterization of a CA-125 producing cell line (OVAS-21) from a clear cell adenocarcinoma of the ovary. *Human cell* 1: 347, 1988. (in Japanese)
15. Nozawa, S., Tsukazaki, K., Sakayori, M., Teng, C., Iizuka, R. Establishment of a human ovarian clear cell carcinoma cell line (RMG-I) and its single cell cloning -with special reference to the stem cell of the tumor-. *Human Cell* 1: 426-435, 1988. (in Japanese)
16. Kikuchi, Y., Hirata, J., Kita, T., Imaizumi, E., Tode, T., Nagata, I. Enhancement of antiproliferative effect of cis-diamminedichloropratinum (II) by clomiphene and tamoxifen in human ovarian carcinoma cells. *Gynecol. Oncol.* 49: 365-372, 1993.
17. Nishida, M., Kohno, K., Nishide, K. Knacks and problems on chemosensitivity tests, especially MTT assay. *Human Cell* 5: 87-98, 1992. (in Japanese)
18. Twentyman, P. R., Luscombe, M. A study of some variables in a tetrazolium dye (MTT) based assay for cell growth and chemosensitivity. *Br. J. Cancer* 56: 279-285, 1987.
19. Tattersall, M. H. N., Sodergren, J. E., Sengurpta, S.K., Trites, D. H., Modest, E. J., Frei, E., III. Pharmacokinetics of actinomycin D in

patients with malignant melanoma. *Clin.Pharmacol.Ther*. 17: 701-708, 1975.

20. Ohno, T., Shimoyama, T., Kimura, K., Yamada, H. Pharmacokinetics of epirubicin in cancer patients. *Jap. J. Cancer & Chemo*. 13: 1881-1886, 1986. (in Japanese)
21. Hirabayashi, K., Okada, E. Combination chemotherapy with 254-S, ifosfamide, and peplomycin for advanced or recurrent cervical cancer. *Cancer* 71: 2769-2775, 1993.

PART III

THE OTHER FACTORS RELATED TO THE MECHANISM OF CDDP RESISTANCE

CHAPTER 13

COMPLEXITY OF CIS-DIAMMINEDICHLOROPLATINUM(II) RESISTANCE MECHANISM IN HUMAN OVARIAN CANCER CELLS*

Yoshihiro Kikuchi,[1] Junko Hirata, Kenji Ishii, Tsunekazu Kita and Ichiro Nagata

Department of Obstetrics and Gynecology, National Defense Medical College, Namiki 3-2, Tokorozawa, Saitama 359, Japan

ABSTRACT

Various factors that have seemed to play some roles in cisplatin (CDDP) resistance mechanisms were examined in human ovarian cancer cell lines sensitive (KF, TYK and KK), with acquired resistance (KFr and TYK/R) or with intrinsic resistance (MH) to CDDP. Concentrations of CDDP required for 50% inhibition of proliferation (IC_{50}) of each cell line were 0.38, 0.31 and 0.76 μM for KF, TYK and KK cells, respectively while KFr, TYK/R and MH showed about 3.4-fold, 3.0-fold and 4.2-fold IC_{50} to the respective paired cell line. The CDDP uptake by MH cells showing highest CDDP resistance with regard to the IC_{50} was lowest and followed by KFr, TYK/R and KK cells. Expression of mRNA of topoisomerase I (topo I) by TYK/R was most marked and followed by

---

* Address for reprints and correspondence: Yoshihiro Kikuchi, MD., Department of Obstetrics and Gynecology, National Defense Medical College, Namiki 3-2, Tokorozawa Saitama 359, Japan. Tel; 0429-95-1687 Fax; 0429-96-5213 e-mail; QWL04765@niftyserve.or.jp

TYK and MH, while KK, KF and KFr showed only a weak expression. Although expression of mRNA of topo II was more marked in KFr and MH cells than in KF and KK, that in TYK/R was weaker rather than that in TYK. In addition, expression of mRNA of γ-glutamylcystein synthetase (γ-GCS) was more marked in CDDP resistant cell lines than in the paired cell lines. Expression of mRNA of glutatione S-transferase (GST-π) in TYK, TYK/R, KK and MH cells was marked with the same degree, while that in KF and KFr cells was only trace. These results were almost consistent with those of the cellular glutathione (GSH) contents. KF, KFr and KK cells did not express mRNA of human metallothionein (hMT), while in TYK and MH cells its expression was observed with marked expression in TYK/R cells. Nuclear mutant p53 protein was highest in the TYK/R cells and followed by TYK, KK and MH cells.

These results suggest that although a decrease of CDDP uptake and an increase in expression of γ-GCS mRNA seemed to be factors common to CDDP resistance, the other factors examined in this study were varied without a consistent pattern between the respective paired cells, showing complexity of CDDP resistance.

INTRODUCTION

Resistance to available chemotherapeutic drugs is a major obstacle to effective, potentially curative chemotherapy in ovarian cancer. Although aggressive treatment of advanced ovarian cancer patients with a platinum containing combination chemotherapy regimen is associated with a 40% to 60% clinical complete response rate, chemotherapy is rarely curative [1]. Thus, the majority of ovarian cancer patients are destined to die from their disease. Virtually, all of these patients die with chemotherapy-refractory cancer. From this perspective, drug resistance may be considered an integral aspect of ovarian cancer biology. A major drawback to cisplatin (CDDP) therapy is that many tumor either are intrinsically resistant to the compound or develop resistance over the course of treatment [2, 3]. Extensive studies in this area have demonstrated a number of mechanism which can contribute to CDDP resistance. Among these are reduced drug accumulation, increased levels of detoxifying agents like glutathione (GSH), and increased repair of the adducts [4-7]. In addition, DNA topoisomerase II (topo II) is increased in some CDDP-resistant human ovarian cancer cell lines [8, 9] and in a CDDP-resistant murine leukemia cell line [10]. In contrast, little attention has been paid on a possible role for topo

I in CDDP-resistance except for a recent study [11]. The most of studies mentioned above have been made by using cell lines with acquired but not intrinsic resistance to CDDP.

Thus, we have established a series of CDDP-resistant cell lines (KFr and TYK/R) by treating the respective parent cell line (KF and TYK) with incremental, increasing concentrations of CDDP and clinically intrinsic CDDP-resistant cell lines (KK and MH) [12-15]. In order to more fully elucidate the multiple mechanisms responsible for CDDP-resistance, we attempted to determine a role not only of drug accumulation, drug detoxification or DNA repair but also of topo I and II in the acquired and intrinsic CDDP-resistance.

MATERIALS AND METHODS

Drugs and Chemicals. CDDP was obtained from the Brystol-Myers Squibb Co., Tokyo, Japan. All other drugs and chemicals not specifically mentioned were purchased from Sigma (St. Louis, MO).

Cell Culture and Establishment of CDDP-resistant Cell Lines. The KF cell line was established from tissue of a patient with serous cystadenocarcinoma of the ovary [16]. The CDDP-resistant KFr cell line was obtained after repeated exposure of the parent KF cell line to escalating doses of CDDP [12]. Similarly, the TYK/R was an acquired CDDP-resistant cell line from the parent TYK cell line [15]. The KK or MH cell line was established from ascites of a patient with clear cell carcinoma of the ovary or serous cystadenocarcinoma of the ovary, respectively. The patients from whose ovarian carcinomas KK and MH cells were derived died of progressive disease, with no effective response to CDDP-based chemotherapy, suggesting intrinsic resistance to CDDP [13, 14]. The cells were grown as monolayer cultures in RPMI 1640 medium supplemented with 10% fetal bovine serum, 2 mM glutamine, 100 units penicillin/ml, and 100 μg streptomycin/ml (Grand Island Biological Co., Grand Island, NY) in a humidified atmosphere of 5% CO_2 at 37 and were usually subcultured once a week with 0.25% trypsin. To examine concentrations of CDDP required for 50% inhibition of each cell proliferation in vitro (IC_{50}), we seeded 10^4 cells for KF and KFr, 2 x 10^4 cells for TYK and TYK/R, and 10^5 cells for KK and MH in the multidishes and added CDDP at the concentrations indicated. After 4 days of culture without replenishment of CDDP, cells were harvested and counted with a hematocytometer. The degree of resistance to CDDP was compared using the IC_{50} value. Living cells grown in culture dishes were examined with a phase-contrast microscope.

Platinum Assays. The cultured cells in a preconfluent state were harvested using a rubber policeman after incubating with a small amount of 0.25% trypsin and counted with a hematocytometer. The cell number was adjusted to 10^7 cells/ml with RPMI 1640 medium and CDDP was added to obtain a final concentration of 100 μM in the medium. After 3 h incubation, cells were harvested, washed three times with fresh medium, and resuspended in 1 ml of medium. The cell viability was examined by using the trypan blue dye exclusion test. The incubation time at this cell density did not affect the cell viability. The cell suspension was sonicated (50% duty cycle for 3 min) using a W-225 sonicator (Heat Systems-Ultrasonics, Inc., Farmingdale, NY). After centrifugation at 30,000 g for 1 h, the supernatants were taken for platinum assay. The platinum assay was performed as described previously [17] with a Perkin-Elmer Model 603 atomic absorption spectrometer equipped with a heat graphite atomizer on which the temperature control had been modified to produce a gradual increase in temperature. Protein was determined with a protein microassay (Bio-Rad, Richmond, CA) [18].

GSH Content. Cells (5-10 x 10^6) at preconfluent state were lysed by sonication at 4 in 1 ml of phosphate buffered saline (PBS). The supernatant was obtained for assay after centrifugation (10,000 g for 10 min at 4). The protein was precipitated by adding 12% 5-sulfosalicylic acid (SSA) (1 vol. of SSA to 3 vol. of sample). After standing on ice for 1-4 h, the samples were centrifuged (10,000 g for 10 min). The SSA extract was assayed by an enzymatic recycling method published elsewhere [19]. Values are the mean of 2 independent experiments. Results were normalized according to the numbers of cells.

Northern Blot Analysis. The total RNA was extracted using the acid guanidium isothiocyanate-phenol-chloroform method [20] from the exponentially growing cells. Human DNA topo I cDNA, human DNA topo II cDNA, and human GST-π cDNA were used as probes [11]. Human MT-II, which encoded hMT-II [21], was obtained from the American Type Culture Collection (Rockville, MD). A human kidney γ-GCS probe (1.7 kilobases) was used to screen human ovarian carcinoma cDNA library in λ-ZAP II. RNA (15 μg) was subjected to electrophoresis in a 1% agarose gel containing 2.2 M formaldehyde and then was transferred to a nylon membrane (Hybond N^+;

Amersham Japan, Tokyo, Japan). The filter was hybridized with each ^{32}P-labeled cDNA probe in 50% deionized formamide, 10x Denhardt's buffer, 5x SSC (1x SSC = 0.15 M NaCl-0.015 M sodium citrate, pH 7.0), and 0.1% SDS at 30 for 36 h. The filter was then washed twice in 2x SSC and 0.1% SDS at room temperature. Autoradiography was performed for 12 h with an intensifying screen at -70. The intensity of the autoradiograms obtained was quantified by densitometric scanning.

Nuclear Mutant p53 Protein Assay. The cells in a preconfluent state were harvested and adjusted to 10^7 cells/ml with fresh medium. The cell suspension was washed 3 times with ice-cold PBS. The cell pellets were resuspended in 5x ice-cold swelling buffer (20 mM Tris-HCl, 5 mM EDTA, 1 mM PMSF, pH 8.0) and incubated on ice for 30 min with gently mixing. Tween-20 was added to be a final concentration of 1% (v/v) into the cell suspension. After an additional 30 min incubation, NaCl was added to be a final concentration of 0.5 M and the suspensions were incubated for 15 min. After centrifugation at 70,000 g for 30 min at 4, the resultant supernatants were taken for mutant p53 protein assay. Mutant p53 protein was determined by p53 mutant selective quantitation ELISA assay kit (Oncogene Science, Inc., Manhasset, NY) using antibody reactive with a conformationally sensitive epitope, located approximately between amino acids 155 and 215 [22]. Results were normalized according to the cellular protein contents and showed the mean from three separate experiments.

RESULTS

Sensitivity to CDDP and Intracellular Platinum Accumulation. As shown in Table 1, KFr, TYK/R and MH cells showed 3.37-, 2.97- and 4.21-fold higher resistance to CDDP than KF, TYK and KK cells with regard to the IC_{50} value, respectively. The intracellular platinum content of KFr and MH cells was significantly decreased than that of KF and KK cells, whereas that of TYK/R was not significantly different from that of TYK.

Expression of Topo I and II mRNA and CDDP Resistance. The CDDP-acquired resistant KFr cell line which was derived from the parent KF cell line was characterized by markedly higher expression of topo II (but not topo I) mRNA, while the CDDP resistant TYK/R cell line derived from TYK cells

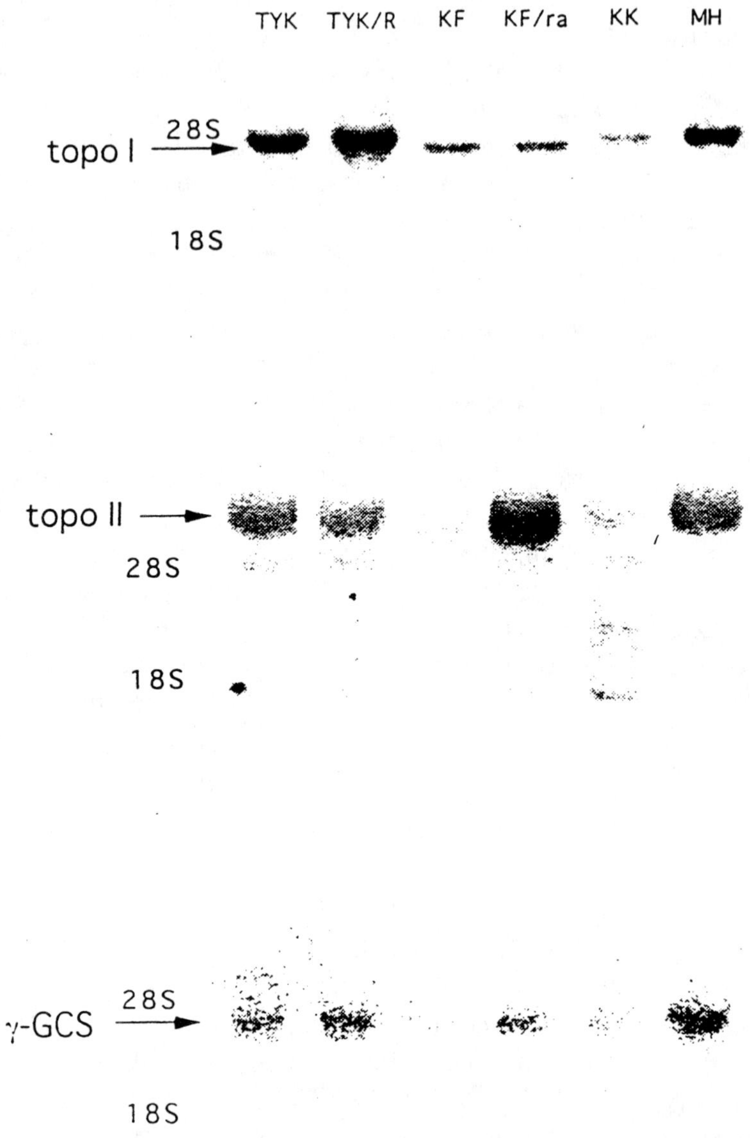

Fig. 1. Northern blot analysis of DNA topo I and II, and γ-GCS mRNA. Samples of total RNA (15 μg) extracted from various ovarian cancer cell lines were all subjected to electrophoresis in a 1% agarose gel containing 2.2 M formaldehyde, transfered to a nylon membrane, and hybridized with ^{32}P-labeled cDNA probe.

showed higher expression of topo I (but not topo II) mRNA than the TYK cell line. On the other hand, the MH cell line with higher natural resistance to CDDP than the KK cell line had markedly higher expression of both topo I and II mRNAs, compared to the KK cell line (Figs. 1 and 3).

Intracellular GSH Content and Expression of GSH-related Enzyme mRNAs. Although the intracellular GSH content and the degree of CDDP resistance seemed to correlate between KF and KFr cell lines, the GSH content of TYK/R and MH with higher CDDP resistance was significantly decreased rather than increased, compared to that of TYK and KK (Table 2). As shown in Figs. 1 and 3, expression of γ-GCS mRNA by the CDDP-resistant cell lines was more marked than that by the paired CDDP-sensitive cell lines. However, expression of GST-π mRNA in TYK, TYK/R, KK and MH cells was marked with the same degree, while that in KF and KFr cells was only trace (Figs. 2 and 3).

Expression of hMT mRNA and CDDP Resistance. Any expression of hMT mRNA was not observed in KF, KFr and KK cell lines, while its expression in TYK and MH cell lines was observed with marked expression in the TYK/R cell line (Figs. 2 and 3).

Mutant p53 Protein and CDDP Resistance. The KFr and TYK/R cell lines produced significantly higher mutant p53 protein than the parent KF and TYK cell lines, while the degree of production by TYK and TYK/R was about 48- and 84-fold higher than that by KF and KFr, respectively. However, MH cells with higher CDDP-resistance than KK cells produced only one-fifth mutant p53 protein of KK cells (Table 3).

DISCUSSION

Various mechanisms have been proposed for the development of CDDP resistance including an altered efflux of the drug, improved drug detoxification by elevated hMT or GSH levels, enhanced DNA repair capacity or decreased DNA accessibility [2, 3]. It has also been proposed that changes in oncogene expression may mediate repair of CDDP-induced DNA damage [23, 24]. Of these various mechanisms, a reduced accumulation of CDDP has seemed to be the most common observation in CDDP-resistant cancer cells. We have also demonstrated that the mechanism of acquired CDDP-resistance in human ovarian cancer cells involves a decrease of CDDP accumulation in the tumor

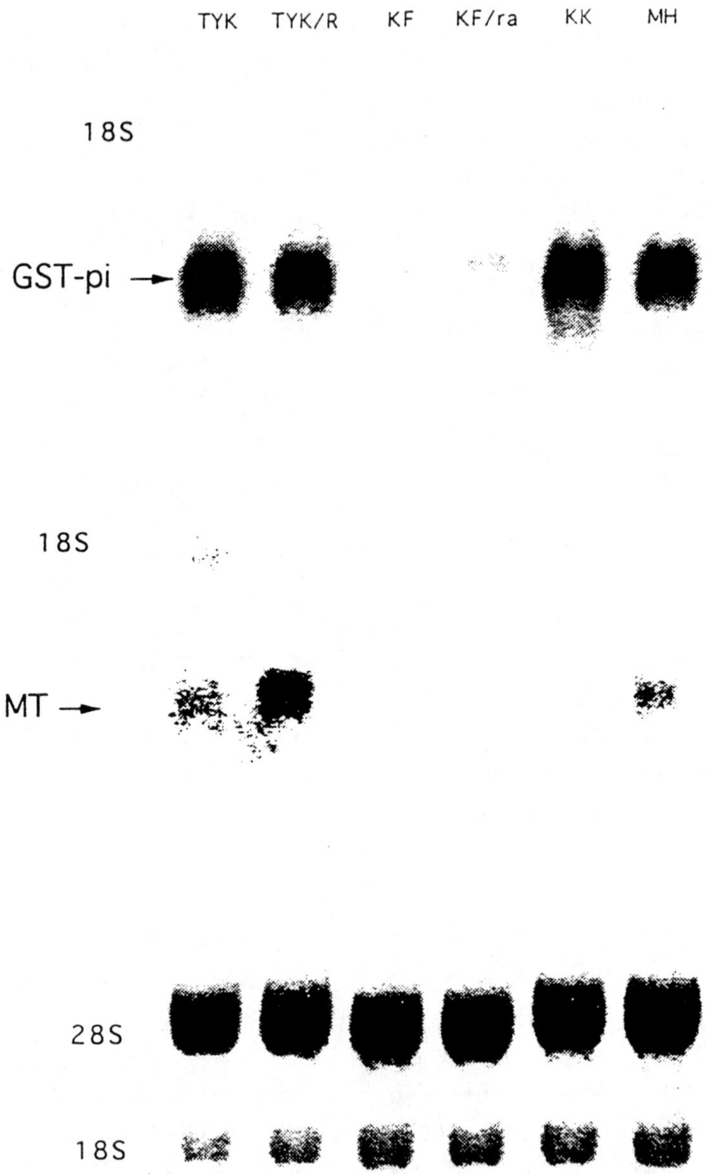

Fig. 2. Northern blot analysis of human GST-π and MT mRNA. As described in Fig. 1, electrophoresis was performed.

Table 1. The sensitivity of various ovarian cancer cell lines to CDDP and its cellular accumulation

Cell lines	IC_{50} CDDP(μM)	CDDP uptake (ng/mg protein)
KF	0.38 ± 0.04	86.6 ± 18.7
KFr	1.28 ± 0.11	53.6 ± 8.6
	(3.37)[a,c]	(61.9)[b,c]
TYK	0.31 ± 0.03	99.1 ± 20.1
TYK/R	0.92 ± 0.08	89.2 ± 13.2
	(2.97)[a,c]	(90.0)[b]
KK	0.76 ± 0.08	160.0 ± 30.4
MH	3.20 ± 0.27	47.3 ± 7.5
	(4.21)[a,c]	(29.6)[b,c]

Note. After each cell line was exposed to various concentrations of CDDP for 4 days, the IC_{50} values were calculated. The CDDP uptake was measured by the atomic absorption method after exposure of each cell line to 100 μM CDDP for 3 h. The mean values (±SD) for each cell line were derived from three separate experiments. [a] Relative resistance to KF, TYK and KK. [b] Percent of CDDP uptake to KF, TYK and KK. [c] P<0.01, compared to each paired cell line (unpaired Student's t test).

Table 2. Intracellular GSH content

Cell lines	GSH content ($nmol/10^7$cells)[a]
KF	24.3 ± 5.8
KFr	41.2 ± 6.9[b]
TYK	164.0 ± 15.3
TYK/R	101.8 ± 10.6[c]
KK	283.2 ± 29.3
MH	102.0 ± 14.7[d]

[a]Mean ± SD from five separate experiments. [b]P<0.01, compared to KF, [c]P<0.01, compared to TYK and cP<0.01, compared to MH (unpaired Student's t test).

cells [25, 26]. In the present study, although the intracellular platinum accumulation not only in the acquired CDDP-resistant cell lines (KFr and TYK/R) but also in the natural CDDP-resistant cell line (MH) were significantly decreased, the extent of the decrease did not seem to be sufficient to account for the resistance of each cell lines (especially TYK/R), suggesting involvement of the other mechanisms (Table 1).

Resistance to anticancer agents is often attributed to changes in cytosolic thiol groups [27]. Several investigators have demonstrated that the intracellular GSH content also increased with increasing CDDP-resistance [28, 29]. However, it has been reported that the GSH content in CDDP-resistant cell lines derived from Chinese hamster ovary cells [30] or bladder cancer cells [11] was not changed. Thus, the role of GSH in the CDDP-resistance remains still unclear. In the present study, the intracellular content of GSH was significantly increased in the CDDP-resistant KFr cell line. However, the GSH levels of the CDDP-resistant TYK/R and MH cell lines were significantly lower than those of the CDDP-sensitive TYK and KK cell lines (Table 2). Thus, there was no consistent correlation between the GSH content and the extent of CDDP-resistance in our ovarian cancer cell lines. Since we determined only the GSH contents in this study, it is necessary to be explored whether the total sulfydryl contents may be involved in the CDDP-resistance of our cell lines.

The GSTs have been intensively investigated as potential mediators of drug resistance. These enzymes catalyze the conjugation of GSH to electrophilic substances, thus rendering them more water soluble. The observation by Batist et al. [31] that a multidrug resistant human breast cancer cell line overexpressed the isoenzyme of GST led to increased interest in this isoenzyme as a potential marker of drug resistance. Numerous groups have found increased expression of GST-π in cell lines and clinical samples which are resistant to platinum compounds [30, 32, 33]. We also measured the expression of GST-π mRNA in the CDDP-resistant cell lines (KFr, TYK/R and MH) [Figs. 2 and 3]. There were no significant differences in the expression of GST-π mRNA between the CDDP-resistant lines and the paired CDDP-sensitive lines, while GST-α and GST-μ were not expressed either in any of the cell lines. Therefore, GSTs do not appear to be involved in the CDDP-resistance of our human ovarian cancer cell lines.

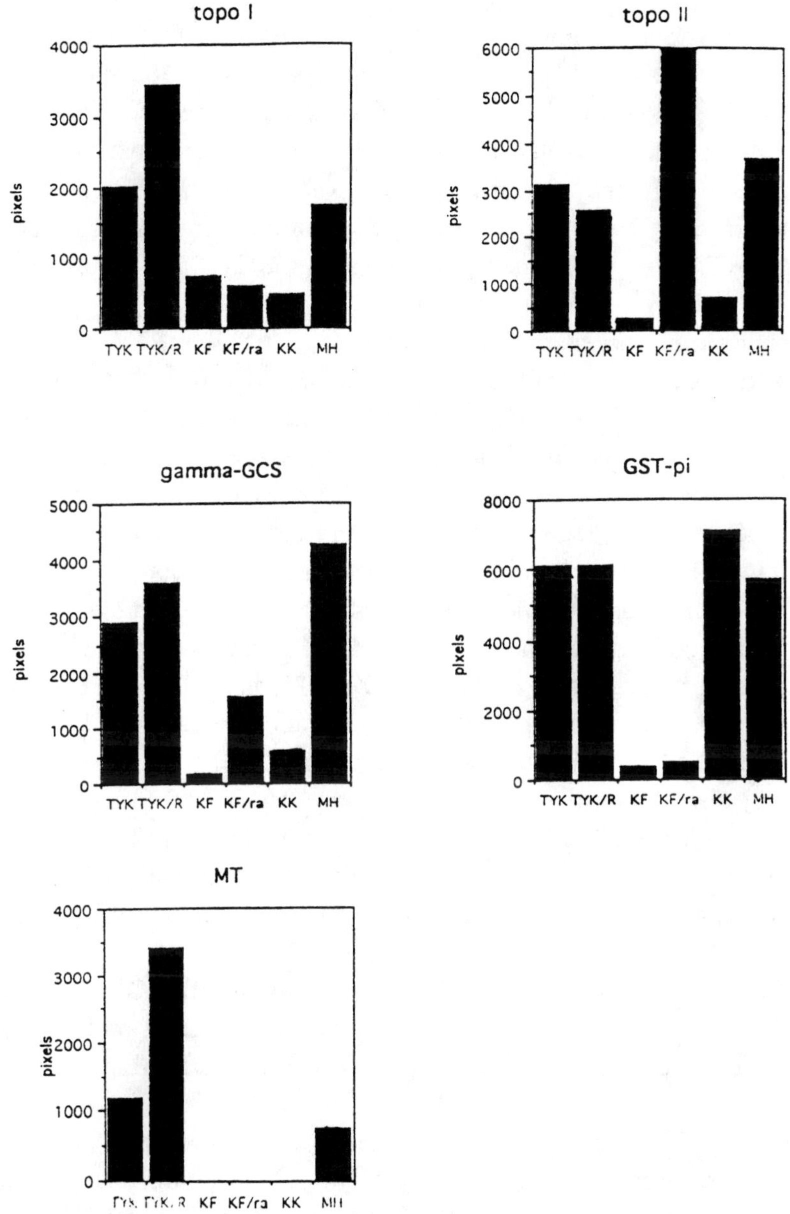

Fig. 3. Densitometric scanning of the autoradiograms obtained by Northern blot analysis.

Since γ-GCS is an important catalyst for the synthesis and salvage pathway of GSH metabolism [34], it would be expected that the enzyme would be increased in resistant cells. Since GSH synthetase does not catalyze the rate-limiting step of GSH synthesis, increased levels of this enzyme would not be expected nor were they found [28]. However, the mRNA level of γ-GCS was increased in the CDDP-resistant cell lines examined in this study, compared to the paired CDDP-sensitive cell lines [Figs. 1 and 3]. Similar observations have also been made by Godwin et al. [28].

In addition, we examined expression of hMT mRNA to evaluate the relationship between CDDP-resistance and hMT expression in our established ovarian cancer cell lines. The KFr cell line selected in vitro for CDDP resistance as well as the parental KF cell line showed no expression of hMT mRNA at our level of detection, while the TYK/R cell line selected similarly in vitro for CDDP resistance showed more marked expression of hMT mRNA, compared to the parental TYK cell line. The relatively CDDP-resistant MH cell line had detectable expression level of hMT mRNA while not detectable in the relatively CDDP-sensitive KK cell line (Figs. 2 and 3). Andrews et al. [35] reported that cadmium chloride-resistant cell lines, 2008/MT and COLO/MT showed cross-resistance to CDDP and that MT levels were elevated 23-fold in 2008/MT and 9.4-fold in COLO/MT compared to their parental cell lines. Similarly, Kasahara et al. [36] also demonstrated that the expression of MT mRNA was inversely correlated with the sensitivity to CDDP. Schilder et al. [37] reported that only two of five cell lines with in vitro induced resistance to CDDP had detectable MT mRNA, while the other CDDP resistant cell lines as well as the parental A2780 ovarian cancer cell line showed no expression of MT mRNA and that there was variable expression of MT mRNA among the OVACAR cell lines. These results were consistent with our present observations and suggest that the CDDP-resistance can be acquired with or without induction of MT gene by CDDP.

Topos I and II are nuclear enzymes which are novel targets of cancer chemotherapy. Because DNA topos catalyze DNA conformational changes, a change in the cellular levels of topos I and II would be expected to modulate the cellular sensitivity to the DNA-targeting agent CDDP. Because DNA topo I can substituted for topo II in most functions, topo I might also be expected to contribute to CDDP resistance. However, little attention has been paid for a

Table 3. Mutant p53 protein content

Cell lines	Mutant p53 protein (ng/10^7cells)
KF	0.125 ± 0.002[a]
KFr	0.189 ± 0.005[b]
TYK	6.02 ± 0.31
TYK/R	15.88 ± 1.52[c]
KK	3.71 ± 0.50
MH	0.691 ± 0.020[d]

Note. After nuclear protein was extracted as described in MATERIALS AND METHHODS, the mutant p53 nuclear protein in each cell line was determined. [a]Mean ± SD from three separate experiments. [b]$P<0.01$, compared to KF, [c]$P<0.01$, compared to TYK and [d]$P<0.01$, compared to KK (unpaired Student's t test).

possible role of topo I in CDDP resistance. In our present study, it was revealed that the acquired CDDP-resistant TYK/R (but not KFr) and the intrinsic CDDP-resistant MH overexpressed DNA topo I mRNA, suggesting some role in CDDP resistance mechanisms. Similar observations have also been made by Kotoh et al. [11]. It has been reported that DNA topo II also plays a role in the production of CDDP resistance in cancer cell lines [8-10]. In the present study, the overexpression of topo II mRNA in the KFra (but not TYK/R) and the MH cells was also observed. Namely, the intrinsic CDDP-resistant cell line (MH) showed overexpression of not only topo II mRNA but also of topo I mRNA, whereas the acquired CDDP-resistant cell lines (KFra and TYK/R) had overexpression of either topo I or topo II mRNA, suggesting that overexpression of topo I and/or topo II mRNA might be involved in the CDDP-resistance (Figs. 1 and 3).

Mutations in the p53 gene are among the most common genetic changes in human carcinomas. The association between p53 mutation and poor patient prognosis has been reported [38, 39], suggesting the relevance of p53 mutation to drug resistance in human tumors. Thus, we examined the contents of nuclear mutant p53 protein in the acquired and intrinsic CDDP-resistant cell lines by using p53 mutant selective quantitation ELISA assay kit. As shown in Table 3, the KFr and TYK/R cell lines selected in vitro for CDDP resistance had significantly higher nuclear mutant p53 protein levels than the respective parental KF and TYK cell lines. However, the MH cell line with intrinsic CDDP-resistance had lower those rather than the relatively sensitive KK cell line. These results support a recent proposal that acquired mutations in p53, which may occur during treatment with CDDP, are associated with acquired CDDP-resistance [40].

REFERENCES

1. Ozols, R. F., and Young, R. C. Chemotherapy of ovarian cancer. *Semin. Oncol.*,11:251-263, 1984.
2. Andrews, P. A., and Howell, S. B. Cellular pharmacology of cisplatin: perspectives on mechanisms of acquired resistance. Cancer Cells, 2:35-43, 1990.
3. Timmer-Bosscha, H., Mulder, N. H., and deVries, E. G. E. Modulation of cis-diamminedichloroplatinum(II) resistance: a review. Br. J. Cancer, 66:227-238, 1992.
4. Hromas, R. A., North, J. A., and Burns, C. P. Decreased cisplatin uptake by resistant L1210 leukemia cells. Cancer Lett., 36:197-201, 1987.
5. Waud, W. R. Differential uptake of cis-diamminedichloroplatinum(II) by sensitive and resistant murine L1210 leukemia cells. Cancer Res., 47:6549-6555, 1987.
6. Chen, G., and Zeller, W. J. In vitro investigations on induction and reversal of cisplatin resistance in a rat ovarian tumor cell line. J. Cancer Res. Clin. Oncol., 116:443-447, 1990.
7. Eastman, A., and Schulte, N. Enhanced DNA repair as a mechanism of resistance to cis-diamminedichloroplatinum(II). Biochemistry, 27:4730-4734, 1988.
8. Sriram, R., Ali-Osman, F., Livington, R., Ellis, G., Needle, M. N., and Stein, D. Modulation of topoisomerase (Topo) II on the kinetics of formation and repair of cis-platinum (cis-DDP) induced DNA-interstrand cross links (DNA-ISC) in human tumor cells sensitive and resistant to cis-DDP. Proc. Am. Assoc. Cancer Res., 31:335, 1990.

9. deJong, S., Zijlstra, J. G., Mulder, N. H., and deVries, E. G. E. Lack of cross-resistance to fortriecin in a human small-cell lung carcinoma cell line showing topoisomerase II-related drug resistance. Cancer Chemother. Pharmacol., 28:461-464, 1991.
10. Waud, W. R., Harrison, S. D. J., Gilbert, K. S., Laster, W. R. J., and Griswold, D. P. J. Antitumor drug cross-resistance in vivo in a cisplatin-resistant murine P388 leukemia. Cancer Chemother. Pharmacol., 27:456-463, 1991.
11. Kotoh, S., Naito, S., Yokomizo, A., Kumazawa, J., Asakuno, J., Kohno, K., and Kuwano, M. Increased expression of DNA topoisomerase I gene and collateral sensitivity to camptothecin in human cisplatin-resistant bladder cancer cells. Cancer Res., 54:3248-3252, 1994.
12. Kikuchi, Y., Miyauchi, M., Kizawa, I., Oomori, K., and Kato, K. Establishment of a cisplatin-resistant human ovarian cancer cell line. J. Natl. Cancer Inst., 77:1181-1185, 1986.
13. Kikuchi, Y., Hirata, J., Kita, T., Imaizumi, E., Tode, T., and Nagata, I. Enhancement of antiproliferative effect of cis-diamminedichloroplatinum(II) by clomiphene and tamoxifen in human ovarian cancer cells. Gynecol. Oncol., 49:365-372, 1993.
14. Hirata, J., Kikuchi, Y., Kita, T., Imaizumi, E., Tode, T., Ishii, K., Kudoh, K., and Nagata, I. Modulation of sensitivity of human ovarian cancer cells to cis-diamminedichloroplatinum(II) by 12-O-tetradecanoylphorbol-13-acetate and D,L-buthionine-S,R-sulphoximine. Int. J. Cancer, 55:521-527, 1993.
15. Yoshiya, N. Establishment of a cell line from human ovarian cancer (undifferentiated carcinoma of FIGO classification) and analysis of its cell-biological characteristics and sensitivity to anticancer drugs. Acta Obstet. Gynec. Jpn., 38:1747-1753, 1986 (in Japanese).
16. Kikuchi, Y., Iwano, I., and Kato, K. Effects of calmodulin antagonists on human ovarian cancer cell proliferation in vitro. Biochem. Biophys. Res. Commun., 123:385-392, 1984.
17. Litterst, C. L., Gram, T. E., Dedrick, R. L., Leroy, A., and Guarino, A. M. Distribution and disposition of platinum following intravenous administration of cis-diamminedichloroplatinum(II) (NSC119875) to dogs. Cancer Res., 36:2340-2344, 1976.

18. Bradford, M. M. A rapid and sensitive method for the quantitation of microgram quantities of protein utilizing the principle of protein-dye binding. Anal. Biochem., 72:248-254, 1976.
19. Griffith, O. W. Determination of glutathione and glutathione disulfide using glutathione reductase and 2-vinyl pyridine. Anal. Biochem., 106:207-212, 1980.
20. Chomozynski, P., and Sacchi, N. Single-step method of RNA isolation by acid guanidium thiocyanate-phenol-chloroform extraction. Anal. Biochem., 162:156-159, 1987.
21. Krain, M., and Richards, R. I. Human metallothionein genes - primary structure of the metallothionein-II gene and related processed gene. Nature (Lond.), 227:680-685, 1970.
22. Gannon, J. D., Greaves, R., Iggo, R., and Lane, D. P. Activating mutations in p53 produces a common conformational effect. A monoclonal antibody specific for the mutant form. EMBO J., 9:1595-1602, 1990.
23. Scanlon, K. J., Kashani-Sabet, M., Miyachi, H., Sowers, L. C., and Rossi, J. Molecular basis of cisplatin-resistance in human carcinomas: model systems and patients. Anticancer Res., 9:1301-1312, 1989.
24. Langton-Webster, B. C., Xuan, J-A., Brink, J. R., and Salomon, D. S. Development of resistance to cisplatin is associated with decreased expression of the gp185c-erb-2 protein and responses to therapy in an ovarian tumor cell line. Cell Growth Differ., 5:1367-1372, 1994.
25. Kikuchi, Y., Iwano, I., Miyauchi, M., Kita, T., Oomori, K., Kizawa, I., Sugita, M., and Tenjin, Y. The mechanism of acquired resistance to cisplatin by a human ovarian cancer cell line. Jpn. J. Cancer Res., 79:632-635, 1988.
26. Kikuchi, Y., Iwano, I., Miyauchi, M., Kita, T., Sugita, M., Tenjin, Y., and Nagata, I. Possible mechanisms of resistance to cis-diamminedichloroplatinum(II) of human ovarian cancer cells. Jpn. J. Cancer Res., 81:701-706, 1990.
27. Louie, K. G., Behrens, B. C., Kinsella, T. J., Hamilton, T. C., Grotzinger, K. R., Mckoy, W. M., Winkler, M. A., and Ozols, R. F. Radiation survival parameters of antineoplastic drug-sensitive and -resistant human ovarian cancer cell lines and their modification by buthionine sulfoximine. Cancer Res., 45:2110-2115, 1985.

28. Godwin, A. K., Meister, A., O'Dwyer, P. J., Huang, C. S., Hamilton, T. C., and Anderson, M. E. High resistance to cisplatin in human ovarian cancer cell lines is associated with marked increase of glutathione synthetase. Proc. Natl. Acad. Sci. USA., 89:3070-3074, 1992.
29. Oldenburg, J., Begg, A. C., vanVugt, M. J. H., Ruvekamp, M., Schronagel, J. H., Pinedo, H. M., and Los, G. Characterization of resistance mechanisms to cis-diamminedichholoroplatinum(II) in three sublines of the CC531 colon adenocarcinoma cell line in vitro. Cancer Res., 54:487-493, 1994.
30. Saburai, Y., Nakagawa, M., Ono, M., Sakai, M., Muramatsu, M., Kohno, K., and Kuwano, M. Increased expression of glutathione S-transferase gene in cis-diamminedichloropltinum(II)-resistant variants of a Chinese hamster ovary cell line. Cancer Res., 49:7020-7025, 1989.
31. Batist, G. M., Tulpale, A., Sinha, B., Kataoka, A. G., Myers, C. E., and Cowan, K. H. Overexpression of a novel anionic glutathione transferase in multi-drug resistant human breast cancer cells. J. Biol. Chem., 261:15544-15549, 1986.
32. Teicher, B. A., Holden, S. A., Kelly, M. J., Shea, T. C., Cucchi, C. A., Rosowsky, A., Henner, W. D., and Frei, E., III. Characterization of a human squamous carcinoma cell line resistant to cis-diamminedichloroplatinum(II). Cancer Res., 47:388-393, 1987.
33. Nakagawa, K., Yokota, J., Wada, M., Sasaki, Y., Fujiwara, Y., Sakai, M., Muramatsu, M., Terasaki, T., Tsunokawa, Y., Terada, M., and Saijo, N. Levels of glutathione S-transferase mRNA in human lung cancer cell lines correlate with the resistance to cisplatin and carboplatin. Jpn. J. Cancer Res., 79:301-304, 1988.
34. Anderson, M. E., and Meister, A. Transport and direct utilization of -glutamylcysteine for glutathione synthesis. Proc. Natl. Acad. Sci. USA., 80:707-711, 1983.
35. Andrews, P. A., Murphy, M. P., and Howell, S. B. Metallothionein-mediated cisplatin resistance in human ovarian carcinoma cells. Cancer Chemother. Pharmacol., 19:149-154, 1987.
36. Kasahara, K., Fujiwara, Y., Nishio, K., Ohmori, T., Sugimoto, Y., Komiya, K., Matsuda, T., and Saijo, N. Metallothionein content correlates with the sensitivity of human small cell lung cancer cell lines to cisplatin. Cancer Res., 51:3237-3242, 1991.

37. Schilder, R. J., Hall, L., Monks, A., Handel, L. M., Farnace, A. J., Jr., Ozols, R. F., Fojo, A. T., and Hamilton, T. C. Metallothionein gene expression and resistance to cisplatin in human ovarian cancer. Int. J. Cancer, 45:416-422, 1990.
38. Horio, Y., Takahashi, T., Kuroishi, T., Hibi, K., Suyama, M., Niimi, T., Shimokata, K., Yamakawa, K., Nakayama, Y., Ueda, R., and Takahashi, T. Prognostic significance of p53 mutations and 3p deletions in primary resected non-small cell lung cancer. Cancer Res., 53:1-4, 1993.
39. Thorlacius, S., Borresen, A-L., and Eyfjord, J. E. Somatic p53 mutations in human breast carcinoma in Icelandic population: A prognostic factor. Cancer Res., 53:1637-1641, 1993.
40. Lowe, S. W., Bodies, S., McClatchey, A., Remington, L., Ruley, H. E., Fisher, D. E., Housman, D. E., and Jacks, T. P53 status and the efficacy of cancer therapy in vivo. Science, 266:807-810, 1994.

CHAPTER 14

LOCALIZATION OF NUCLEAR DNA IN CDDP TREATED OVARIAN CARCINOMA CELL LINES BY OPTICAL SECTIONING WITH CONFOCAL LASER SCANNING MICROSCOPE(CLSM)

Michio Sugita', Tadashi Sugishita,Yoshio Tenjin, Yoshihiro Kikuchi, Ichiro Nagata.

Dept. of Obstet. & Gynecol., Chiba University, Schoolof Medicine, Dept. of Gynecology, Sasaki Institute, Kyoundo Hospital, Dept.of Obstet. & Gynecol., Natlional Defense Medical College 1-8-1, Inohana, Chuo-Ku, Chiba, 260, Japan

Key words: CLSM, Propidium Iodide, CDDP,Morphology Apoptosis

INTRODUCTION

In recent years, Confocal Laser Scanning Microscopy (CLSM) has been introduced and applied in cell biology and clinical use as a new technology.[1-3] CLSM is expected to provide much new optical information and advantages for defining the structure and function of many kinds of cells.

Compared to conventional optical microscopy, we can get higher resolution, optical sectioning, and reconstructed three-dimensional images of a single cell without mechanical slicing.[4,5] It is easy to understand why CLSM is sometimes called the "CT SCAN" of the single cell.

Moreover high contrast views are obtained even in overlapped cells. In other words, strong cell dispersion procedures for aggregated cells are not always needed.[6]

The direct target of many chemotherapeutic agents is the nucleus. Therefore, it is very useful to evaluate the initial effect by detecting the initial change of nuclear DNA distribution by chemotherapy. Recently we have been applied CLSM analysis for this purpose.

In this paper, the basic studies on the localization of nuclear fluorescence stained with propidium iodide (PI) and changes of topographical DNA distribution of the ovarian carcinoma cell lines treated with CDDP will be discussed.

INSTRUMENTATION

A OLYMPUS LSM-GB200 equipped with argon ion laser and two galvanometer scanner mirrors was utilized for all studies (Fig.1). A conventional fluorescence microscopy is included to this CLSM system and used for screening the target cells before CLSM analysis to minimize bleaching fluorescence. Serial optical sections at 0.1 mm intervals along the z-axis are possible by using Piezo Z stage.

Fig. 2 shows the schematic diagram for the confocal mode. In CLSM, the object is illuminated with a limited, small spot derived from a focused laser beam at the focal point, and transports information from this point.

By moving this focus point on the focal plane we are able to obtain a good contrast and high resolution image, because in a CLSM image most unnecessary light (above or below focal plane) can be deleted from the contrast image. For instance, light intensity at point B which is apart from focal point A is so weak that the scattered light from point B doesn't disturb the information from point A seriously.

Furthermore in confocal mode the light coming from in-focus plane is detected through the pinhole, while the light from out-of-focus plane is eliminated by the pinhole in front of the photodetector.[6-8] The thickness of tomogram in confocal mode is determined by the diameter of the pinhole. The used laser wavelength was 488nm for the excitation of FITC and PI. The confocal or nonconfocal images were digitalized and saved in magnet-optical discs through an IBM computer system.

MATERIALS & METHODS

1) COMPARISON BETWEEN NONCONFOCAL AND CONFOCAL IMAGES

KK cells (ovarian clear cell adenocarcinoma cell line)[9} were used. Cells were harvested at confluent growth and fixed with 70% ethanol, then stored at 4°C before use. Cells were washed twice by centrifugation in PBS. It was suspended in the fluorescent dye solution which consisted of PI (1.0 μg/ml) in PBS.

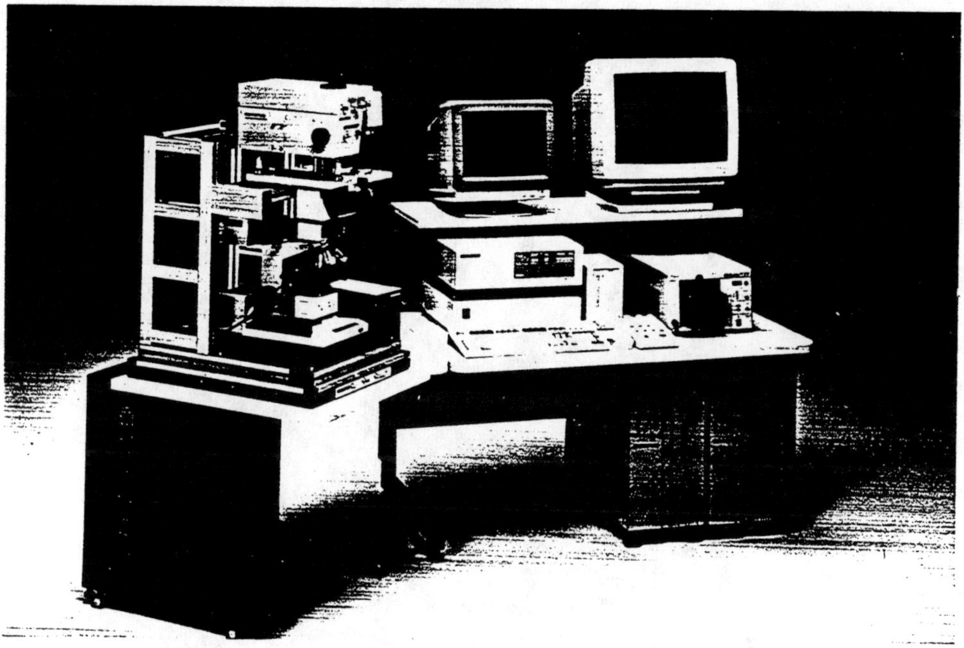

Figure 1. Total view of LSM-GB200 (OLYMPUS)

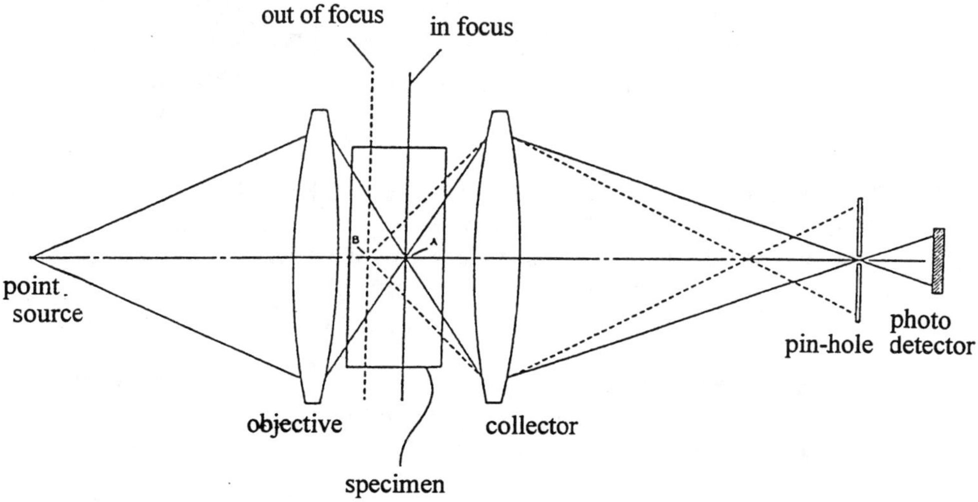

Figure 2. Schematic diagram for the confocal mode. A: Focus B: Defocus

3A

3B

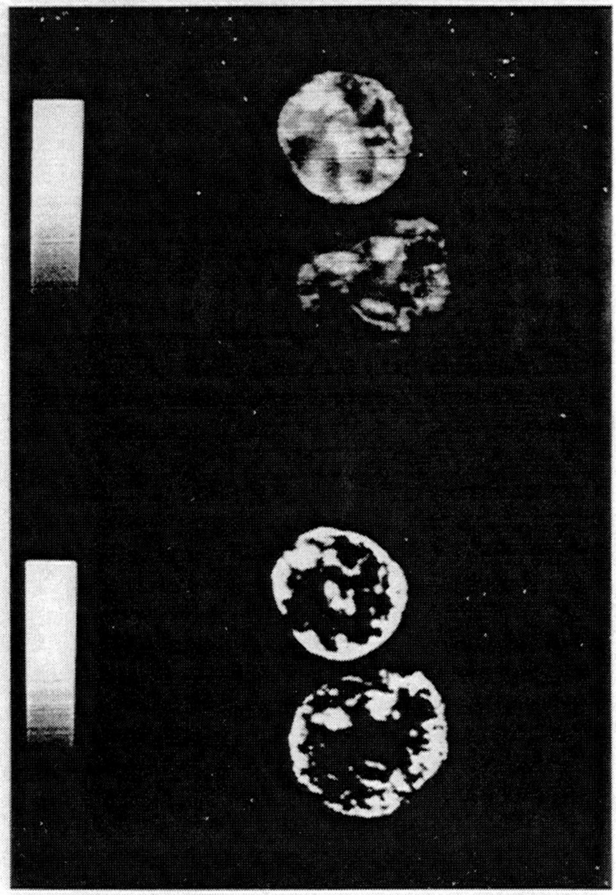

Figure 3 Confocal view and nonconfocal view in KK cell. 3A: nonconvocal image (above). 3B: confocal image (below). 3A resembles conventional fluorescence microscope image. Note the higher resolution and absence of out-of-focus blur in confocal image.

First, cells were searched by the conventional fluorescent microscopy system, and scanned without the pinhole nonconfocally. Next, the same cells were observed with the pinhole confocally (Fig. 3).

2) Nucleolus

Normal endometrial (EM) cells were scraped with a cytobrush after the hysterectomy and fixed with 70% ethanol. Cells were washed in PBS and stained with PI(5.0 μg/ml) & FITC (50 μg/ml) simultaneously. Serial confocal tomograms were examined for fluorescent localization of nucleolus (Fig. 4).

3) PI concentration

Normal endometrial cells were scraped with a cytobrush after the hysterectomy and fixed with 70% ethanol as material for this study.

First, cells stained with 100 μg/ml PI were observed 15 minutes and 2 hours after staining (Fig. 5). Next, the diameter of the pinhole was compared (Fig. 6). Then the concentration of PI (1.0 - 50 μg/ml) was compared to determine the optimal concentration for observation of nuclear DNA distribution by CLSM(Fig. 7-10).

4) KK cells and MH cells (ovarian serouscyst adenocarcinoma cell line) treated with CDDP

KK and MH cells [9] at exponential growth were treated with CDDP (1.0 mM to 10 mM) for 36 hours. Cells were harvested and fixed as described above, and stained with PI (5.0 μg/ml) then observed at sequential confocal tomograms at 0.3 to 0.8mm intervals along the z-axis to detect the morphological effect (Fig. 11-18).

Results

1) Comparison between Nonconfocal and Confocal Images

Greater resolution and good contrast views were obtained in confocal view (Fig.3b) compared to the blurred nonconfocal image (Fig.3a). In the confocal mode, the marked heterogeneity of DNA(PI) distribution at the focal plane in the nucleus was revealed.

2) Nucleolus

Much FITC accumulated like a ball inside the nucleus (Fig.4a). Strong PI fluorescence localized around the FITC ball (Fig. 4b).

3) PI concentration

Diffuse PI fluorescence all over the nucleus of focal plane was observed both 15 min.and 2hrs. after 100 μg/ml PI staining (Fig.5).

A

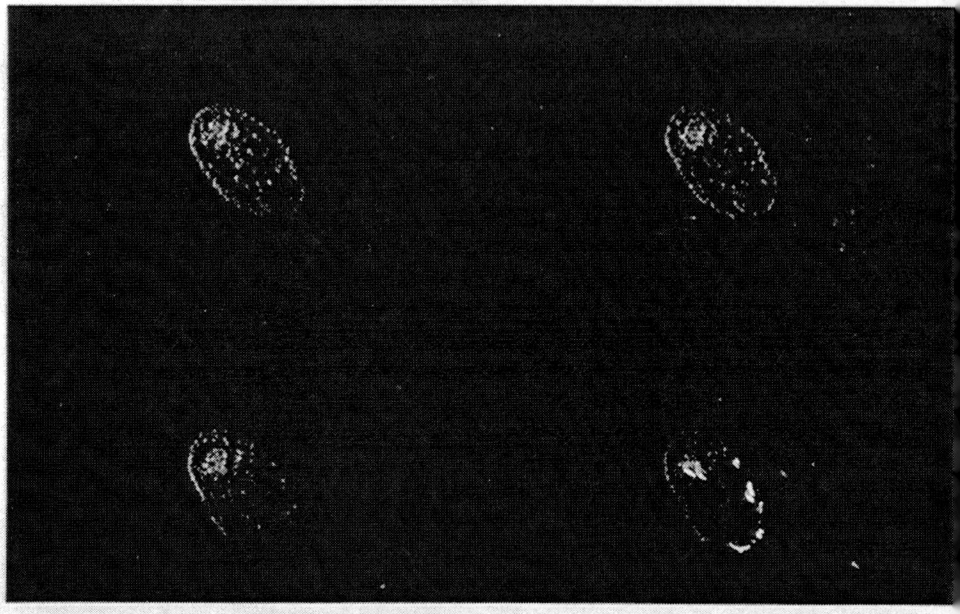

B

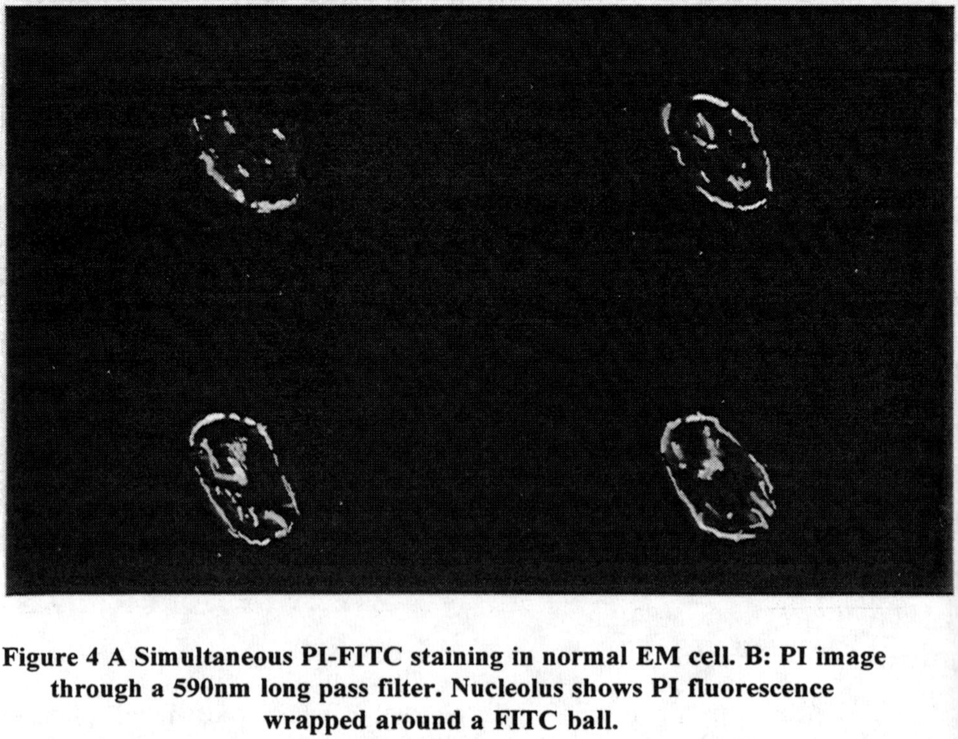

Figure 4 A Simultaneous PI-FITC staining in normal EM cell. B: PI image through a 590nm long pass filter. Nucleolus shows PI fluorescence wrapped around a FITC ball.

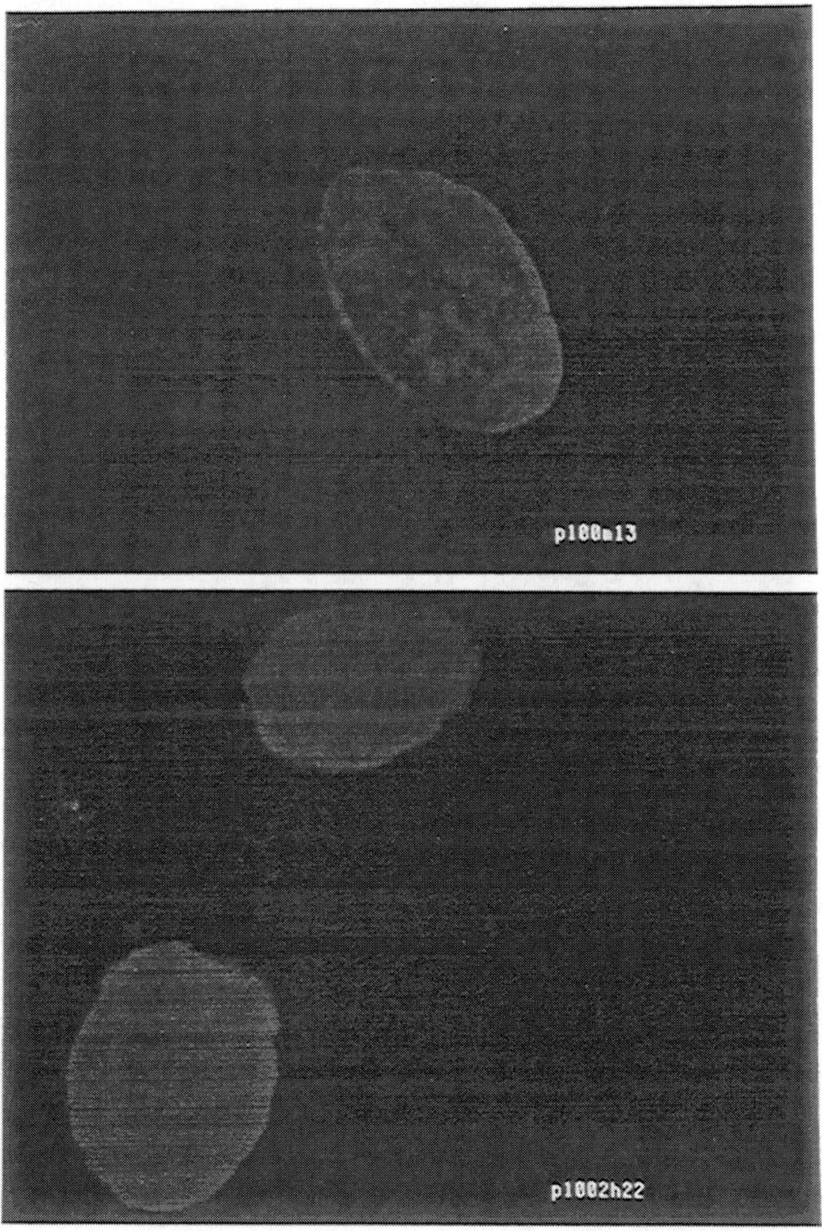

Figure 5 Top: normal EM cells 15 minutes after staining with 100μg/ml PI. Bottom: normal EM cells 2 hours after staining with 100μg/ml PI. Both show diffuse PI fluorescence all over the nucleus. The earlier observation gets relatively better views.

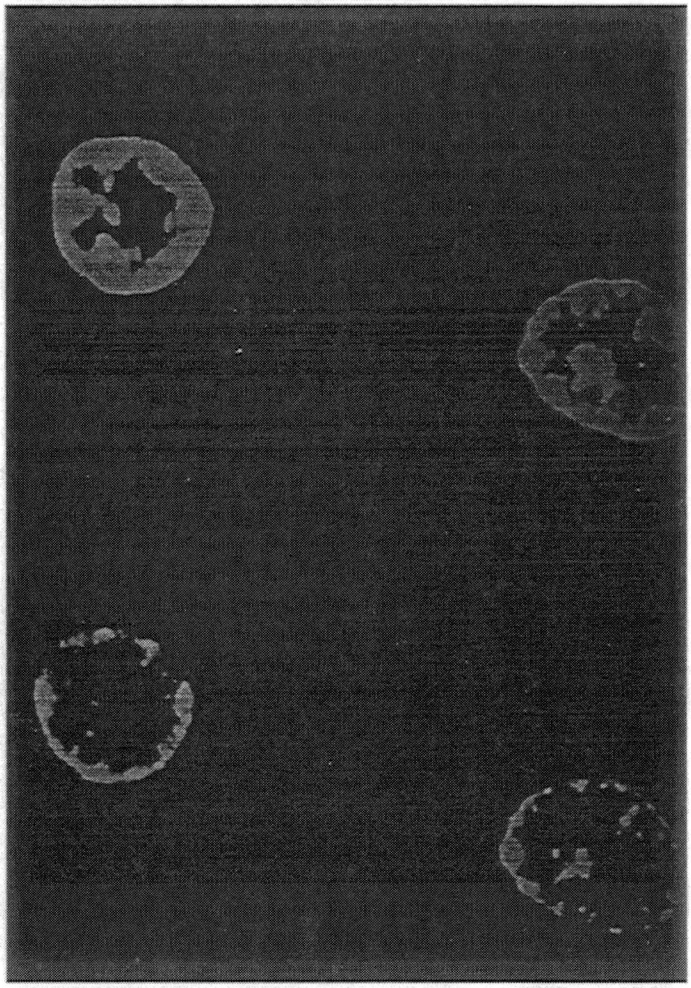

Figure 6 Top: large pinhole. Bottom: small pinhole. Both are same normal EM cells in confocal mode. Note the thickness of tomograms in confocal mode is determined by the diameters of the pinhole.

As the diameter of the pinhole was correlated well with depth of tomogram, smaller pinhole would provide better contrast images as long as the fluorescence is not weak (Fig.6). Diffuse PI fluorescence all over the nucleus was observed in the concentration over 10 μg/ml (Fig.7,8). In the concentration of 1.0 μg/ml, a strong fluorescence along the nuclear membrane and around the nucleolus was localized heterogeneously(Fig. 9,10).

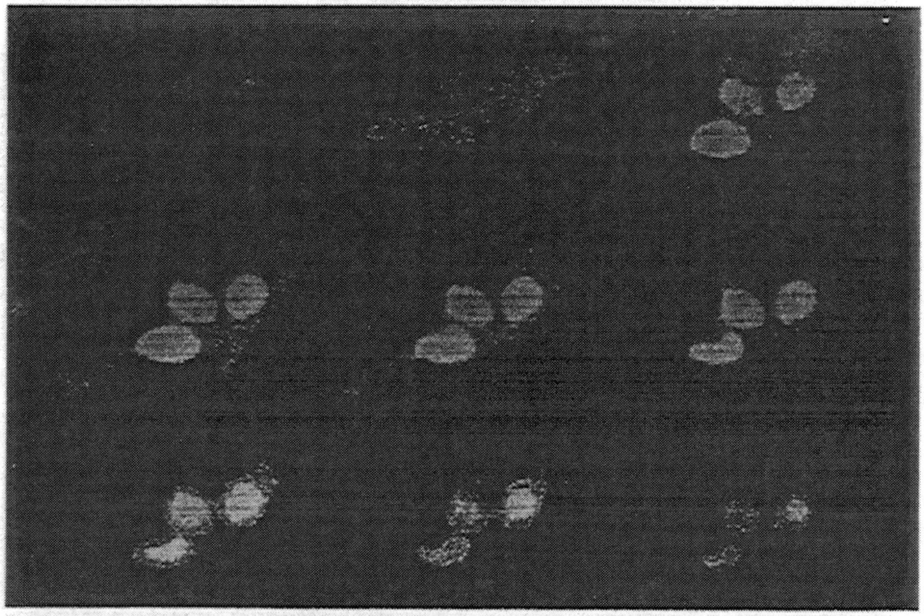

Figure 7: PI 50 μg/ml (normal EM cells). Serial confocal tomograms at 1.0 μm interval along the z-axis in confocal mode. Diffuse PI fluorescence all over the nucleus was observed.

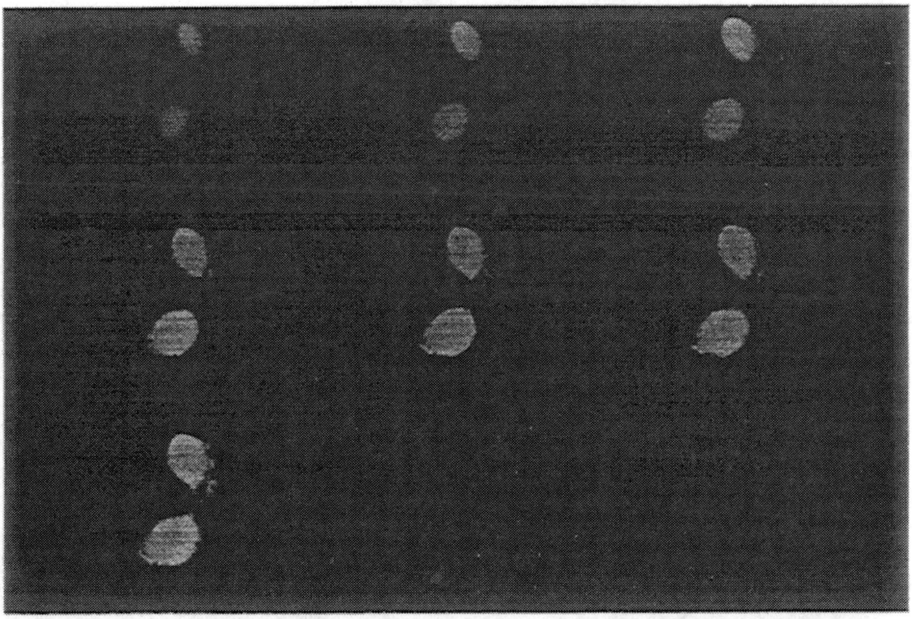

Figure 8: PI 10 μg/ml (normal EM cells). Serial confocal tomograms at 1.0 μm interval along the z-axis in confocal mode. Diffuse PI fluorescence all over the nucleus was observed.

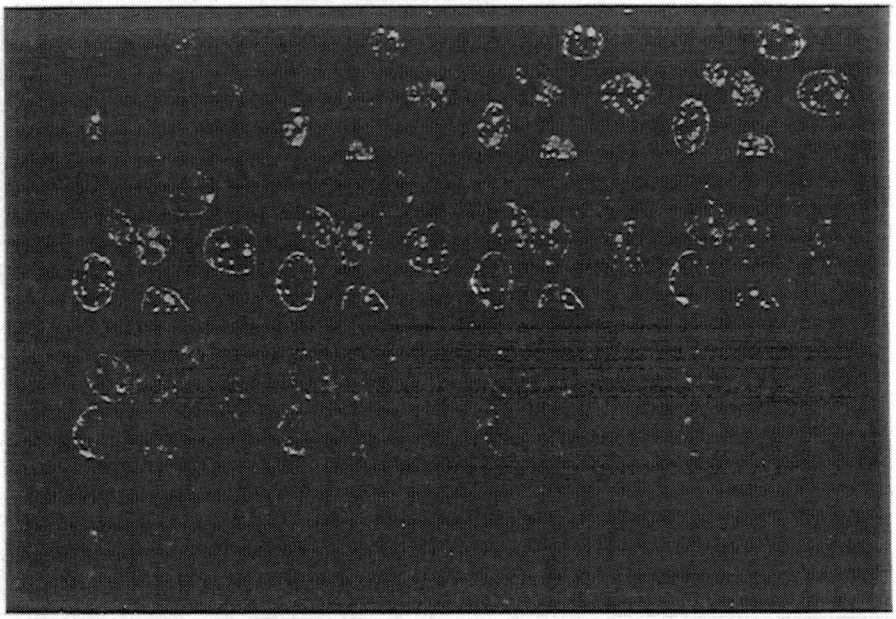

Figure 9: PI 1.0 μg/ml (normal EM cells). Serial confocal tomograms at 0.8 μm interval along the z-axis in confocal mode. Note the very high degree of resolution and good contrast.

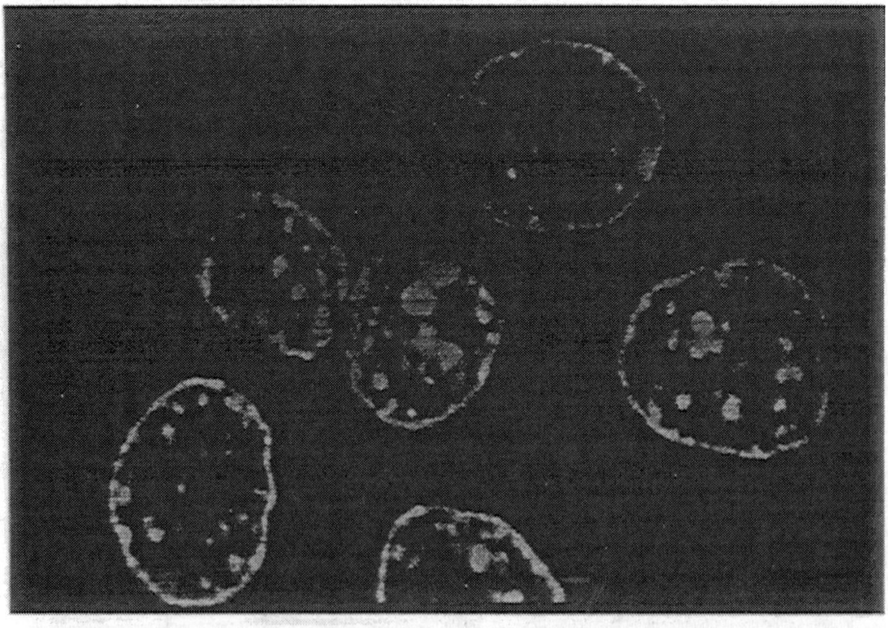

Figure 10: An enlarged view of serial confocal tomograms in Fig. 9

4) KK cells and MH cells (ovarian serouscyst adenocarcinoma cell line) treated with CDDP

Both KK cells and MH cells showed similar morphological changes with CDDP treatment. Cells treated with CDDP showed nuclear swelling, irregular fluorescence distribution, and karyorrhexis (Fig. 11-18).

Croissant or doughnut shaped findings were often recognized stereoscopically. While the nuclear swelling or giant nucleus was noticeable in lower concentration, karyorrhexis was conspicuous in high concentration.

Discussion

CLSM provides good contrast, rejection of signals from out-of-focus, improved resolution images, individual continuous cellular tomograms without mechanical slicing, and stereographic views that are observed by three-dimensional reconstruction.

CLSM has been applied for defining structure and function in various research fields and organs.[10-18]

It is quite an easy and useful technique for comparative study of cell function and nuclear DNA distribution with PI staining. Moreover high contrast views are obtained even in overlapped cells. In other words, strong cell dispersion procedures for aggregated cells are not always needed.

We applied CLSM analysis for the basic studies on the localization of nuclear fluorescence stained with PI and changes of topographical DNA distribution of the ovarian carcinoma cell lines treated with CDDP.

1) Comparison between nonconfocal and confocal images

In nonconfocal mode or conventional fluorescence images, signals from above and below the plane of focus make the images degraded. In confocal mode by using a pinhole, the unnecessary light from out-of-focus plane is eliminated. When compared to blurred nonconfocal image, the confocal view shows a very high degree of resolution and good contrast.

2) Nucleolus

Nucleolus contain high concentration of RNA and proteins. Nucleolus

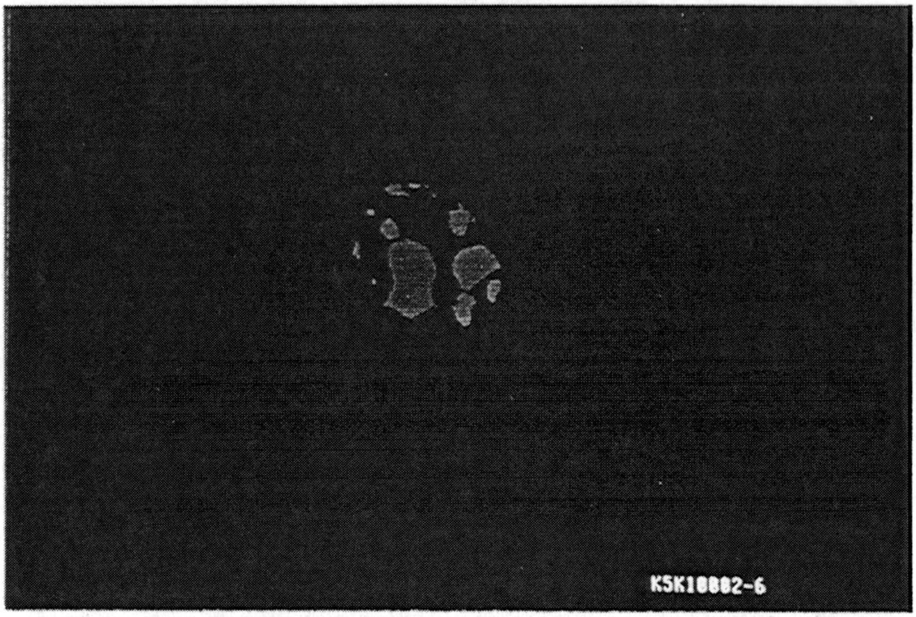

Figure 11: CDDP (5μM) treated KK cells in serial confocal mode. Note the marked karyorrhexis or chromatin clumps.

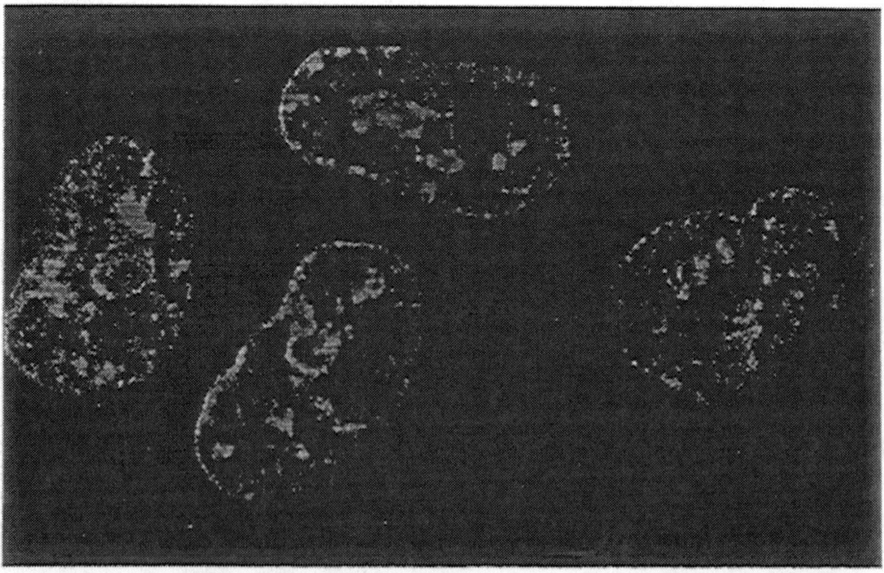

Figure 12: CDDP (2.5μM) treated KK cells in serial confocal mode. Note the giant nucleus.

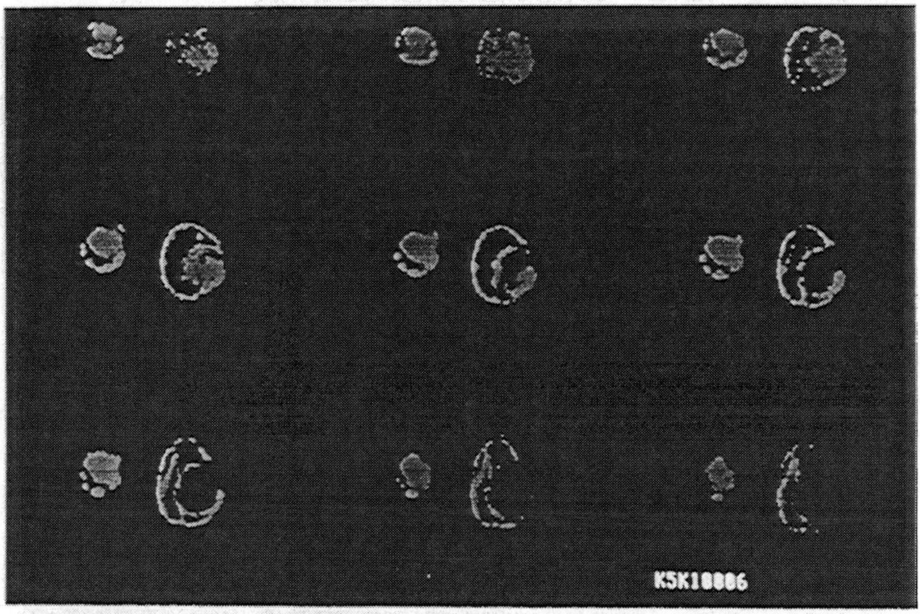

Figure 13: CDDP (5μM) treated KK cells. Croissant shaped cell.

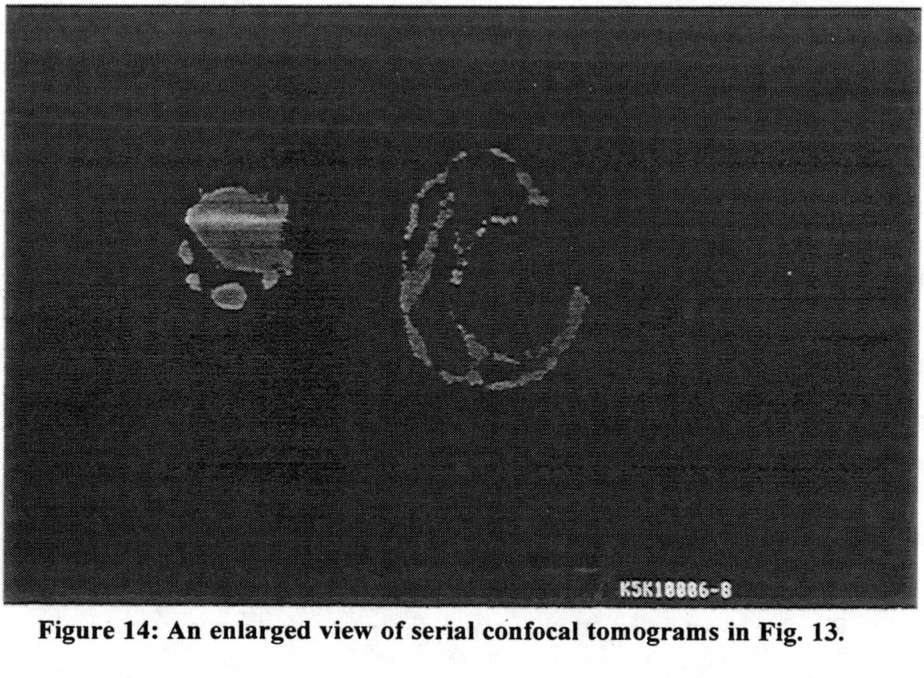

Figure 14: An enlarged view of serial confocal tomograms in Fig. 13.

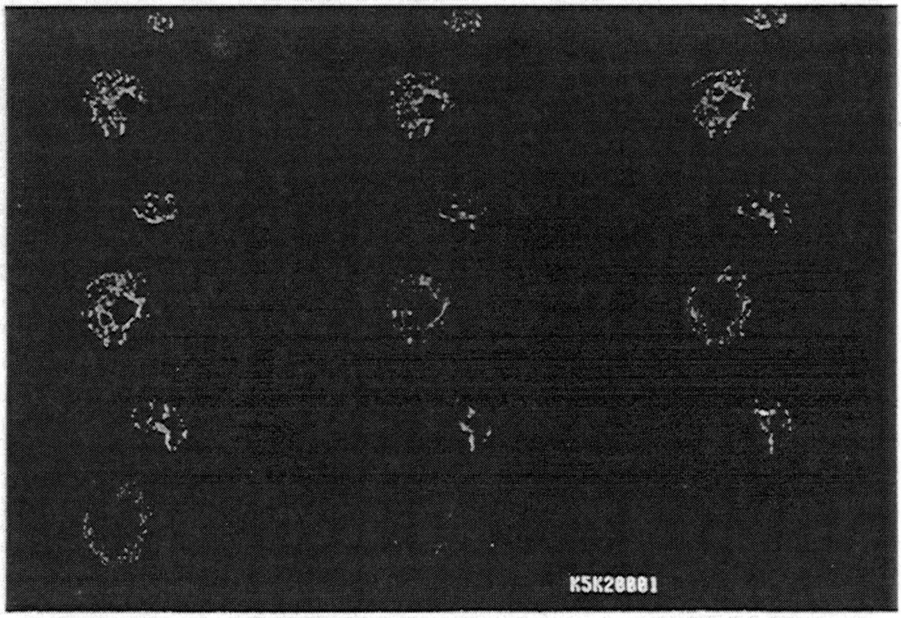

Figure 15: CDDP (5μM) treated KK cells. Doughnut shaped cell.

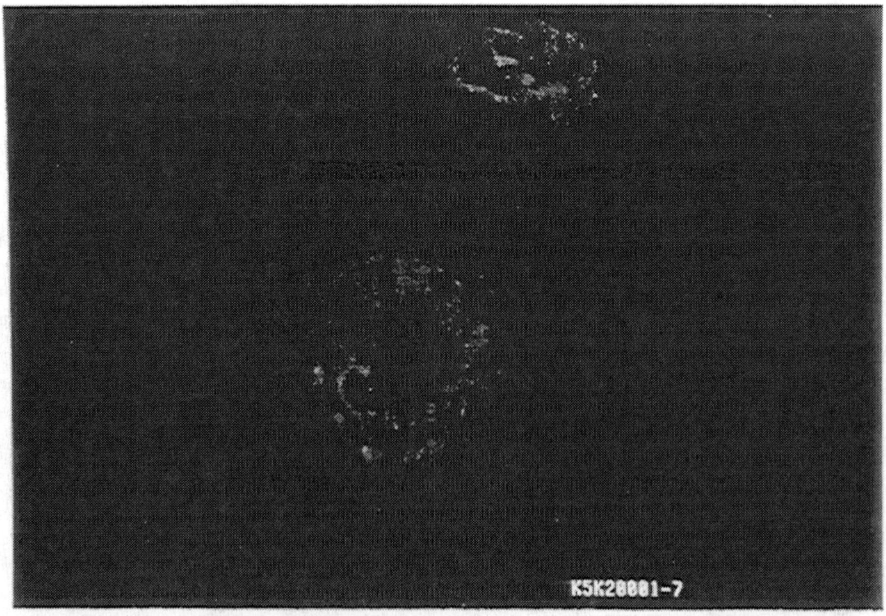

Figure 16: An enlarged view of serial confocal tomograms in Fig. 15.

shows PI fluorescence wrapped around a FITC ball in our confocal images. Therefore it is relatively easy to detect nucleolus even by single PI staining without PI-FITC double staining. Consequently nucleolus show a PI ball which is empty inside.

3) PI CONCENTRATION

Although 50μg/ml of PI concentration is widely applied to flow cytometry, [19] high concentration of PI(over 10μg/ml) often makes confocal images dim and difficult to evaluate.

The earlier observation(within 30 min.) after staining sometimes makes it possible to evaluate DNA distribution. However it usually takes 30min. to an hour per sample to observe and save the data. As the stainability is stable in lower PI concentration, a more precise and improved detail was obtained. Consequently the best concentration of PI to observe nuclear inner structure in confocal mode was 1.0 to 10 μg/ml.

4) KK CELLS TREATED WITH CDDP

Most of direct target of chemotherapeutic agents is the nucleus, especially nuclear DNA or enzymes related to DNA. Therefore, it is very useful to evaluate the earlier effect of nuclear DNA distribution after chemotherapy by CLSM analysis.

In our study both KK cells and MH cells showed similar morphological changes with CDDP. Cells treated with CDDP showed nuclear swelling, croissant or doughnut shaped findings, irregular fluorescence distribution, and karyorrhexis.

While the nuclear swelling or giant nucleus was noticeable in lower concentration, karyorrhexis was conspicuous in high concentration. Stereoscopical croissant or doughnut shaped findings were often recognized in 3 to 5 mM of CDDP. These findings suggest morphological changes in apoptotic process. Smith GJ et al. [10] describe that nuclear swelling precedes brightly stained chromatin clumps near the margin of the nucleus in apoptotic process. We assume that the nuclear swelling is the initial feature, then croissant or doughnut shaped findings appear, and finally the clumps of chromatin along nuclear membrane are found as apoptosis progresses.

As CLSM analyses are applied to cytopathologic fields more often, 3-dimensional expressions for morphological findings like croissant or doughnut will become widely accepted.

ACKNOWLEDGMENT

This work was supported in part by the Grant-in-Aid for Cancer Research (5-31) from the Ministry of Health and Welfare.

REFERENCES

1. White JG, Amos WB, Fordham M. An evaluation of confocal versus conventional imaging of biological structures by fluorescence light microscopy. *J Cell Biology* 1987;105:41-48
2. Shotton DM. Confocal scanning optical microscopy and its application for biological specimens. *J Cell Science* 1989;94:175-206.
3. White JG, Amos WB. Confocal microscopy comes of age. *Nature* 1987;328:183-184.
4. Ohtani Y, Ohtani O, Nakatani T. Microanatomy of the rat diaphragm: A scanning electron and confocal laser scanning microscopic study. *Arch. Histol. Cytol.* 1993;56:317-328.
5. Sugita M, Sugishita T, Tenjin Y. Localization of nuclear DNA by optical sectioning with confocal laser scanning microscope(CLSM). *Cytometry* 1993; Supplement 6:23.
6. Sugita M, Tenjin Y. The application of confocal laser scanning microscope(CLSM) in cell biology. *Nippon Rinsho.* 1993;51:1108-1113.(in Japanese)
7. Takamatsu T, Fujita S. Microscopic tomography by laser scanningmicroscopy and its three-dimensional reconstruction. *J Microscopy* 1987;149:167-174.
8. Suzuki T, Horikawa Y. Development of a real-time scanning laser microscope for biological use. Appl. Opt. 1986;25:4115-4121.
9. Sasa H, Kikuchi Y, Hisano A. et al. Cytokinetic effects of cisplatin on cisplatin-resistant ovarian cancer cell line. *Human Cell* 1992;5:384-391
10. Smith GJ, Bagnell R, Bakewell WE et al. Application of confocal scanning laser microscopy in experimental pathology. *J Electron Microscopy Technique* 1991;178:38-49.
11. Streck RJ, Rolf MM, Barret KE et al. Utility of confocal laser scanning microscopy for defining the expression and topographical distribution of activation-and/or proliferation-associated antigens on human leukocytes. *Focus* 1991;13:74-78.
12. Deitch JS, Smith KL, Lee CL et al. Confocal scanning laser microscope images of hippocampal neuron intracellularly labeled with biocytin. *J Neuroscience Methods* 1990;33:61-76.

13. Bakewell WE, Viviano CJ, Dixon D et al. Confocal laser scanning immunofluorescence microscopy of lamellar bodies and pulmonary surfactant protein A in isolated alveolar type II cells. *Laboratory Investigation* 1991;65:87-95.
14. Fairbairn D, O'Neill KL, Standing MD. Application of confocal laser scanning microscopy to analysis of H_2O_2-induced DNA damage in human cells. *Scanning* 1992;15:136-139.
15. Niggli E, Piston DW, Kirby MS et al. A confocal laser scanning microscope designed for indicators with ultraviolet exception wavelengths. *Am. J. Physiol.* 1994;266: C303-C310.
16. Sasano H, Date F, Itakura Y et al. Confocal laser scanning microscopy in cytopathology. *Modern Pathology* 1993;6:625-629.
17. Williams DA. Quantitative intracellular calcium imaging with laser-scanning confocal microscopy. *Cell Calcium* 1990;11:589-597.
18. Lizard G, Chignol MC, Chardonnet Y et al. Detection of human papillomavirus DNA in CaSki and HeLa cells by fluorescent in situ hybridization. *J Immunological Methods* 1993;157:31-38.
19. Shotton DM. Confocal scanning optical microscopy and its application for biological specimens. *J Cell Science* 1989;94:175-206.
20. Krishan A. Rapid flow cytofluorometric analysis of mammalian cell cycle by propidium iodide staining. *J Cell Biology* 1975;66:188-193.

CHAPTER 15

CDDP RESISTANCE AND HEAT SHOCK PROTEIN 60[1]

Eizo Kimura, Yoshiteru Terashima, Stephen B. Howell
*Department of Obstetrics and Gynecology, Jikei University School of Medicine
Department of Medicine and the Cancer Center, University of California, San Diego

Heat shock proteins (hsp) are a unique set of highly conserved proteins induced by exposure to heat and a variety of other types of stress (Lindquist, 1989). It is commonly accepted that the function of the hsp is either to protect cells against subsequent heat stress, or to enhance the ability of cells to recover from the toxic effects of heat or other types of stress. Transcriptional activation of heat shock genes is mediated by the binding of heat shock factor to a conserved nucleotide sequence (the heat shock element) present in the promoter of heat-inducible genes (Lindquist, 1989; Sorger, 1991). The heat shock element sequence for eukaryotes is rotationally symmetric, C--GAA--TTC--G, and is generally located on the coding strand of DNA upstream from the TATA box (Lindquist, 1989; Sorger 1991; Pelham 1982). However, not all heat shock genes induced by one type of stress are necessarily induced by other forms of stress, and the pattern of heat shock protein response to various agents can be quite different and complex (Carper et al., 1987).

The heat shock response was originally described as a phenomenon of inducible gene expression in *Drosophila* and it is a well-studied biological effect that is common to all living cells and organisms (Morimoto et al., 1990). The heat shock genes and their encoded proteins are highly conserved through

---

1 All correspondence to; Eizo Kimura, M.D. Dept. of OB/GYN, Jikei University School of Medicine, 3-25-8, Nishishinbashi Minatoku, Tokyo 105, Japan, Tel: 81-3-3433-1111 Ext.3521, FAX: 81-3-3433-1111 Ext.3527

evolution. Recent studies suggested that expression of heat shock proteins may be prognostically important. Investigation of breast cancer specimens has indicated that the over-expression of a 27kD heat shock protein, hsp27, is associated with an increased risk of disease recurrence (Tandon et al., 1990; Chamness et al., 1989; Thor et al., 1991).

Mielo et al. have examined heat shock protein expression in human ovarian cancer. They demonstrated that hsp70 and hsp90 were expressed at low levels in normal ovary and benign tumors, but at higher levels in the more advanced stages of ovarian cancer (Mielo et al., 1990). hsp60 (also referred to as hsp58 or the GroEL homolog) is one member of the heat shock protein family. It is present within the mitochondria of all mammalian cells so far examined where, in combination with hsp70, it serves as a chaperonin and assists in the correct folding of newly synthesized proteins (Lunger et al., 1992).

SURVIVAL OF OVARIAN CANCER PATIENTS AND HSP60 MRNA EXPRESION

There is marked heterogeneity in the expression of hsp60 mRNA, detected by Northern blot analysis, both amongst normal tissues in the adult and fetus, and between tumor samples from patients with testicular, colon and ovarian cancers (Kimura et al., 1991). More recently, it was reported that the level of hsp60 mRNA expression is a valuable prognostic factor for patients with epithelial ovarian cancer treated with platinum compounds (Kimura et al., 1993a). Patients whose tumors over-express hsp60 mRNA have a much shorter survival than patients whose tumors express very low levels. But except for the fact that it can be induced by exposure to heat, little is known about regulation of hsp60 expression in comparison to the other major heat shock proteins.

HSP60 MRNA EXPRESSION IN DDP-SENSITIVE 2008 CELLS AND DDP-RESISTANT 2008/C13*5.25 CELLS

When comparing the expression of hsp60 in parental human ovarian carcinoma 2008 cells and a subline, 2008/C13*5.25, selected in vitro for 11-fold resistance. Expression of hsp60 mRNA was increased by 1.7-fold in 2008/C13*5.25 cells relative to 2008 cells. Despite the small increase in steady-state mRNA level, there was a larger difference (3.8-fold) between the two types of cells in the expression of hsp60 at the protein level (Kimura et al., 1993b).

INDUCTION OF HSP60 MRNA EXPRESSION BY DDP IN 2008 CELLS

Heavy metals have been reported to induce a variety of stress-related genes. A 5 day exposure of 2008 cells to an IC_{50} concentration of DDP caused a 1.5-fold increase in hsp60 mRNA expression and the incresed expression persisted for at least 8 hours after the end of DDP exposure. On the other hand, such treament had no effect on metallothionein II_A ($MTII_A$) mRNA level. A 1 hour exposure of 2008 cells to an IC_{50} concentration of DDP (3.5μM) increased hsp60 mRNA by 1.8-fold at 8 hours and 1.3-fold at 12 hours after exposure. In contrast, incubation of 2008 cells with IC_{50} concentrations of either $CdCl_2$ or $ZnCl_2$ for 8 hours had no effect hsp60 mRNA levels, but under the same conditions of exposure, $CdCl_2$ and $ZnCl_2$ produced a 5.9-fold and an 11.6-fold induction of $MTII_A$ mRNA, respectively. Thus, hsp60 expresion was induced to a greater extent by DDP than by $ZnCl_2$ and $CdCl_2$. This result suggests that eiher the hsp60 promoter does not contain the metal-responsive elements found in the $MTII_A$ promoter or the elements fail to activate transcription (Kimura et al., 1993b).

EFFECT OF FACTORS THAT MODURATE DDP SENSITIVITY ON HSP60 MRNA CONTENT OF 2008 CELLS

If the expression of hsp60 is a determinant of sensitivity to DDP, then one might expect things that are known to alter the DDP sensitivity of 2008 cells to regulate hsp60 mRNA level. The DDP sensitivity of 2008 cells can be enhanced by depletion of glutathionine following treatment with buthionine sulfoximin (BSO) (Andrews et al., 1986; Andrews et al., 1988a), activation of protein kinase A with forskolin (Mann et al., 1991) or protein kinase C with 12-O-tetradecanoylphorbol-13-acetate (TPA) (Isonishi et al., 1990), or exposure of cells to epidermal growth factor (EGF) (Christen et al., 1990). In contrast, DDP sensitivity can be reduced by pre-treating the cells with ouabain (Andrews et al., 1988b; Andrews et al., 1991). Northern blot analysis comparing the hsp60 mRNA levels in 2008 cells treated with ouabain, forskolin, BSO, EGF, and TPA under conditions known to affect the sensitivity to DDP revealed that none of these treatments altered hsp60 mRNA expression. TPA had no effect on hsp60 expression but did markedly increase expression of $MTII_A$ (Kimura et al., 1993b). Thus, in 2008 cells the hsp60 message levels were not responsive to activators of signal-transduction pathways known to infulence DDP sensitivity.

MEDIAN EFFECT ANALYSIS OF THE INTERACTION BETWEEN DDP AND HEAT SHOCK

To determine whether the interaction was synergistic, only additive, or even antagonistic, the mathematically rigorous technique of median effect analysis is useful (Chou et al., 1986). Median effect analysis permits calculation of the combination index (CI). CI values of >1 indicate antagonism, a value of 1 indicates additivity, and values of <1 indicate synergy. The magnitude of the difference from a value of 1 reflects the magnitude of the synergy or antagonism. Median effect analysis using a 1 hour exposure to DDP and varying times of concurrent exposure to hyperthermia yielded CI values very close to 1 over the 2 log range of cell kill examined, indicating only additivity. When examined the nature of the interaction under conditions where cells were exposed first to hyperthermia for various periods of time, and then incubated at 37°C for 4 hours to allow full induction of the heat shock genes before being treated with DDP for 1 hour, there was a very small degree of antagonism in these conditions between hyperthermia and DDP. This indicates that the fully integrated heat shock response does not offer significant protection against DDP cytotoxicity by 4 hours (Kimura et al., 1993c).

PROSPECTS FOR THE FUTURE

Little information is available on the factors that regulate expression of hsp60, or on the actual role that the product of this gene plays in determining cellular sensitivity to DDP. However, one way that hsp60 can reliably be induced is with heat shock. This adds a new dimension to the issue of the nature of the interaction between hyperthermia and DDP, since it raises the possibility that heat shock serves to induce a gene that may confer DDP resistance. To investigate it more directory, we need to confirm that the cells acquire the DDP-resistant phenotype when hsp60 gene is transfected into the DDP-sensitive cells.

REFERENCES

1. Andrews PA, Murphy NP, Howell SB (1986) Differential sensitization of human ovarian carcinoma and mouse L1210 cells to cisplatin and melphalan by glutathione depletion. *Mol Pharmacol* 30 :643
2. Andrews PA, Schiefer MA, Murphy NP, Howell SB (1988a) Enhanced potentiation of cisplatin cytotoxicity in human ovarian carcinoma cells by prolonged glutathione depletion. *Chem Biol Interactions* 65 :51
3. Andrews PA, Velury S, Mann SC, Howell SB (1988b) *cis*-diamminedichloroplatinum(II) accumulation in sensitive and resistant human ovarian carcinoma cells. *Cancer Res* 48 :68
4. Andrews PA, Mann SC, Huynh HH, Albright KD (1991) Role of Na+, K+-adenosine triphosphatase in the accumulation of *cis*-diamminedichloroplatinum(II) in human ovarian carcinoma cells. *Cancer Res* 51 :3677
5. Carper SW, Duffy JJ, Gerner AW (1987) Heat shock proteins in thermotolerance and other cellular processes. *Cancer Res* 47 :5249
6. Chamness GC, Ruiz A, Fulcher G, et al (1989): Estrogen-inducible heat shock protein hsp27 predicts recurrence in node-negative brest cancer. *Proc Am Assoc Cancer Res* 30:252
7. Chou TC, Talalay P (1986) Quantitative analysis of dose-effect relationships: the combined effects of multiple drugs or enzyme inhibitors. *Adv Enzyme Reg* 22 :27
8. Christen RD, Hom DK, Porter DC, Andrews PA, Macleod CL, Hafstrom L, Howell SB (1990) Epidermal growth factor regulatesthe in vitro sensitivity of human ovarian carcinoma cells to cisplatin. *J Clin Invest* 86 :1632
9. Isonishi S, Andrews PA, Howell SB (1990) Increased sensitivity to cis-diamminedichloroplatinum(II) in human ovarian carcinoma cell sin response to treatment with 12-0-tetradecanoylphorbol-13-acetate. *J Biol Chem* 265 :3623
10. Kimura E, Enns RE, Hom DK, Arboleda MJ, Slamon DJ, Howell SB (1991) Expression of the carboxy-terminal portion of P1 mitochondrial chaperonin (CTP-1) in normal and cancer tissues. *Proc Am Soc Clin Oncol* 10 :101
11. Kimura E, Enns RE, Arboleda MJ, Slamon DJ, Howell SB (1993a) Correlation of the survival of ovarian cance patients with mRNA expression of the 60-kD heat-shock protein HSP-60. *J Clin Oncol* 11 :891-898
12. Kimura, E. Enns RE, Thiebaut, F, Howell, SB (1993b) Regulation of HSP60 mRNA expression in a human ovarian carcinoma cell line. *Cancer Chemother Pharmacol* 32 :279-285

13. Kimura, E, Howell, SB, (1993c) Analysis of cytotoxic interaction between cisplatin and hyperthermia in a human ovarian carcinoma cell line. *Cancer Chemother Pharmacol* 32 :419-424
14. Lindquist S (1989) The heat-shock response. Ann Rev Biochem 55 :1151
15. Lunger T, Lu C, Echols H, et al: Successive action of DnaK, DnaJ and GroEL along the pathway of chaperone-mediated protein folding. *Nature* 356:683-689, 1992
16. Mann SC, Andrews PA, Howell SB (1991) Modulation of cis-diamminedichloroplatinum(II) accumulation and sensitivity by forskolin and 3-isobutyl-1-methylxanthine in sensitive and resistant human ovarian carcinoma cells. *Int J Cancer* 48 :866
17. Mileo AM, Fanuele M, Battaglia F, et al: Selective over-expression of mRNA coding for 90KDa stress-protein in human ovarian cancer. *Anticancer Res* 10:903-906, 1990
18. Morimoto RI, Tissieres A, Georgopoulos C (1990): The stress response, function of the proteins, and perspectives, in Morimoto RI, Tissieres A, Georgopoulos C (eds): *Stress proteins in biology and medicine*. Cold Spring Harbor, NY, Cold Spring Harbor Laboratory Press, pp1-pp36
19. Pelham HRB (1982) A regulatory upstream promoter element in the Drosophila hsp heat-shock gene. *Cell* 30 :517
20. Sorger PK (1991) Heat shock factor and the heat shock response. *Cell* 65 :363
21. Tandon AK, Clark GM, Chamness GC, et al (1990): Heat shock/stress response protein: Biological and clinical significance in breast cancer. *Proc Am Soc Clin Oncol* 9:23
22. Thor A, Benz C, Moore D II, et al (1991): Stress response protein (srp-27) determination in primary human breast carcinomas: Clinical, histological, and prognostic correlations. *J Natl Cancer Inst* 83:170-178

CHAPTER 16

CISPLATIN-RESISTANCE AND DNA REPAIR IN HUMAN OVARIAN CANCER CELL LINES*

Yasuhiko Kiyozuka[1], Haruo Nishimura[2], Shunsuke Imai[3] and Minoru Morimatsu[4]

Second Department of Pathology[1], Kansai Medical College, Moriguchi, Osaka, Department of Obstetrics and Gynecology[2], Kurume University School of Medicine, Kurume, Fukuoka, Department of Obstetrics and Gynecology[3], Nara Medical College, Kashihara, Nara and Second Department of Pathology[4], Kurume University School of Medicine, Kurume, Fukuoka, Japan

INTRODUCTION

Ovarian cancer is the most common fatal tumor affecting women in developed countries. The long term prognosis for advanced ovarian cancer patients is still poor in spite of development of combined treatment modality with surgery and the introduction of active chemotherapeutic agents [1]. Of them, cis-diamminedichloroplatinum(II) (cisplatin) has been the most important anticancer drug in the past decade for ovarian cancer patients. A present urgent clinical problem is that its efficacy is often limited by the development of resistance. Understanding the molecular basis of cisplatin-resistance may lead to strategies to circumvent this frequent clinical problem. The mechanism for

* Address for reprints and correspondence: Yasuhiko Kiyozuka, MD., The Second Department of Pathology, Kansai Medical College, 10-15 Fumizonochou, Moriguchi, Osaka 570, Japan Tel: 06-992-1001 Fax: 06-992-5023

cisplatin-resistance are thought to be complex involving several components simultaneously: i) decreased drug accumulation [2], ii) detoxification in the cytosol by direct binding to a non-protein thiol such as glutathione (GSH) or to a protein thiol such as metallothionein [3, 4], iii) increased enzymatic inactivation by glutathione S-transferase (GST), and iv) an increased capacity to remove cytotoxic DNA by acitvated DNA repair enzymes [5-7].

To date, the only DNA lesions which could be reliably quantitated in mammalian cells exposed to cytotoxically relevant concentrations of the drug have been considered to be interstrand cross-links in the N7 sites of adjacent guanines and DNA-protein cross-links, which should be quite effective for blocking transcription [8-10]. Several reports demonstrated that the number of interstrand cross-links induced by cisplatin is correlated with its cytotoxicity [11]. The decreased ability to remove these cross-links in some repair-deficient mammalian cells with hypersensitivity to cisplatin support the hypothesis that DNA cross-links are important cytotoxic lesions [12]. Inhibition of DNA repair has been shown to restore sensitivity to cisplatin in cisplatin-resistant tumors both in vitro and in vivo [11]. Based on these observations, some clinical trials to circumvent cisplatin-resistance are proposed and ongoing [13]. The observation that resistance to cisplatin or other bifunctional alkylating agents is associated with enhanced enzymatic detoxification pathways as well as increased DNA repair capacity has led to the clinical evaluation of inhibitors of these enzymes. Evaluation of aphidicolin in combination with cisplatin in an in vivo model of cisplatin refractory human ovarian cancer seemed to support the clinical development [14].

In the present study, we established four kinds of ovarian cancer cell lines with different sensitivity to cisplatin and attempted to determine ability of various DNA polymerase inhibitors, such as aphidicolin, caffeine, AZT and Ara-C to enhance sensitivity to cisplatin.

MATERIALS AND METHODS

OVARIAN CANCER CELL LINES

Human ovarian serous cystadenocarcinoma (SHIN-3) and fibrosarcoma (KEN-3) cell lines were established from the tumor tissue before treatment with cisplatin of patients who developed resistance to cisplatin [15, 16]. MN-1 and EC cell lines were developed from mucinous cystadenocarcinoma of the ovary and endodermal sinus tumor of the ovary before treatment with cisplatin of patients who responded well to cisplatin-based chemotherapy, respectively [17, 18]. These cell lines were incubated in Dulbecco's minimum essential medium (DMEM) supplemented with 10% fetal calf serum (FCS) (GIBCO, Grand Island, NY), 100 units/ml penicillin, and 0.3 mg/ml glutamine at 37 in a humidified atmosphere of 5% CO_2 in air.

CHEMICAL AGENTS

Cisplatin (Nippon Kayaku Co., Ltd., Tokyo, Japan) was dissolved in distilled water at a concentration of 500 μg/ml. Aphidicolin (Wako Junyaku Co., Ltd., Osaka, Japan) was dissolved in a steril dimethyl sulfoxide (DMSO) at a concentration of 10 mg/ml. Cytosine-1-ß-D-arabinofuranoside (Ara-C) (Sigma Chemical Co., St. Louis, MO), 3'-azido-3'-deoxythymidine (AZT) (Wako Junyaku Co., Ltd., Osaka, Japan) and caffeine (Sigma Chemical Co., St. Louis, MO) were dissolved in distilled water to be 100 mg/ml, 10 mg/ml and 20 mg/ml, respectively. These stock solutions were diluted with DMEM containing 10% FCS to be final concentrations prior to use. Cisplatin was stored at 4, while other stock solutions were stored at -20. The final concentration of DMSO in the culture medium was adjusted to be less than 1.0% (v/v), which was confirmed in preliminary studies to have no antiproliferative effect.

MTT ASSAY

MTT (3-[4,5-dimethylthiazol-2-yl]-2,5-diphenyltetrazolium bromide) assay was performed as described previously [19, 20]. The number of cells ($5x10^3$ to $1x10^4$ per 50 μl of culture medium) plated into 96-well microtiterplates was determined after preliminary experiments so that the untreated cells were in the exponential growth phase during the experiment. After preincubation for 12 hr, cisplatin and/or other agents were added into the each well to be desired concentrations. After culture for 1 or 4 hr in the presence of drugs followed by postincubation for 48 hr without drugs, 13 µl (5 mg/ml) of MTT (Sigma Chemical Co., St. Louis, MO) diluted with phosphate-buffered saline (PBS, pH 7.6) was added to each well and incubated at 37 for 4 hr. The medium was then aspirated from each well using an automatic plate washer (Eimax 601, Fujirebio Inc., Shizuoka, Japan). To solubilize the formazan, 150 µl of DMSO was added to each well using a multichannel pipette, and the plates were placed on a plate shaker (Timer mixer MB-1, Torika Corp., Tokyo, Japan) for 2 min. Absorbance was read immediately at 540 nm on a scanning multiwell spectrophotometer (Eimax A-4, Fujirebio Inc. Shizuoka, Japan).

Intracellular Accumulation of Cisplatin

An equal number of $5x10^5$ cancer cells in 20 ml of medium were inoculated into 75 cm^2 culture flasks. After preincubation for 24 hr, 10 µg/ml of cisplatin was added. After 4 hr-incubation with cisplatin, cells in culture flasks were harvested with trypsin and washed three times in cold PBS. Cells were suspended in 2 ml of PBS and the intracellular content of cisplatin was determined with a flameless atomic absorption spectrometer (SPQ 6500, Seiko, Tokyo, Japan). The platinum content per cell was expressed as $\mu g/10^7$ cells. The results are presented as the mean of triplicate samples. To determine the efflux rate of cisplatin from cells, the cells were further incubated for 72 hr after removal of cisplatin from culture and the cisplatin content retained in the cells was also determined. The efflux rate (%) was calculated as follows; Efflux rate (%) = [(cisplatin content after exposure with cisplatin for 4 hr – cisplatin content after cisplatin-free incubation for 72 hr)/cisplatin content after exposure with cisplatin for 4 hr] x 100.

COMBINED EFFECTS OF CISPLATIN AND DNA POLYMERASE INHIBITORS

We examined the effects of cisplatin on the cell proliferation, using various concentrations of cisplatin based on the IC_{50} as determined by preliminary studies. The cells were continuously exposed with cisplatin for 1 hr or 4 hr, and followed by cisplatin-free incubation for 48 hr. Thereafter, the cell-number in each well was determined by MTT assay. The IC_{50} value shows the concentration of cisplatin that produced a 50% reduction of absorbance in control untreated cells at 540 nm. The final concentrations of Ara-C, AZT, caffeinee and aphidicolin used were the range of 0.001-1000 µg/ml, 1-50 µg/ml, 0.01-1 mg/ml and 0.05-50 µM, respectively. After continuous exposure with above-mentioned drugs for 48 hr, IC_{10} or IC_{20} values for each cell line were determined. To examine combined effects of cisplatin and DNA polymerase inhibitors, cells preincubated with cisplatin for 1 or 4 hr were washed with PBS and exposed with IC_{10} or IC_{20} concentrations of aphidicolin, caffeinee, AZT or Ara-C for 48 hr. Results show the mean of the 8 wells. The ability of each DNA polymerase inhibitor to enhance cisplatin sensitivity was determined as follows; Enhancement rate (%) = [(IC_{50} of cisplatin alone – IC_{50} of cisplatin in combined treatment of cisplatin and DNA polymerase inhibitors)/IC_{50} of cisplatin alone] x 100.

RESULTS

DIFFERENT SENSITIVITIES TO CISPLATIN

IC_{50} values of cisplatin-sensitive MN-1 cells to cisplatin were 5.6 µg/ml with exposure for 1 hr and 1.0 µg/ml with exposure for 4 hr. Similarly, IC_{50} values of EC cells relatively sensitive to cisplatin were 15.5 µg/ml for 1 hr and 2.6 µg/ml for 4 hr. On the other hand, SHIN-3 and KEN-3 cells relatively resistant to cisplatin had more than 5-fold higher IC_{50} values than MN-1 or EC cells, showing IC_{50} of 70.0 µg/ml for 1 hr or 16.0 µg/ml for 4 hr in SHIN-3 cells and IC_{50} of 120.0 µg/ml for 1 hr or 27.0 µg/ml for 4 hr in KEN-3 cells (Table 1). These cell lines with different sensitivity to cisplatin may be useful for elucidation of the mechanism of cisplatin-resistance.

Table 1. Comparison of the IC_{50} values and the cellular accumulation of cisplatin in various human ovarian cancer cell lines

Cell lines	IC_{50} values (μg/ml)		Platinum content ($\mu g/10^7$ cells)		Efflux rate (%)
	1 hr[a]	4 hr	4 hr[b]	72 hr[c]	
MN-1	5.6	1.0	36.1	17.5	51.5
EC	15.5	2.6	47.6	26.4	44.6
SHIN-3	70.0	16.0	16.7	7.1	57.2
KEN-3	120.0	27.0	1.6	1.5	7.9

[a]Contact time with cisplatin.
[b]Platinum contents incorporated 4 hr after exposure with 10 μg/ml of cisplatin.
[c]Retained platinum contents when incubated for 72 hr after removal of cisplatin.
Results show the mean value of 8 samples. MN-1 and EC cells are relatively sensitive to cisplatin, while SHIN-3 and KEN-3 cells are relatively resistant to cisplatin.

Intracellular Cisplatin Accumulation

As shown in Table 1, when EC cells were incubated with 10 μg/ml cisplatin for 4 hr the cellular platinum content was highest among these four cell lines, showing 47.6 $\mu g/10^7$ cells. MN-1 cells with highest sensitivity to cisplatin also showed higher uptake of cisplatin, compared to SHIN-3 and KEN-3 cells with less sensitivity to cisplatin. Especially, platinum-uptake by KEN-3 cells was extremely low and seemed to be sufficient to account for the mechanism of cisplatin-resistance. Efflux rates of SHIN-3, MN-1 and EC cells were 57.2%, 51.5% and 44.6%, respectively. In KEN-3 cells with lowest intracellular accumulation of platinum, the efflux rate was slowest as far as it is observed within 72 hr of incubation.

Combined Effects of Cisplatin and DNA Polymerase Inhibitors

As shown in Table 2, MN-1 cells seemed to be most sensitive to aphidicolin, caffeine and Ara-C among four cell lines examined, suggesting correlation between sensitivities to cisplatin and these drugs. However, SHIN-3 cells with

Table 2. Comparison of IC_{10} or IC_{20} values to DNA polymerase inhibitors in various human ovarian cancer cell lines

Cell	Aphidicolin (μM)		Caffeine (mg/ml)		AZT (μg/ml)		Ara-C (μg/ml)	
line	IC_{10}	IC_{20}	IC_{10}	IC_{20}	IC_{10}	IC_{20}	IC_{10}	IC_{20}
MN-1	0.025[a]	0.1	0.053	0.14	11.0	30.0	0.03	0.1
EC	4.0	23.0	0.12	0.33	18.0	70.0	30.0	80.0
SHIN-3	1.2	2.4	0.10	0.21	9.5	20.0	1.0	10.0
KEN-3	15.0	40.0	0.095	0.15	100.0	230.0	350.0	800.0

[a]Data are the mean values from 8 samples. Exposure time was 4 hr.

less sensitivity to cisplatin were more sensitive to all DNA polymerase inhibitors used than EC cells with higher sensitivity to cisplatin. It is noteworthy that cisplatin-resistant KEN-3 cells showed extremely low sensitivity to all DNA polymerase inhibitors except for caffeine. Fig. 1. shows effects of cisplatin alone or combined effects with aphidicolin on the proliferation of SHIN-3 cells. The IC_{50} value of cisplatin alone was 7.1 μg/ml. When cisplatin was combined with aphidicolin, the IC_{50} of cisplatin reduced to 3.0 μg/ml with IC_{10} of aphidicolin and to 1.1 μg/ml with IC_{20} of aphidicolin, showing 57.7% and 84.5% of enhancement rate, respectively. Similarly, we determined the enhancement rate (%) of sensitivity to cisplatin by DNA polymerase inhibitors in all cell lines used (Fig. 2). Figs. 2a and 2b show the enhancement rate by aphidicolin, Figs. 2c and 2d by caffeine, Figs. 2e and 2f by AZT and Figs. 2g and 2h by Ara-C, repectively. As shown in Figs. 2a and 2b, the sensitivity of cisplatin-resistant SHIN-3 cells to cisplatin by 1 or 4 hr exposure with cisplatin was most markedly enhanced by aphidicolin, while that of more cisplatin-resistant KEN-3 cells was hardly enhanced by a IC_{10} dose of aphidicolin. Although the sensitivity of cisplatin-sensitive MN-1 cells to cisplatin by 1 hr exposure with cisplatin was only modestly enhanced, that by 4 hr exposure with cisplatin was markedly increased. On the other hand, it is noteworthy that the sensitivity of KEN-3 with marked resistance to cisplatin was increased to more than 50% in the enhancement rate. In addition, the sensitivity of the other cell lines was remarkably enhanced especially when IC_{20} dose of caffeine was used (Figs. 2c

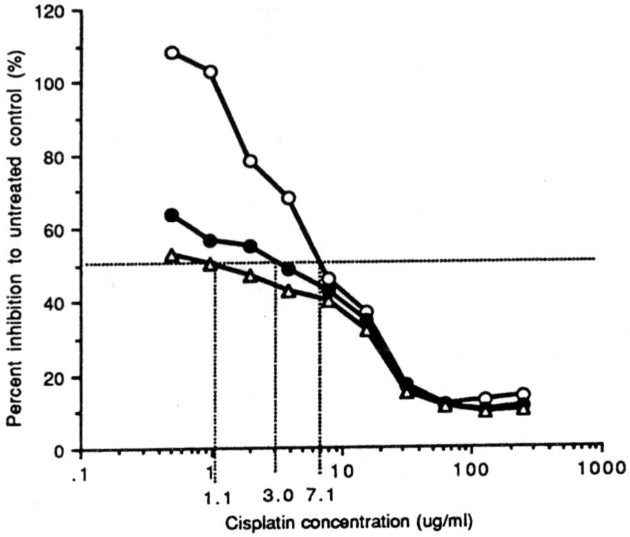

Fig. 1. Combined effects of aphidicolin to cisplatin on SHIN-3 cell proliferation. Cells were incubated with cisplatin for 1 hr and after removal of cisplatin from the cell culture, cells were incubated in the absence or presence of aphidicolin for 48 hr. ○–○; cisplatin alone, ●–●; cisplatin followed by IC_{10} of aphidicolin, Δ–Δ; cisplatin followed by IC_{20} of aphidicolin.

and 2d). In 1 hr-exposure to cisplatin, sensitization effect to cisplatin by AZT was observed only in EC cells, while under condition of 4 hr-exposure with cisplatin, the enhancement rate by AZT showed around the range of 20-60% in all cell lines (Figs. 2e and 2f). The general figure of 1 hr exposure to cisplatin followed by Ara-C resembled that of 4 hr exposure to cisplatin followed by aphidicolin (Fig. 2g). However, the degree of its sensitization by Ara-C after 4 hr exposure to cisplatin was similar to each other cells (Fig. 2h). Taken together, SHIN-3 cells relatively well responded for sensitization of cisplatin by all DNA polymerase inhibitors except for AZT, while KEN-3 cells were sensitized only by caffeine. Caffeine and aphidicolin generally possessed more ability to enhance the sensitivity to cisplatin than AZT and Ara-C.

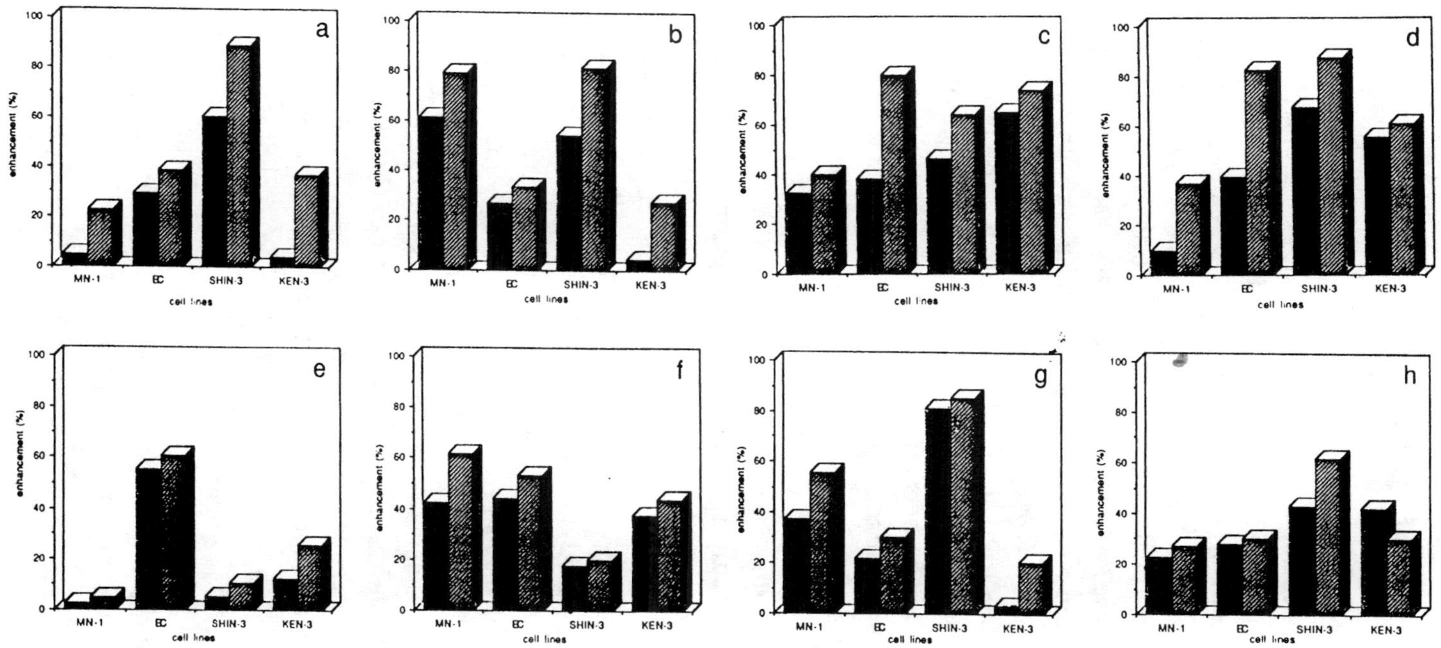

Fig. 2. Enhancement effects by various DNA polymerase inhibitors on the cisplatin- sensitivity of MN-1, EC, SHIN-3 and KEN-3 cells. a, 1 hr exposure to cisplatin followed by IC_{10}; ■ or IC_{20}; ▒ of aphidicolin. b, 4 hr exposure to cisplatin followed by IC_{10}; ■ or IC_{20}; ▒ of aphidicolin. c, 1 hr exposure to cisplatin followed by IC_{10}; ■ or IC_{20}; ▒ of caffeine. d, 4 hr exposure to cisplatin followed by IC_{10}; ■ or IC_{20}; ▒ of caffeine. e, 1 hr exposure to cisplatin followed by IC_{10}; ■ or IC_{20}; ▒ of AZT. f, 4 hr exposure to cisplatin followed by IC_{10}; ■ or IC_{20}; ▒ of AZT. g, I hr exposure to cisplatin followed by IC_{10}; ■ or IC_{20}; ▒ of Ara-C. h, 4 hr exposure to cisplatin followed by IC_{10}; ■ or IC_{20}; ▒ of Ara-C.

DISCUSSION

As cisplatin has been a key drug in chemotherapy for ovarian cancer, resistance to cisplatin is a major problem for gynecologic oncologists. Among several mechanisms proposed for the acquired resistance, the cellular DNA repair functions have been focussed because it is well established that DNA is a critical intracellular target of platinum compounds. There are several evidences that enhanced DNA repair is involved in cisplatin resistance mechanisms [21-23]. Masuda et al. [6] showed that DNA repair pathway was increased about 3-fold in the acquired cisplatin-resistant 2780cp ovarian cancer cell line than in the parental cisplatin-sensitive A2780 cells, confirming enhanced removal of platinum from DNA in 2780cp cells by atomic absorption spectrophotometry. Lai et al. [24] also demonstrated a 2 to 3-fold increase of DNA repair using PE01 and PE04 cell lines, which developed cisplatin-resistance during treatment. The increased platinum removal from total genomic DNA was found to be associated with the increased cisplatin-resistance, using a panel of cisplatin-resistant cell lines developed by continuous and incremental exposure of the A2780 cells to cisplatin [25]. The present study was performed using ovarian cancer cell lines with different degree of intrinsic resistance to cisplatin. According to the cisplatin-sensitivity test, the sensitivity decreased in order of MN-1, EC, SHIN-3 and KEN-3 (Table 1). The sensitivity of each cell line to cisplatin was 2.6 and 2.8-fold (with 1 hr and 4 hr exposure to cisplatin) for EC cells, 4.5 and 16.0-fold for SHIN-3 cells, and 21.4 and 27.0-fold for KEN-3 cells lower than that of MN-1 cells, respectively. Intracellular accumulation of cisplatin in these cells after 4 hr exposure to 10 μg/ml cisplatin did not correlate with the sensitivity to cisplatin. Efflux rate of cisplatin was higher in the cisplatin-sensitive cell lines rather than the cisplatin-resistant cell lines. These results seem to suggest that the cisplatin-resistance mechanisms are complex including alterations in drug transport, enhanced detoxification, and increased repair of DNA damage. As for DNA polymerases, three prokaryotic DNA polymerases, designated I, II, and III, have been identified in E. coli by Kornberg and others [26, 27]. It is well-known that higher organisms possess at least five DNA polymerases, designated α, β, γ, δ and ε [28, 29]. Although several lines of evidence initially implicated DNA polymerase α as the primary replication enzyme of eukaryotes, its processibility is only moderate, so that the enzyme is expected to polymerize only 100 to 200 nucleotides before releasing [30]. DNA polymerase δ is characterized by very high processibility and having the 3'5' exonuclease activity required for proofreading [31]. DNA polymerase γ was primarily found in association with mitochondria in eukaryotic cells, and is thought to be specialized for DNA replication in these organelles. Polymerase ε, which has structure and properties similar to polymerase δ, has been implicated in DNA repair [32]. DNA polymerase β may work in coordination with polymerase α and ε in DNA repair. In vitro studies using cultured cell lines have documented the increased activity in some of these enzymes involved in the DNA repair process. Fornace et al. [33] revealed increased levels of DNA replication and repair enzymes, such as DNA polymerase α and β, thymidilate synthetase, thymidine kinase, and dihydrofolate reductase in a cisplatin-resistant cell line. Perez et al. [34] examined the effects of aphidicolin, which is an inhibitor of DNA polymerase α and γ, on unscheduled DNA synthesis following cisplatin treatment in A2780 and the cisplatin-resistant 2780cp cell lines and revealed that aphidicolin inhibits the DNA repair in both cell lines to 70% and results in a 3.5-fold enhancement of cisplatin sensitivity in 2780cp cells. Synergistic effect of Ara-C, another inhibitor of DNA polymerase α, to cisplatin was presented by Synder et al. [35, 36]. Similarly, Scanlon et al. [37] have reported that cytotoxicity to cisplatin was significantly enhanced when cisplatin-resistant colon cancer cell lines were treated with cisplatin and azidothymidine, which is an inhibitor of DNA polymerase β and γ. Sciano et al. [38] demonstrated a marked increase in cytotoxicity of cisplatin by caffeine or pentoxyfillin, which is an inhibitor of DNA polymerase α and β, using a cisplatin-resistant ovarian cancer cell line (BG-1). As shown in Fig. 2, all DNA polymerase inhibitors used in this study enhanced more or less cisplatin-cytotoxicity to human ovarian cancer cell lines, suggesting that DNA polymerases play an important role in the cisplatin-sensitivity.

Recently, the human DNA repair genes ERCC1 and ERCC2 have been cloned and characterized, and their relative abilities to confer resistance to a variety of DNA-damaging agents have been demonstrated [39, 40]. ERCC1 and ERCC2 are human DNA repair genes that are associated with in vitro resistance to selected DNA-damaging agents. ERCC1 expression levels in human tumor tissue may have a role in clinical resistance to platinum compounds. ERCC1 serves as an excision nuclease, whereas ERCC2 serves as a helicase [40]. Another DNA repair gene, human xerodermia pigmentosum group A correcting gene (XPAC gene), may also play a role in clinical resistance to cisplatin in ovarian cancer tissue [41]. In addition, ERCC1 expression was directly related to cisplatin-DNA adduct repair capability as well as cisplatin resistance, suggesting a primary role for ERCC1 in affecting DNA repair [42, 43]. Thus, our established human ovarian cancer cell lines with different sensitivity to cisplatin may be useful for further elucidating a role of such DNA repair genes in the mechanisms of cisplatin-resistance.

REFERENCES

1. Young RC, Fuks A, and Hoskins WJ.: Cancer of the ovary. In VT Devita Jr, et al (ed) *Cancer-principles and practice of oncology*, J.B. Lippincott, Philadelphia, p1162-1196, 1989.
2. Teicher BA, Holden SA, Kelly MJ, Shea TC, Cucchi CA, Rosowsky A, Henner WD, and Frei E, .: Characterization of a human squamous carcinoma cell line resistant to cis-diamminedichloroplatinum(II). *Cancer Res* 47:388-393, 1987.
3. Hamilton TC, Winker MA, Louie KG, Batist G, Behrens BC, Tsuruo T, Grotzinger KR, Mckoy WM, Young RC, and Ozols RF.: Augementation of adriamycin, melphalan, and cisplatin cytotoxicity in drug-resistant and -sensitive human ovarian carcinoma cell lines by buthionine sulfoximine mediated glutathione depletion. *Biochem Pharmacol* 34:2583-2589, 1985.
4. Kelly SL, Basu A, Teicher BA, Hacker MP, Hamer DH, and Lazo JS.: Overexpression of metallothionein confers resistance to anticancer drugs. Science 241:1813-1815, 1988.
5. Eastman A, and Schulte N.: Enhanced DNA repair as a mechanism of resistance to cis-diamminedichloroplatinum(II). *Biochemistry* 27:4730-4734, 1988.
6. Masuda H, Tanaka T, Matsuda H, and Kusaba I.: Increased removal of DNA-bound platinum in a human ovarian cancer cell line resistant to cis-diamminedichloroplatinum(II). *Cancer Res* 50:1863-1866, 1990.
7. Parker RJ, Eastman A, Bostick-Bruton F, and Reed E.: Acquired cisplatin resistance in human ovarian cancer cells is associated with enhanced repair of cisplatin-DNA lesions and reduced drug accumulation. *J Clin Invest* 87:772-777, 1991.

8. Lippard SJ.: New chemistry of an old molecule: cis$(PtNH_3)_2Cl_2$. *Science* 218:1075-1082, 1982.
9. Kohn KW, Spears CL, and Doty P.: Inter-strand crosslinking of DNA by nitrogen mustard. *J Mol Biol* 19:266-288, 1966.
10. Brookers P, and Lawley PD.: The reaction of mono and bifunctional alkylating agents with nucleic acids. *Biochem J* 80:496-503, 1961.
11. Zhen W, Link CJ Jr, O'Connor PM, Reed E, Parker R, Howell SB, and Bohr VA.: Increased gene-specific repair of cisplatin interstrand cross-links in cisplatin-resistant human ovarian cancer cell lines. *Mol Cell Biol* 12:3689-3698, 1992.
12. Sherman S, and Lippard SJ.: Structural aspects of platinum anticancer drug interactions with DNA. *Chem Rev* 87:1153-1181, 1987.
13. Sessa C, Zucchetti M, Davoli E, Califano R, Cavalli F, Frutaci S, Gumbrell L, Sulkes A, Winograd B, and D'Incaci M.: Phase I and clinical pharmacological evaluation of aphidicolin glycinate. *J Natl Cancer Inst* 83:1160-1164, 1991.
14. O'Dwyer PJ, Moyer JD, Sulffness M, Harrison SD Jr, Cysyk R, Hamilton TC, and Plowman J.: Antitumor activity and biochemical effects of aphidicolin glycinate (NSC 303812) alone and in combination with cisplatin in vivo. *Cancer Res* 54:724-729, 1994.
15. Imai S, Kiyozuka Y, Maeda H, Noda T, and Hosick HL.: Establishment and characterization of a human ovarian serous cystadenocarcinoma cell line that produces the tumor marker CA-125 and tissue polypeptide antigen. *Oncology* 47:177-184, 1990.
16. Kiyozuka Y, Nishimura H, Iwanaga S, Yakushiji M, Ito K, Nakano S, Tamori N, and Adachi S.: Establishment and characterization of human ovarian fibrosarcoma cell line and its sensitivity to anticancer agents. *Acta Obstet Gynecol Jpn* 44:461-468, 1992 (in Japanese).
17. Yoshida M, Kiyozuka Y, Noda T, Imai S, and Ichijo M.: Establishment and characterization of human cell line derived from mucinous cysadenocarcinoma of ovary. *J Jpn Soc Clin Cytol* 32:1-8, 1993 (in Japanese).
18. Imamura K, Kiyozuka Y, Nishimura H, and Yakushiji M.: Novel germ cell tumor cell line established from a testicular feminization syndrome. *Oncol Rep* 2:17-25, 1995.

19. Mossman T.: Rapid clorimetric assay for cellular growth and survival: Application to proliferation and cytotoxic assays. *J Immunol Methods* 65:55-63, 1983.
20. Twentyman PR, and Luscombe M.: A study of some variables in a tetrazolium dye (MTT) based assay for cell growth and chemosensitivity. *Br J Cancer* 56:279-285, 1987.
21. Fox M, and Roberts J.: Drug resistance and DNA repair. *Cancer Metast Rev* 6:261-281, 1987.
22. Sekiya S, Oosaki T, Andoh S, Suzuki N, Akabori M, and Takamizawa H.: Mechanisms of resistance to cis-diamminedichloroplatinum(II) in a rat ovarian carcinoma cell line. *Eur J Cancer Clin Oncol* 25:429-437, 1989.
23. Torres-Garcia SJ, Cousineau L, Caplan S, and Panasci L.: Correlation of resistance to nitrogen mustards in chronic lymphocytic leukemia with enhanced removal of melphalan-induced DNA cross-links. *Biochem Pharmacol* 38:3122-3123, 1989.
24. Lai G, Ozols RF, Smyth J, Young RC, and Hamilton TC.: Enhanced DNA repair and resistance to cisplatin in human ovarian cancer. *Biochem Pharmacol* 37:4597-4600, 1988.
25. Johnson SW, Perez RP, Godwin AK, Yeung AT, Handel LM, Ozols RF, and Hamilton TC.: Role of platinum-DNA adduct formation and removal in cisplatin resistance in human ovarian cancer cell lines. *Biochem Pharmacol* 47:689-697, 1994.
26. Kornberg A, and Baler TA.: *DNA replication*, 2nd ed. New York: W.H. Freeman, 1992 (Chapter 4 and 6 describe DNA polymerases; Chapter 9 describes DNA ligase; Chapter 21 covers the enzymology of DNA repair).
27. McHenry C.: DNA polymerase III holoenzyme; components, structure, and mechanism of a true replicative complex. *J Biol Chem* 266:19127-19130, 1988.
28. Sancar A, and Sancar G.: DNA repair enzymes. *Ann Rev Biochem* 57:29-67, 1987.
29. DePamphilis ML.: Transcriptional elements as components of eukaryotic origins of DNA replication. *Cell* 52:635-638, 1988.
30. Burgers PMJ.: Eukaryotic DNA polymerase and : conserved properties and interactions, from yeast to mammalian cells. *Prog Nucleic Acid Res Mol Biol* 37:236-280, 1989.

31. Bambara RA, and Jessee CB.: Properties of DNA polymerase δ and ε, and their roles in eukaryotic DNA replication. *Biochem Biophys Acta* 1088:11-24, 1991.
32. Syvaoja JE.: DNA polymerase epsilon: the latest member in the family of mammalian DNA polymerases. *Bioess* 12:533-536, 1990.
33. Fornace A, Alamo I, and Hollander C.: DNA damage-inducible transcripts in mammalian cells. *Proc Natl Acad Sci* USA 85:8800-8804, 1988.
34. Perez RP, Godwin AK, Hamilton TC, and Ozols RF.: Ovarian cancer biology. *Semin Oncol* 18:186-204, 1991.
35. Snyder R, Carrier W, and Regan J.: Application of arabinofuranosyl cytosine in the kinetic analysis and quantitation of DNA repair in human cells after ultraviolet radiation. *Biophys J* 35:339-350, 1981.
36. Zittoun J, Marquet J, David JC, Maniey D, and Zittoun R.: A study of the mechanisms of cytotoxicity of Ara-C on three human leukemic cell lines. *Cancer Chemother Pharmacol* 24:251-255, 1989.
37. Scanlon KJ, Kashani-Sabet M, and Sowers LC.: Overexpression of DNA replication and repair enzymes in cisplatin-resistant human colon carcinoma HCT8 cells and circumvention by azidothymidine. *Cancer Commun* 1:269-275, 1989.
38. Sciano MA, Sevin BU, Perras J, Ramos R, Wolloch EH, and Averette HE.: In vitro enhancement of cis-platinum antitumor activity by caffeine and pentoxyfillin in a human ovarian cell line. *Gynecol Oncol* 43:37-45, 1991.
39. Hoeijmakers JHJ, Weeda G, Troelstra C, van Duin M, Westerveld A, van der Eb A, and Bootsma D.: Molecular genetic dissection of mammalian excision repair. In *DNA Repair Mechanism and Their Biological Implications in Mammalian Cells*, Edited by M.W. Lambert and J. Laval, Plenum Press, New York p563-574, 1993.
40. Dabholker M, Bostick-Bruton F, Weber C, Bohr V, Egwuagu C, and Reed E.: ERCC1 and ERCC2 expression in malignant tissues from ovarian cancer patients. *J Natl Cancer Inst* 84:1512-1517, 1992.
41. Dabholker M, Vionnet J, Bostick-Bruton F, Yu JJ, and Reed E.: Messenger RNA levels of XPAC and ERCC1 in ovarian cancer tissue correlate with response to platinum-based chemotherapy. *J Clin Invest* 94:703-708, 1994.
42. Dabholker M, Parker R, and Reed E.: Determination of cisplatin sensitivity in non-malignant, non-drug-selected human T cell lines . *Mut Res* 274:45-56, 1992.

43. Dabholker M, Vionnet J, Parker RJ, Bostick-Bruton F, Dobbins A, and Reed E.: Expression of an alternatively spliced ERCC1 mRNA species, is related to reduced DNA repair efficacy in human T lymphocytes. *Oncol Rep* 2:209-214, 1995.

CHAPTER 17

CISPLATIN (CDDP) RESISTANCE AND MULTIDRUG RESISTANCE: ARE THEY REALLY NOT ASSOCIATED?

Shinji Arao[1,3], Wun-Jae Kim[1,2,4], Wen-Jeng Wu[1,2,5], Yoshiyuki Kakehi[2], Osamu Yoshida[2], Hitoshi Okamura[3], Hiroshi Hiai And Manabu Fukumoto[1,6]

Departments of [1]Pathology and [2]Urology, Faculty of Medicine, Kyoto University, Sakyo-ku, Kyoto 606, Japan, [3] Department of Obstetrics and Gynecology, School of Medicine, Kumamoto University, Kumamoto 860, Japan, [4] Present address : Department of Urology, College of Medicine, Chungbuk National University, MT.48 Kaeshin-Dong, Cheongju, Chungbuk, 360-763, Korea, [5] Present address : Department of Urology, Kaohsiung Medical College, Kaohsiung 80708, Taiwan, R.O.C., [6] Corresponding Author

Some hematological malignancies and childhood solid tumors can be cured by combination chemotherapy in the majority of patients (Frei 1985). For the treatment of solid tumors such as ovarian, testicular and small cell lung cancer, cisplatin (CDDP) is a key agent (Loherer and Einhorn, 1984). However, chemotherapy for advanced cancer remains suboptimal and has had little impact on the survival of patients with solid tumors. The resistance, inherent or acquired, to cytotoxic drugs is the major obstacle to chemotherapy (Young 1990). The primary reason for the failure of chemotherapy in cancer patients is cross-resistance of tumor cells to a wide variety of functionally and structurally unrelated antitumor agents.

Multidrug resistance (MDR) is characterized by cross-resistance within a single class of unrelated drugs (Biedler and Riehm 1970). Drugs associated with MDR are generally amphipathic, lipophilic natural substances including Adriamycin and vincristine. Classical MDR is closely correlated with overexpression of the 170-kDa plasma membrane glycoprotein, termed P-glycoprotein (P-gp) (Juliano & Ling, 1976), which is encoded by the mdr1 gene in humans (Ueda et al., 1986). Although the exact physiological function of P-gp remains unknown, overproduced P-gp pumps drugs out of cells resulting in a decrease of drugs in MDR cells.

MDR which is not attributed to P-gp overproduction is termed atypical MDR. Topoisomerase (Topo) II catalyzes DNA strand breaks and is a target of Adriamycin and VP-16 which are MDR drugs. Both qualitative and quantitative decreases in activity of the enzyme induce MDR (Fernandes et al., 1993). Recently another class of protein, MRP (multidrug resistance-associated protein) which is responsible for the MDR phenotype has been demonstrated (Cole et al., 1992). The MRP protein is 190-kDa and is a member of the ATP-binding cassette superfamily of membrane transport proteins like, but distinctively different from, P-gp. Although MRP protein is distributed mainly in the endoplasmic reticulum and to a lesser degree in plasma membranes (Krishnamachary and Center, 1993), its role in causing MDR remains unknown.

Various mechanisms for CDDP resistance are reported : decreased intracellular drug accumulation, altered drug metabolism, increased repair of DNA damage and altered drug targets (See other chapters in this book). However, the major mechanism responsible for CDDP resistance remains unelucidated. Although CDDP resistance is not considered to be associated with MDR, CDDP resistant cells occasionally acquire cross-resistance to other unrelated drugs including MDR drugs (Hamaguchi et al., 1993). Therefore, investigating the relationship between CDDP resistance and MDR will give insight into ways to improve cancer chemotherapy.

DEVELOPMENT OF DRUG RESISTANT CELL LINES

Human renal cell carcinoma cell lines Caki-1, NC65 and ACHN, and a bladder carcinoma cell line 5637 were obtained from American Type Culture Collection. Their CDDP resistant sublines, Caki-1/CDDP, NC65/CDDP and ACHN/CDDP of up to 5mg/ml of CDDP were isolated by a multiple step selection. An Adriamycin resistant subline 5637/DR5.5 of up to 55 ng/ml of Adriamycin was also obtained by multiple stepwise selection. Caki-1/CDDP, NC65/CDDP and ACHN/CDDP cells were maintained in 5 μg/ml of CDDP, and 5637/DR5.5 cells were maintained in 55 μg/ml of Adriamycin in RPMI1640 medium supplemented with 10% fetal calf serum. The drug sensitivity of each cell line measured by dye exclusion test using trypan blue is shown in Fig. 1. Comparing IC50 values, Caki-1/CDDP, NC65/CDDP and ACHN/CDDP were 70-fold, 32-fold and 10-fold more resistant to CDDP than their parental cell lines, respectively. 5637/DR5.5 were 5-fold more resistant to Adriamycin.

Assay for Gene Expression

Polymerase chain reaction (PCR) after reverse transcription (RT-PCR) was performed to measure gene expression. Northern blot analysis usually requires at least 10 mg of total RNA to detect transcripts and is not sensitive enough to detect mdr1 gene expression of clinical materials. Slot (or dot) blot analysis is more sensitive but less quantitative and less reliable compared with Northern analysis because of higher background hybridization. On the other hand, RT-PCR needs less than 1 mg of total RNA for more than 40 assays. Conditions of PCR have to be determined: whether the PCR product is the target sequence to be analyzed or not and whether the PCR cycle, at which gene expression is compared, is within the numbers which reflect the amount of PCR products in proportion to copy numbers of the transcript or not. The amount and quality of RNA have to be normalized. However, RT-PCR is a simple, sensitive and highly quantintative method to assess gene expression. Moreover we can pick up the exact portion of tissues necessary from the clinical samples because enough RNA for RT-PCR analysis can be extracted from several collected thin sections of frozen tissues.

Fig.2A is a typical autoradiogram of RT-PCR showing mdr1 and MRP gene expressions. A cell line K562 was derived from chronic myelogenous leukemia (CML) cells and its Adriamycin resistant derivative K562/ADM cells were used as negative and positive controls for mdr1 gene expression, respectively. Another CML cell line KYO-1 was used as control for moderate expression of the mdr1 gene. On the autoradiogram at this exposure level, a band from mdr1 transcript could be seen only in Caki-1 cells among the 3 cell lines examined and their CDDP resistant derivatives. Interestingly mdr1 gene expression is not observed even in 5637/DR5.5 cells despite the fact that Adriamycin is an MDR drug. Certain intensity of bands from MRP transcripts is demonstrated in all the cell lines examined. Fig. 2B shows mdr1 and MRP gene expressions presented by the relative yield of the target sequence to b2-microglobulin (b2m). Radioactivity incorporated into PCR products was

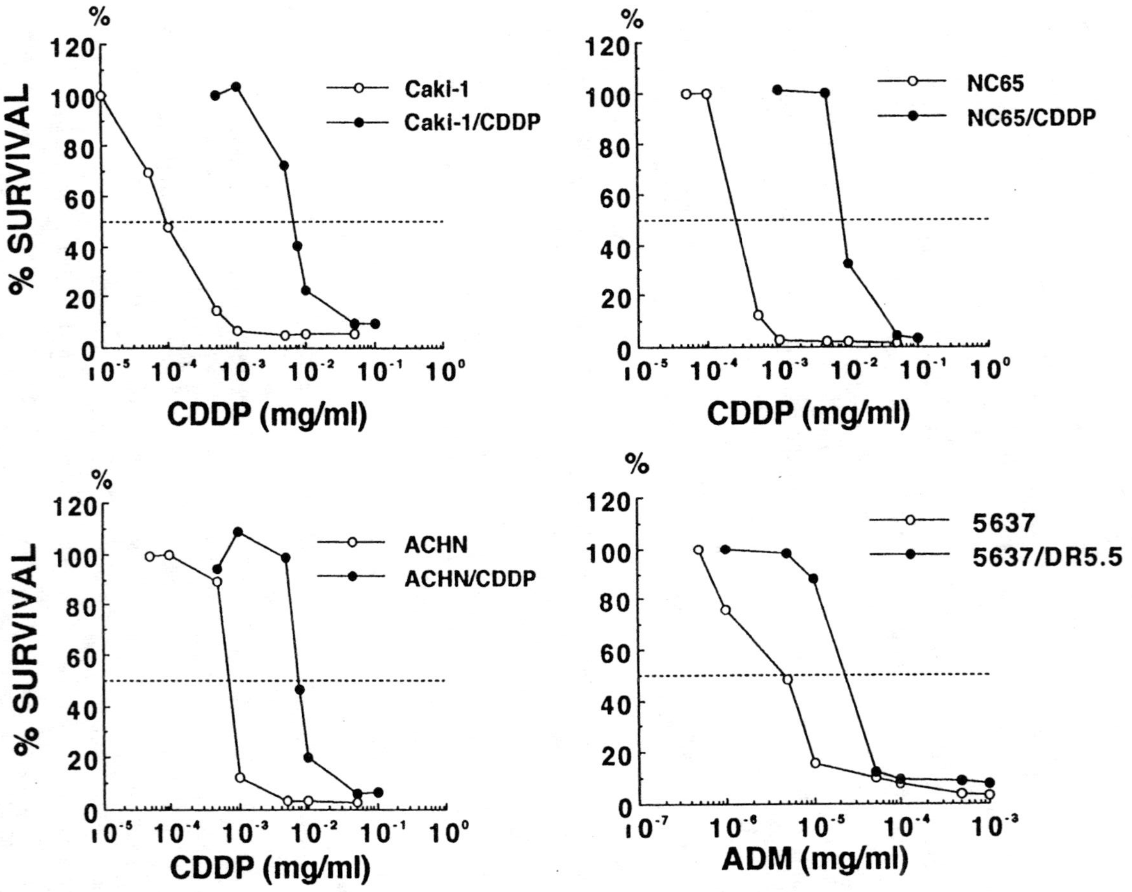

Fig.1 Survival of drug resistant and parental cells in vitro.
5x103 cells were treated with various concentrations of drugs for 72 hr. Cytotoxicity was assayed principally by Biedler and Riehm (1970). The results are expressed as the surviving fraction from treated groups compared to untreated controls. Each point is the mean of triplicate experiments.

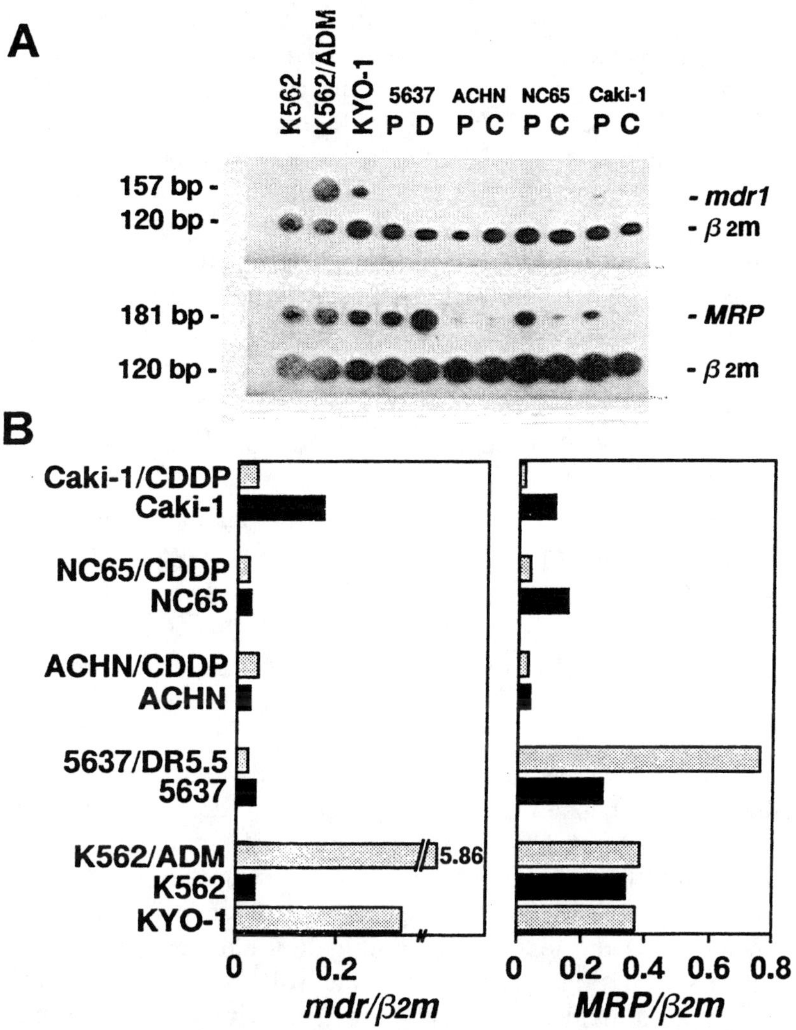

Fig. 2 Expressions of the mdr1 and the MRP genes. Typical autoradiogram of RT-PCR (A) and normalized expressions (B).

Experimental procedure for quantification of mdr1 gene expression was described else where (Arao et al., 1994). A pair of primers for MRP expression was designed to amplify nucleotides between 1380-1541 of the MRP cDNA (Cole et al., 1992) and was confirmed not to amplify MRP of genomic DNA. Primers for b2-microglobulin (b2m) were used for control of the whole procedure including reverse transcription and PCR. Each gene expression is the mean value of triplicate experiments after being normalized against b2m expression. P, parental cells; D, Adriamycin resistant cells; C, CDDP resistant cells

determined using a Bioimaging Analysis System, BAS 2000 (Fujix, Japan). Compared with K562, all the cell lines examined except Caki-1 were practically negative for mdr1 expression. CDDP resistant cell lines tended to show less mdr1 gene expression than their corresponding parental cell lines. 5637/DR5.5 cells revealed only slightly higher expression of the mdr1 gene. The expression levels of the MRP gene were relatively higher than those of the mdr1 gene, suggesting that MRP expression is more ubiquitous than mdr1/P-gp expression. All the CDDP-resistant cell lines examined showed lower MRP gene expression level than their parental lines. 5637/DR5.5 showed 2.8-fold higher expression of the MRP gene compared with its parental cell line.

Immunocytochemical Staining of P-Glycoprotein.

As shown in Fig. 3, Caki-1/CDDP cells were stained stronger than Caki-1 cells. Other cell lines were faintly positive for P-gp. These results were consistent with mdr1 gene expressions.

Conclusion

CDDP so far is one of the most efficient and widely administrated chemotherapeutic agents. Although the higher the dose of CDDP is, the more effective the chemotherapy is, the amount of the drug is limited because of the side effects. Therefore, to characterize the relationship of resistances among various chemotherapeutic agents is necessary for assessment of the most effective and the least toxic combination chemotherapy.

To date conflicting data exist on the role of Topo II in resistance to CDDP : increased incidence of low Topo II activity in CDDP treated ovarian cancers (van der Zee et al., 1991) and enhanced Topo II activity in a CDDP resistant cell line (de Jong et al., 1990). On the other hand, CDDP resistance has not been thought to influence mdr1 gene expression, presumably because a method sensitive enough to detect minute differences of gene expression was not applied to measure mdr1 gene expression. The present study showed that CDDP resistance causes down regulation of MRP gene expression remarkably and mdr1/P-gp expression partly. These suggest that CDDP resistance does not share cross-resistance with MDR drugs but rather

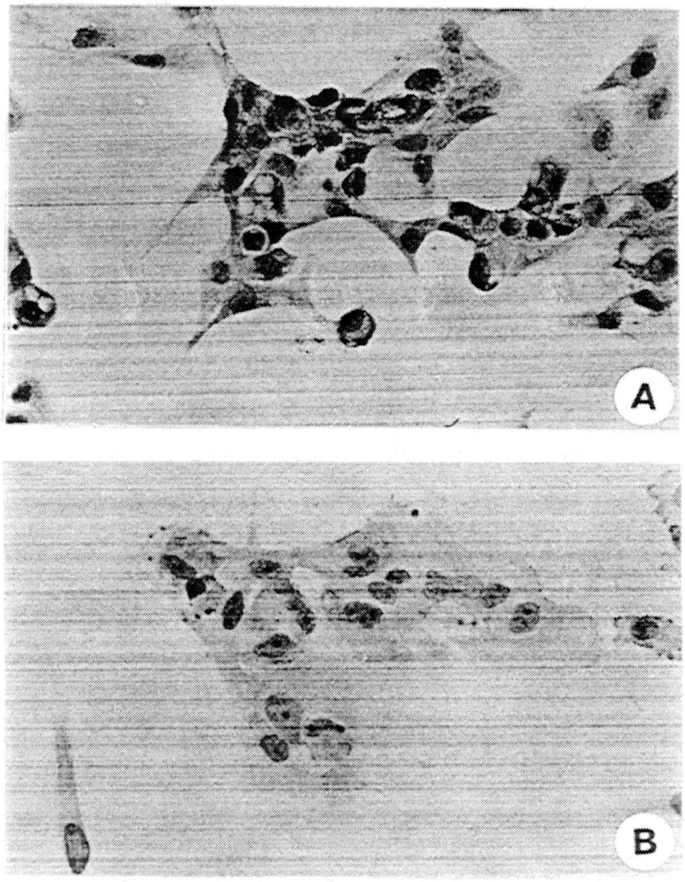

Fig. 3. Immunocytochemical staining of P-glycoprotein (P-gp) Cells grown in Lab-tek chamber slides (Miles Scientific, IL) were fixed with 4% paraformaldehyde. Immunocytochemical staining was performed using a monoclonal antibody, MRK16 against P-gp and Vectastain Elite ABC kit (Vector Lab., CA). Caki-1/CDDP cells (A) especially at the part of agglutination were intensively positive for P-gp, whereas Caki-1 cells (B) were slightly positive.

reciprocal resistance to MDR drugs. Although the mechanisms which cause this reciprocal phenomenon are unclear, this suggests that MDR drugs are effective on CDDP resistant tumor cells.

5637/DR5.5 cells showed only a negligible amount of mdr1 gene expression but showed a remarkable increase of MRP gene expression. An MRP gene transfection study revealed that MRP overexpression confers MDR similar to that formerly associated exclusively with elevated levels of P-gp. Furthermore, MRP overexpression has no effect on expressions of the mdr1 or the Topo II genes and on CDDP resistance (Grant et al., 1994). K562 cells expressed a relatively high level of the MRP gene, similar to K562/ADM cells. However, K562 cells are quite sensitive to MDR drugs (Nishio et al., 1990) and MRP expression seems more ubiquitous and abundant among various organs and tissues. These suggest that MDR results principally from mdr1/P-gp overexpression rather than MRP overproduction.

ACKNOWLEDGMENT

We thank Dr. Takashi Tsuruo for providing K562 and K562/ADM cell lines and the monoclonal antibody, MRK16. This work was partly supported by Grants-in-Aid from the Ministry of Education, Science and Culture to M.F. and Y.K.

REFERENCES

1. Arao, S., Suwa, H., Mandai, M., Tashiro, H., Miyazaki, K., Okamura, H., Nomura, H., Hiai, H. and Fukumoto, M. (1994). Expression of multidrug resistance gene and localization of P-glycoprotein in human primary ovarian cancer. *Cancer Res.* 54:1355-1359.
2. Biedler, J.L. and Riehm, H. (1970). Cellular resistance to Actinomycin D in Chinese hamster cells in vitro: cross-resistance, radioautographic, and cytogenetic studies. *Cancer Res.* 30:1174-1184.
3. Cole, S.P.C., Bhardwaj, G., Gerlach, J.H., Mackie, J.E., Grant, C.E., Almquist, K.C., Stewart, A.J., Kurz, E.U., Duncan, A.M.V. and Deeley, R.G. (1992). Overexpression of a transporter gene in a multidrug-resistant human lung cancer cell line. *Science* 258:1650-1654.
4. Fernandes, D.J., Catapono, C.V. and Townsend, A.J. (1993). Topoisomerase-related mechanisms of drug resistance. In: Teicher, B.A. (ed). Drug resistance in oncology pp479-498. Marcel Dekker, New York.
5. Frei III, E. Curative cancer chemotherapy. (1985). *Cancer Res.* 45:6523-6537.

6. Grant, C.E., Valdimarsson, G., Hipfner, D.R., Almquist, K.C., Cole, S.P.C. and Deeley, R.G. (1994). Overexpression of multidrug resistance-associated protein (MRP) increases resistance to natural product drugs. *Cancer Res.* 54;357-361.
7. De Jong, S., Timmer-Bossha, H., de Vries, E.G.E. and Mulder, N.H. (1990). Increased topoisomerase II activity in a cisplatin resistant cell line. *Proc. Am. Assoc. Cancer Res.* 31:337.
8. Hamaguchi, K., Godwin, A.K., Yakushiji, M., O'Dwyer, P.J., Ozols, R.F. and Hamilton, T.C. (1993). Cross-resistance to diverse drugs is associated with primary cisplatin resistance in ovarian cancer cell lines. *Cancer Res.* 53:5225-5232.
9. Juliano, R.L. and Ling, V. (1976). A surface glycoprotein modulating drug permeability in Chinese hamster ovary cell mutants. *Biochim. Biophys. Acta* 455:152-162.
10. Krishnamachary, N. and Center, M.S. (1993). The MRP gene associated with a non-P-glycoprotein multidrug resistance encodes a 190-kDa membrane bound glycoprotein. *Cancer Res.* 53:3658-3661.
11. Loehrer, P.J. and Einhorn, L.H. (1984) *Cisplatin. Ann. Intern. Med.* 100:704-713.
12. Nishio, K, Sugimoto, Y., Nakagawa, K., Niimi, S., Fujiwara, Y., Bungo, M., Kasahara, K., Fujiki, H. and Saijo, N. (1990) Cross-resistance to tumour promoters in human cancer cell lines resistant to adriamycin or cisplatin. *Br. J. Cancer* 62:415-419.
13. Ueda, K., Cornwell, M.M., Gottesman, M.M., Pastan, I., Roninson, I.B., Ling, V. and Riorden, J.R. (1986). The MDR gene responsible for multidrug-resistance, codes for P-glycoprotein. *Biochim. Biophys. Res. Commun.* 141:956-962.
14. van der Zee, A.G.J., Hollema, H., de Jong, S., Boonstra, H., Gouw, A., Willemse, P.H.B., Zijlstra, J.G. and de Vries, E.G.E. (1991). P-glycoprotein expression and DNA topoisomerase I and II activity in benign tumors of ovary and in malignant tumors of the ovary, before and after platinum/cyclophosphamide chemotherapy. *Cancer Res.* 51:5915-5920.
15. Young, R.C. Mechanisms to improve chemotherapy effectiveness. (1990). Cancer 65:815-822.

CHAPTER 18

LIPOSOME-ENCAPSULATED CDDP FOR MODIFICATION OF PHARMACOKINETICS AND TISSUE-DISTRIBUTION

Hiromitsu Yabushita, M.D.
Department of Obstetrics and Gynecology, Aichi Medical University.

Liposomes are microscopic phospholipid vesicles that target naturally to organs that have fenestrated capillaries and are rich in phagocytes such as the liver, spleen, and bone marrow (1-11). The considerable attention has been paid to liposomes as a drug delivery system *in vivo*, because liposomes have many properties suitable for drug carriers such as their low intrinsic toxicity, biodegradability, and almost no immunogenicity. In our previous work (12-14), various molar ratios of the constituents of sulfatide-containing liposomes (egg phosphatidylcholine, cholesterol, and sulfatide) were examined with respect to liposomal efficiency to entrap anticancer agent and to the tissue distribution. Among the ratios of the constituents examined, liposome composed of egg phosphatidylcholine, cholesterol, and sulfatide in a molar ratio of 5:4:1 was the best in terms of entrapment efficiency for both multilamellar vesicles and small unilamellar vesicles. The blood clearance of drug was significantly reduced when the drug was encapsulated in the above liposomes, especially in the multilamellar vesicles. Incorporation of drug into tumors was increased when the drug was encapsulated in the small unilamellar vesicles. The degrees of cellular uptake of drug and cytotoxicity were somewhat higher in the free or small unilamellar vesicles-encapsulated drug than in the drug encapsulated in multilamellar vesicles. Entrapment of drugs in liposomes modifies their pharmacokinetics, organ distribution, and metabolism. The ability of liposomes to avoid certain organs provides a way to prevent organ specific toxicities such as doxorubicin cardiotoxicity (12-15).

Several liposome anticancer products are currently being tested in human (5-10).

Cisplatin (CDDP) is one of the most widely used anticancer agents in chemotherapeutic treatment of testicular, ovarian, and bladder cancers (16, 17). Its main limiting toxicity is nephrotoxicity which can be prevented in most patients by intensive hydration prior to its administration. Cisplatin is not myelosuppressive, which allows for combination with myelotoxic agents. The use of cisplatin is currently limited by its limited spectrum of activity, its chronically induced neurotoxicity, and the emergence of resistance in originally sensitive tumors. The development of a cisplatin derivative with activity against cisplatin resistant tumors and reduced toxicity would represent a significant step forward.

In *in vivo* murine model, a liposomal-encapsulated lipophilic analogue of CDDP was specifically concentrated in a tumor (18). Steerenberg et al. (19) demonstrated reduced nephrotoxicity from liposome-entrapped CDDP compared to free CDDP. Gondal et al. (20) reported that a liposomal-entrapped CDDP having a higher total drug capsulation demonstrates higher therapeutic efficacy when administered intraperitoneally and maintains reduced nephrotoxicity.

The temperature-sensitive liposomes entrapped CDDP were active against tumor (21-24). The targeting therapy with a combination of temperature-sensitive liposomes entrapped CDDP with localized hyperthermia was a feasible approach. The liposome is a large unilamellar vesicle composed of dipalmitoylphosphatidyl choline and distearoylphosphatidyl choline in a molar ratio of 9:1, and it has a phase transition temperature of 41 to 42°C and the osmotic pressure of the internal aqueous phase is 1.5 or higher than the physiological one. When the temperature-sensitive liposomes entrapped CDDP were administrated to tumor-bearing mice together with tumor heating, the uptakes of CDDP in the tumor were 3 to 5 times greater than those of an aqueous CDDP solution (24). Also, the tumor responses were well correlated with the drug-targeting.

Perez-Soler et al. (25) synthesized and developed cis-bis-neodecanoato-trans-R,R-1,2-diaminocyclohexane platinum (II) (NDDP), which is a cisplatin derivative with a cyclohexane ring attached to the amino groups and has remarkable biological properties, such as reduced nephrotoxicity and a lack of cross-resistance in murine systems (26, 27). NDDP is completely insoluble in water and is a liposome dependent compound since the liposome carrier is required for its intravenously administration and for its biological activity.

NDDP entrapped in liposomes composed of dimyristoylphosphatidylcholine and dimyristoylphosphatidylglycerol at a 7:3 molar ratio

(L-NDDP) was found to be non-nephrotoxic in dogs (25), not cross-resistant with cisplatin *in vitro* and *in vivo* in different tumor cell systems (28), and more effective than cisplatin in the treatment of experimental liver metastases (29). In a phase I study in human, the maximum tolerated dose of L-NDDP was 312.5 mg/m^2. The dose-limiting toxicity was myelosuppression, mainly affecting the white blood cell lineage. Other toxicities were mild and consisted of nausea, vomiting, diarrhea, fever, malaise, and transient elevation of liver enzymes. No nephrotoxicity was observed (30).

In *in vitro* studies with human colon carcinoma LoVo cells and their counterparts with acquired resistance to cisplatin, L-NDDP was significantly more cytotoxic than free NDDP against both cell lines (28). In *in vivo* studies against L1210 and L1210/PDD leukemia (resistant to cisplatin), free NDDP was devoid of anti-cancer activity at the optimal dose of the liposome-entrapped form and was still significantly less active than the liposomal entrapped form at 3- to 4-fold higher doses (28). These suggested that NDDP was a liposome-dependent anticancer agent and the liposome dependency of NDDP was either due to changes in pharmacokinetics or cellular pharmacology secondary to liposome incorporation or due to an increased or decreased stability of the compound related to a protective or activating effect of the liposomal carrier (31).

In conclusion, the L-CDDP and L-NDDP have a reduced nephrotoxicity, mild other toxicities, small cross-resistance to CDDP and higher therapeutic efficacy compared to free CDDP as shown in Table 1.

Table 1 Characteristics of liposome-encapsulated CDDP and NDDP

	L-CDDP	L-NDDP
Therapeutic efficacy (uptakes in tumor compared to free CDDP)	about 3-4 folds	about 3-5 folds
Cross-resistance to CDDP	small	none
Nephrotoxicity	mild	none
Other side effects	mild	mild

REFERENCES

1. Perez-Soler, R. Liposomes as carriers of antitumor agents: toward a clinical reality. *Cancer Treat. Rev.*, 16: 67-82, 1989.
2. Weinstein, J. N., and Leserman, L. D. Liposomes as drug carriers in cancer chemotherapy. *Pharmacol. Ther.*, 24: 207-233, 1984.
3. Ryman, B. E., and Tyrell, D. A. Liposomes-bags of potential. *Essays Biochem.*, 16: 49-98, 1980.
4. Patel, H. M., and Ryman, B. E. Systemic and oral administration of liposomes. In: Knight (ed.), *Liposomes: From Physical Structure to Therapeutic Applications*. pp. 409-441. Amsterdam: Elsevier/North-Holland Biochemical Press, 1981.
5. Presant, A. F., Turner, A. F., Nadel, H., Wiseman, C., Kennedy, P., et al. Tumor targeted liposomes: implications of liposome (Vescan) imaging of primary and metastatic tumors for liposomal chemotherapy. *Proc. Am. Soc. Clin. Oncol.*, 8: 10, 1989.
6. Treat, J., Greenspan, A., Forst, D., Maternowski, A., and Rahman, A. Liposome encapsulated doxorubin (LED): phase II trial in recurrent breast cancer. *Proc. Am. Soc. Clin. Oncol.*, 8: 37, 1989.
7. Gabizon, A., Sulkes, A., Brain, S., Amselem, S., and Barenholz, Y. Liposome-associated doxorubicin (L-Dox): a clinical study with an improved preparation. *Proc. Am. Soc. Clin. Oncol.*, 8: 37, 1989.
8. Cowens, J. W., Kanter, P., Brenner, D. E., Ginsberg, R., Meyer, L, et al. Phase I study of doxorubicin encapsulated in liposomes. *Proc. Am. Soc. Clin. Oncol.*, 8: 69, 1989.
9. Hartman, L. C., Steis, R. G., Urba, W. J., Smith, J. W., Creekmore, S., Sznol, M., et al. Phase I study of a muramyl tripeptide derivative, MTP-PE. *Proc. Am Soc. Clin. Oncol.*, 8: 179, 1989.
10. Lam, K., Ahman, F., Hultquist, K., Gschwind, C., and Hersh, E. Phase I study of liposomal muramyl tripeptide-phosphatidylethanolamine (MTP-PE) in cancer patients. *Proc. Am. Soc. Clin. Oncol.*, 8: 185, 1989.
11. Gabizon, A., and Papahadjopoulos, D. Liposome formulation with prolonged circulation time in blood and enhanced uptake by tumors. *Proc. Natl. Acad. Sci.*, 85: 6949-6953, 1988.
12. Ueno, N., Yabushita, H., Noguchi, M., Ishihara, M., Kojima, N., and Yagi, K. Effect of adriamycin entrapped in liposomes on ovarian carcinama cells. *J. Clin. Bichem. Nutr.*, 7: 53-58, 1989.
13. Takano, M., Kojima, N., Ueno, N., Yabushita, H., Noguchi, M., Ishihara, M., and Yagi, K. Improved sulfatide-containing liposomes as carriers of adriamycin. *J. Clin. Biochem. Nutr.*, 4: 223-233, 1988.
14. Kojima, N., Ueno, N., Takano, M., Yabushita, H., Noguchi, M., Ishihara, M., and Yagi, K. Effect of adriamycin entrapped by

sulfatide-containing liposomes on ovarian tumor-bearing nude mice. *Biotechnology and Applied biochemistry*, 8: 471-478, 1986.

15. Herman, E. H., Rahman, A., Ferrans, V. J., Vick, J. A., and Schein, P. S. Prevention of chronic doxorubicin cardiotoxicity in beagles by liposomal encapsulation. Cancer Res., 43: 5427-5432, 1983.
16. Loehrer, P. J., and Einborn, L. Cisplatin. *Ann. Intern. Med*., 100: 704-713, 1984.
17. Zwelling, L. A., and Kohn, K. W. Platinum complexes. *In*: B. A. Chabner (ed.), *Pharmacologic Principles of Cancer Therapy*, pp. 309-338. Philadelphia: W. B. Saunders Co., 1982.
18. Deliconstantinos, G., Gregoriadis, G., Abel, G., Jones, M., and Robertson, D. Incorporation of *cis*-dichloro-*bis*-cyclopentyl-diammine platinum (II) into liposomes enhances its uptake by ADJ/PC GA tumors implanted subcutaneously into mice. *Biochem. Soc. Trans*., 5: 1326-1328, 1977.
19. Steerenberg, P. A., Storm, G., Groot, G., et al. Liposomes as drug carrier system for *cis*-diamminedichloroplatinum (II). *Cancer Chemother. Pharmacol*., 21: 299-307, 1988.
20. Gondal, J. A., Preuss, H. G., Swartz, R., and Rahman, A. Comparative pharmacological, toxicological and antitumoral evaluation of free and liposome-encapsulated cisplatin in rodents. *Eur. J. Cancer*. 29A: 1536-1542, 1993.
21. Yatvin, M. B., Muehlensiepen, H., Porschen, W., Weinstein J. N., and Feinendegen, L. E. Selective delivery of liposome-associated cis-dichlorodiammine platinum (II) by heat and its influence on tumor uptake and growth. *Cancer Res*., 41: 1601-1607, 1981.
22. Iga, K., Ogawa, Y., and Toguchi, H. Heat-induced drug release rate and maximal targeting index of thermosensitive in tumor-bearing mice. *Pharm. Res*. 9: 658-662, 1992.
23. Iga, K., Ogawa, Y., and Toguchi, H. Rates of systemic degradation and reticuloendothelial system (RES) uptake of thermosensitive liposome encapsulating cisplatin in rats. *Pharm. Res*., 10: 1332-1337, 1993.
24. Iga, K., Hamaguchi, N., Igari, Y., Ogawa, Y., Toguchi, H., and Shimamoto, T. Increased tumor cisplatin levels in heated tumors in mice after administration of thermosensitive, large unilameller vesicles encapsulating cisplatin. *J. Pharm. Sci*., 80: 522-525, 1991.
25. Perez-Soler, R., Lautersztain, J., Stephens, L. C., Wright, K., and Khokhar, A. R. Preclinical toxicity and pharmacology of liposome-entrapped *cis-bis*-neodecanoato-*trans-R,R*-1,2-diaminocyclohexa-neplatinum (II). *Cancer Chemoter. Pharmacol*., 24: 1-8, 1989.
26. Prestayko, A. W., Bradner, W. T., Huftalen, J. B., et al. Antileukemic (L1210) activity and toxicity of *cis*-dichlorodiammine-platinum (II) analogs. *Cancer Treat. Rep*., 63: 1503-1507, 1979.

27. Burchenal, J. H., Kelaher, K., O'Toole, T., and Chisholm, J. Lack of cross-resistance between certain platinum coordination compounds in mouse leukemia. *Cancer Res.*, 37: 3455-3457, 1977.
28. Perez-Soler, R., Yang, L. Y., Drewinko, B., Lautersztain, J., and Khokhar, A. R. Increased cytotoxicity and reversal of resistance to *cis*-diamminedichloroplatinum (II) with entrapment of *cis-bis*-neodecanoato-*trans-R,R*-1,2-diaminocyclohexaneplatinum (II) in multilamellar lipid vesicles. *Cancer Res.*, 48: 4509-4512, 1988.
29. Perez-Soler, R., Khokhar, A. R., and Lopez-Berestein, G. Treatment and prophylaxis of experimental liver metastases of M5076 reticulosarcoma with *cis-bis*-neodecanoato-*trans-R,R*-1,2-diaminocycloheaneplatinum (II) encapsulated in multilamellar vesicles. *Cancer Res.*, 47: 6462-6466, 1987.
30. Perez-Soler, R., Lopez-Berestein, G., Lautersztain, J., Al-Baker, S., Francis, K., Macias-Kiger, D., Raber, M. N., and Khokhar A. R. Phase I clinical and pharmacological study of liposome-entrapped *cis-bis*-neodecanoato-*trans-R,R*-1,2-diaminocyclohexaneplatinum (II). *Cancer Res.*, 50: 4254-4259, 1990.
31. Perez-Soler, R., and Khokhar, A. R. Lipophilic cisplatin analogues entrapped in liposomes: Role of intraliposomal drug activation in biological activity. *Cancer Res.*, 52: 6341-6347, 1992.

PART IV

CLINICAL IMPLICATIONS IN CDDP RESISTANCE

CHAPTER 19

CLINICAL INVESTIGATIONS FOR CIRCUMVENTION OF CDDP RESISTANCE

Masayuki Hatae, Yoshitaka Onishi, Yasutaka Maeda
Department of Obstetrics and Gynecology, Kagoshima City Hospital, Kajiya 20-17, Kagoshima city, Kagoshima 892, Japan

USEFULNESS OF CISPLATIN IN CONVENTIONAL COMBINATION CHEMOTHERAPY FOR OVARIAN CANCER

Ovarian cancer is a highly chemosensitive tumor and chemotherapeutic agents from many different classes have shown activity. Clinical trials during past 20 years have revealed that platinum combination chemotherapy was superior to single agent therapy or other combination in overall response rate (1). A recent meta-analysis comparing survival of advanced ovarian cancer treated with single nonplatinum agents or nonplatinum combinations failed to demonstrate a significant advantage for the combination chemotherapy (2).

The demonstration that cisplatin was active in previously treated patients with advanced ovarian cancer led to the evaluation of cisplatin in the combination chemotherapy of previously untreated patients .The largest control trial of a platinum containing regimen versus a nonplatinum regimen was performed by Gynecologic Oncology Group (GOG) in USA. Patients with advanced ovarian cancer were randomized to receive treatment with the combination of doxorubicin plus cyclophosphamide (AC) or cisplatin, doxorubicin and cyclophosphamide (PAC). The latter PAC chemotherapy was superior to the former two drug regimen with regard to complete response rate, median response duration, progression free interval and overall survival(3). Superiority of cisplatin containing regimens in ovarian cancer patients has been established by the other control studies from Netherlands Cancer Institute comparing the CHAP-5 to Hexa-CAF (4) and the Mayo Clinic trial of cyclolophosphamide and cisplatin compared with cyclophosphamide alone (5). These clinical trials have given the basis for the routine use of cisplatin in combination chemotherapy for previously untreated patients with advanced ovarian cancer.

The role of doxorubicin used in combination with cisplatin has also been investigated in several large well controlled clinical trials. The GOG compared cisplatin plus cyclophosphamide (CP) with the PAC combination in 349 patients with advanced disease(6). The pathologically confirmed complete remission (pCR) rates were similar between the two treatment regimens. There was also no significant difference in progression-free interval or overall survival. Similarly, the Netherlands Cancer Institute group failed to demonstrate that in randomized trial comparing two combination chemotherapy regimens (CHAP-5 vs CP) in advanced ovarian carcinoma the CHAP-5 regimen was superior to CP(7). However, after 7 years of follow up, a large clinical trial in Italy comparing PAC with CP has demonstrated a significantly higher pCR rate (62% vs 40%) and a 10-month increase in median survival in patients treated with the doxorubicin containing regimen(8,9). Meta-analyses of these two trials and additional two randomized studies(10-12) demonstrated a benefit of the doxorubicin-containing regimen with regard to prolongation of survival time.

The interpretation of results obtained from clinical trials comparing the CP regimen versus the PAC regimen have been limited because of differences in toxicity and in dose intensity between these two regimens. Equitoxic regimens have not routinely been compared, and in most studies, doxorubicin has merely been added to cisplatin plus cyclophosphamide. This usually led to an increased dose intensity for the PAC regimen(13).

BASIC RESEARCH FOR CDDP DOSE ESCALATION IN OVARIAN CANCER

Gill et al.(14) have used an immunodensitometry assay to measure levels of platinum-DNA damage in nuclei of buccal mucosa cells of patients receiving cisplatin and carboplatin. In the small number of patients studied, adduct levels in buccal mucosa cells were higher in those patients who responded to therapy.

In a blind cohort study of cisplatin and carboplatin -treated patients with 15 different tumor types, Parker et al.(15) measured the formation of platinum-DNA adduct in peripheral blood leukocyte using atomic absorption spectrometry method. The adduct levels in patients who responded to initial therapy were 3-fold higher than those in non-responders ($p=0.0017$). The higher adduct levels in responder, the higher response rates were obtained ($p=0.00011$). These studies provide insight into the biology of resistance to DNA binding agents. It is clear that increased levels of DNA adduct formation are directly related to tumor cell kill. Since the DNA adduct levels in leukocyte were well correlated with clinical tumor response, the adduct levels in leukocytes seemed to reflect indirectly adduct levels in tumor tissues. This finding is also supported by data from autopsy studies where DNA adduct levels in tumor and bone marrow tissues were virtually identical(16).

DOSE INTENSIFICATION OF CDDP

The standard chemotherapeutic regimen for ovarian cancer has been the combination of cisplatin plus cyclophosphamide in United States. In addition, retrospective studies have indicated that the dose intensity of cisplatin is an important factor in achieving optimal results. Several clinical trials have been performed to evaluate therapeutic efficacy of the cisplatin-based combination chemotherapy and found out a substantial clinical improvement as indicated by increased response rate, increased duration of response and increased time to progression. However, overall effect on survival has been modest(17). The dose of cisplatin in these two-drug combinations has ranged from 50 mg/m^2 to 200 mg/m^2 and the median survival has ranged from 21 months to more than 36 months with a general trend for prolonged median survival in patients receiving the higher doses of cisplatin(18).

A retrospective study of 33 published trials demonstrated that cisplatin was the most active single agent for treatment of epithelial ovarian tumors and the clinical outcome in advanced ovarian cancer was correlated with the dose intensity of cisplatin.

Several prospective trials were initiated to elucidate a relationship between dose intensity and the outcome. The Gynecologic Oncology Group in USA similarly performed a prospective randomized study concerning on a population with suboptimally debulked disease ($\geq$1 cm residual disease following laparotomy)(19). In this large study, which evaluated 485 patients, although a trend increasing both progressive-free and overall survival was seen, this did not made a statistical significance. In this study, the high-dose arm received a 2-fold increases in dose intensity, with identical total dose of drug being delivered.

Kaye et al.(20) reported on a randomized study of two doses of cisplatin given with cyclophosphamide. Patients were randomized to receive six doses of cyclophosphamide every 3 weeks with either 50 mg/m^2 or 100 mg/m^2 cisplatin. In this study, patients of the high-dose arm received 1.3 times higher dose than those of the low-dose arm. Additionally, the high-dose arm delivered 66% higher total dose of cisplatin than the low-dose arm. Analysis of this study is further complicated by the fact that a significant number of patients tested had early stage ovarian cancer and were treated in an adjuvant setting.

Pecorelli et al. performed a controlled clinical trial of two different dose intensity induction regimens in advanced ovarian cancer patients. In this study, 306 patients with stage III and IV were randomized to conventional dose (cisplatin 75 mg/m^2 and cyclophosphamide 750 mg/m^2 iv every 3 weeks x 6 courses) or dose intense (cisplatin 50 mg/m^2 every week x 9 courses). The study design allowed a double dose intensity with a similar total dose (450 mg/m^2) and no dose modification of CDDP. Response rate of dose intense regimen was not increased, compared to conventional dose in evaluation at 1993. According to pathological CR, there was no difference in patients with residual tumor >2 cm following laparotomy between both treatment arms in 1994 report. On the contrary, a statistically significant difference ($p=0.004$) in pathological CR was observed in patients with residual tumor ≤2 cm. A longer follow-up is necessary to determine whether the achievement of substantial responses will have any impact on long term results.

CBDCA AND CDDP COMBINATION

In order to increase platinum dose intensity, combined effects of cisplatin and carboplatin have been studied. Due to comparable efficacy and nonoverlapping toxicities, this treatment modality has been proved to be a feasible approach. Two published studies suggest that nearly full doses of each platinum analog can be combined with acceptable toxicity(22,23). This combination allows 1.5 - 2 fold intensity of cisplatin equivalent dose in standard therapy. Although carboplatin followed by cisplatin may lead to higher myelosuppression, this treatment modality potentially decreases the probability of cisplatin induced renal dysfunction. The Copenhagen Ovarian Cancer Study Group reported a phase II study combining carboplatin and cisplatin. They reported an overall pathologic response rate of 62% by combination therapy of 300 mg/m^2 carboplatin followed by 100 mg/m^2 cisplatin given every 4 weeks. Pathological complete response rate in this study was 22% (22). A subsequent study combined cisplatin and carboplatin with ifosfamide showed a pathological complete response rate of 42% in 37 previously untreated patients(24).

The Belgian Study Group performed a phase I/II trial in 30 untreated patients with bulky residual ovarian cancer(23). They used a staring dose of 300 mg/m^2 carboplatin on day 1 and 100 mg/m^2 cisplatin on day 2 with a vigorous 48 hour hydration scheme, and obtained the same potential complete response rate (22%). A number of combined platinum studies have been reported in the literature (14, 25-28). The planned platinum dose intensity for these trials varies between 37.5 and 63 mg/m^2/week. It is clear that due to myelotoxicity frequent dose reductions were necessary, and thus the delivered platinum dose intensity was significantly lower than the optimal dose.

HIGH DOSE CARBOPLATIN

The dose of carboplatin can be increased with the use of cytokines for eliminating bone marrow toxicity. Reed et al.(29) performed a phase I/II trial of high-dose carboplatin 800 mg/m^2 iv every 35 days with escalating doses of recombinant granulocyte macrophage colony stimulating factor (rGM-CSF) in patients with refractory ovarian cancer. The response rate of 35% (2 CRs and 6 PRs) was similar to the results (27.5%) in a previous study of high-dose carboplatin without rGM-CSF. It is well-known that high-dose carboplatin cause thrombopenia and cumulative myelosuppression and subsequently have its limited dose-escalation.

DOSE INTENSIFIED CLINICAL TRIAL IN KAGOSHIMA CITY HOSPITAL

1) CBDCA AND CDDP COMBINATION THERAPY

Although standard chemotherapeutic regimen for ovarian cancer in Kagoshima City Hospital was cisplatin 50 mg/m^2, adriamycin 50 mg/m^2 plus cyclophosphamide 500 mg/m^2 (CAP) iv every 4 week x 6 courses from 1983 to 1987, the regimen was changed to cisplatin 80 mg/m^2 and cyclophosphamide 500 mg/m^2 (CP) iv every 4 week x 6 courses since 1988. In historical comparison between both regimens, we could not find any significant difference in median survival and clinical response rate of previously untreated patients with stage III advanced ovarian cancer. Therefore, we chose a combination chemotherapy consisting of carboplatin 350 mg/m^2 day 1 and cisplatin 80 mg/m^2 day 3 iv (so called JP regimen) every 4 week x 6 courses to increase platinum dose intensity and the total dose as a third regimen for previously untreated patients with stage III ovarian cancer from 1991. Dose intensity and total dose in

CDDP equivalence of this JP regimen are two times in that of our CP standard regimen. From our historical studies, the JP regimen seemed to be superior to the conventional CAP and CP regimens with regard to the response rate and overall survival rate for stage III ovarian cancer. The clinical response rate was 26.7% for CAP, 36.4% for CP and 75.0%. for JP. The pathological response rate was 36.4% for CAP, 40.0% for CP and 72.7% for JP (Table 1). Overall survival in stage III ovarian cancer was 50% for CAP, 50% for CP and 71.2% for JP at 2 years and 33.3% for CAP, 25% for CP and 71.2% for JP at 3 years, respectively (Fig.1). Moreover, it is noteworthy that the JP regimen showed the satisfactory response for stage IV ovarian cancer (Table 2). As shown in Table 3, this JP regimen seemed to be effective for patients who initially responded to CAP or CP regimen, while to be ineffective for patients who did not

Table 1. Clinical evaluation of J-P regimen as first line chemotherapy for stage III and IV cancer

	CAP	CP	JP
CR(pCR)	1(1)	3(3)	5(4)
PR	3	1	4(4)
NC	5	2	2
PD	2	4	1
NE	4	1	3
Total	15	11	15
Clinical response rate	4/15(26.7%)	4/11(36.4%)	9/12(75.0%)
Pathological response rate	4/11(36.4%)	4/10(40.0%)	8/11(72.7%)

Table 2. Response rate of J-P regimen as first line chemotherapy for stage III and IV cancer

	Clinical response	Pathologica response
Stage III	CR 3 PR 2 NC 1 PD 1 NE 3	CR 3 PR 2 NC 2 PD 1
Stage IV	CR 2 PR 2 NC 1	CR 1 PR 2
Total response rate	75.0%	72.7%

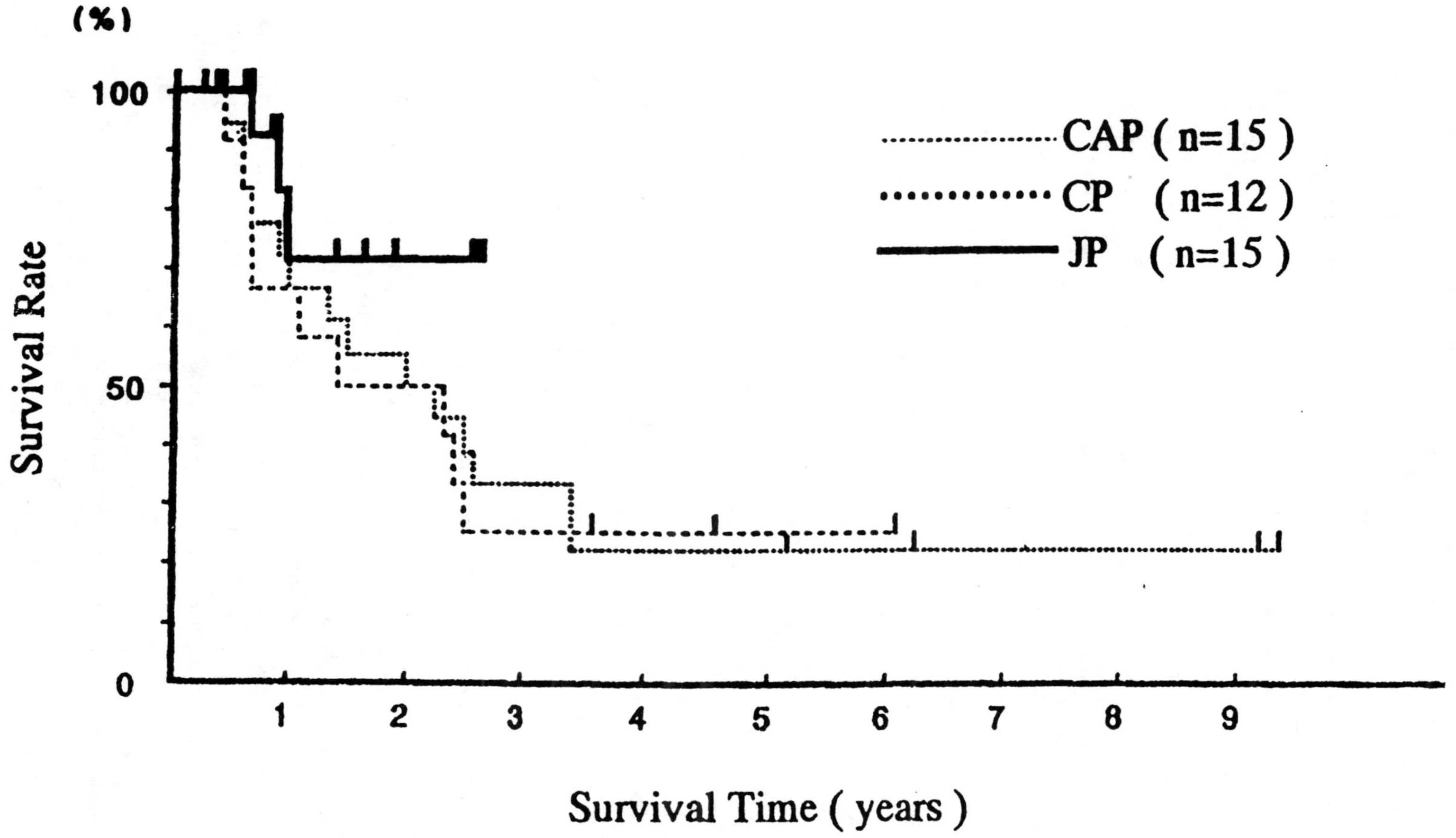

Fig.1 Comparison of survival curves of stage III ovarian cancer patients treated with three different regimens.

Table 3. Clinical evaluation of J-P regimen as second line for ovarian cancer

	case	drug free interval (month)	clinical response
Primary resistance to CP or CAP	1	1	PR
	2	1	PD
	3	1	PD
	4	2	PD
	5	2	PD
	6	2	PD
Recurrence after treatment with CP or CAP	7	13	PD
	8	7	PR
	9	8	NC
	10	8	PR
	11	25	PR
	12	11	NC
SLO positive after treatment with CP or CAP	13	8	CR
	14	6	CR
	15	3	NC

Total response rate (CR+PR); 6/15 (40.0%)
Response rate with drug free interval more than 6 months (CR+PR) ; 4/7 (57.1%)

respond to CAP or CP regimen. Namely, only 1 of 6 patients with primary resistance to CP or CAP regimen had partial response to this JP regimen, while 2 of 3 SLO positive patients who initially responded to CP of CPA regimen had complete response (Table 3).

2) INTRAPERITONEAL (IP) CHEMOTHERAPY

Clinical trials of intraperitoneal chemotherapy in the last decade have been shown to be technically feasible in the majority of patients with ovarian cancer. Although most drugs administered intraperitoneally have a pharmacologic advantage, several questions remain about the role of this treatment modality in patients with ovarian cancer. Intraperitoneal chemotherapy may be ineffective for patients with bulky disease because of the poor drug penetration into tumor masses. Consequently, recent IP trials have focused primarily on the treatment of patients with small volume disease as consolidation after negative second look operation or as second line chemotherapy for patients with minimum residual disease which had respond to initial CDDP containing chemotherapy and have enough treatment free interval over 6 or 12 months after prior chemotherapy.

We assume effectiveness of intraperitoneal chemotherapy as second line chemotherapy because of relative dose-dependency of CDDP and the direct tumor response. After JP treatment for advanced ovarian cancer, IP treatment which consisted of CDDP 100 mg/m^2 and etoposide 200 mg/m^2 with 1500 ml saline every 4 weeks x 6 cycles demonstrated satisfactory clinical effects in two cases who had partial response to initial JP regimen and 6 months treatment free interval. Both two cases have no recurrence for 18 and 22 months respectively after this IP therapy. Fig. 2 shows the clinical course of a patient who had no evidence of disease after JP and IP therapy. Several clinical evidence revealed that the level of resistance to CDDP in clinical treatment was no more than five times except for primary resistance. Markman also confirmed that the salvage CDDP-based IP chemotherapy was effective in patients with small-volume (< 0.5 cm) residual ovarian tumor who responded to initial CDDP-based therapy and /or who relapsed more than 6 months after completing initial systemic chemotherapy(30). The latter evidence may be corresponding to spontaneous reversibility of acquired resistance to CDDP during drug exposure free interval. These interesting clinical evidence may support the reasonable availability of IP salvage chemotherapy for ovarian cancer.

CLINICAL TRIAL IN SUPER HIGH DOSE CHEMOTHERAPY OF CBDCA BASED REGIMEN SUPPORTED BY ABMT OR PBSCT

Based on the results from phase I trials of high-dose chemotherapy with autologous bone marrow transplantation (ABMT), a number of phase II studies have been performed in patients with refractory ovarian cancer. The overall prognosis for patients with refractory ovarian cancer remains to be poor even after high-dose chemotherapy supported by ABMT. Despite high response rates (27 CR and 25 PR in 94 patients, response rate; 55.3%) generated by such treatment, short duration of the response and the high toxicity (including treatment-related deaths) have been obtained. One would predict that ovarian cancer patients with small tumor burden, minimally pretreated and with chemotherapy responsive disease, would have a better outcome to high-dose treatment. Several clinical trials have demonstrated encouraging data in ovarian cancer patients with small volume and chemosensitive persistent disease after front-line treatment (i.e., patients with positive second-look surgery). Little information exists regarding the efficacy and feasibility of high-dose chemotherapy with peripheral blood stem cell transfusion (PBSCT)

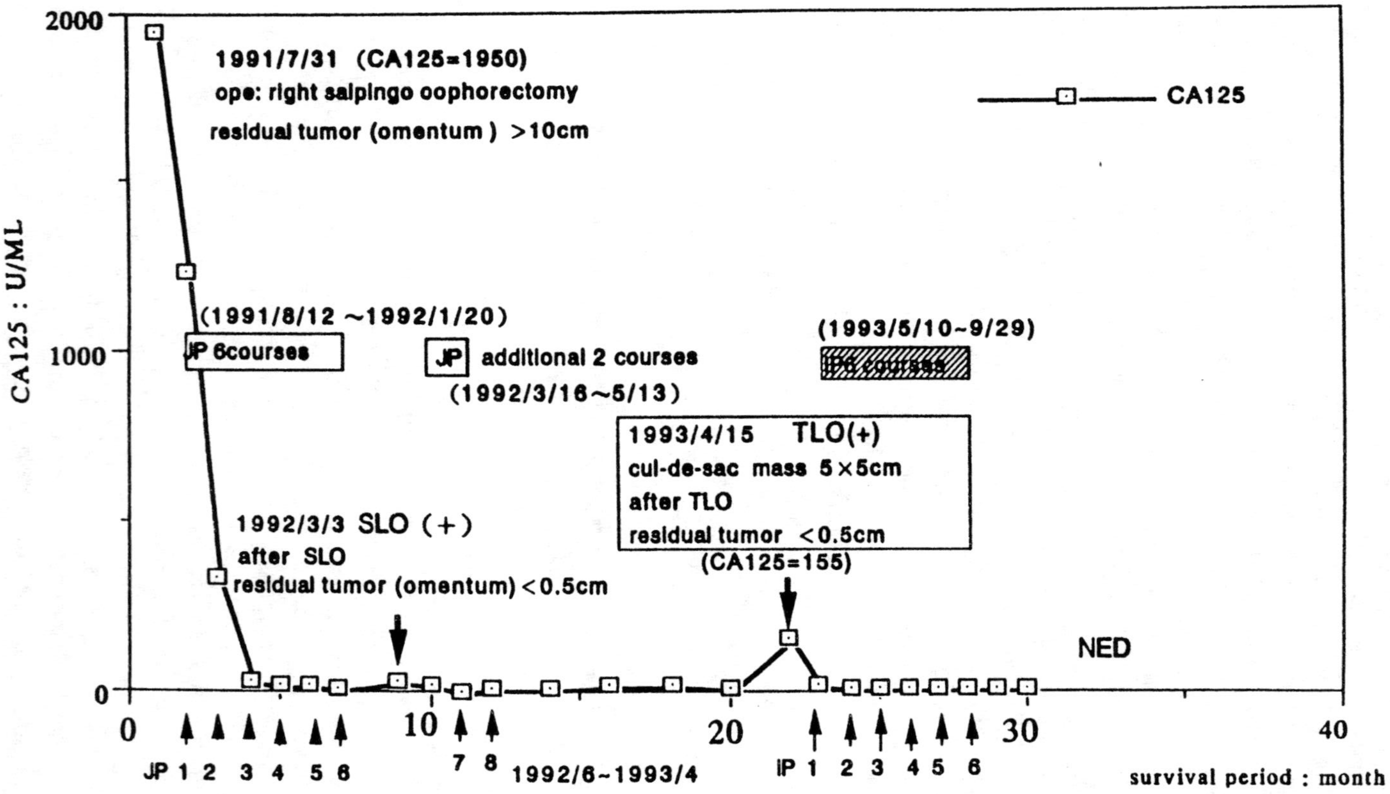

Fig.2 Clinical course of a patient with stage IIIc serous cystadenocarcinoma. She received 6 courses JP treatment after first surgery. Second look operation (SLO) revealed the residual tumor in the omentum (<0.5 cm). After additional 2 courses of JP treatment, tumor mass (5 x 5 cm) in cul-de-sac was removed at third look operation (TLO). After cytoreduction at TLO, she received 6 cycles of i. p. treatment by CDDP and is alive with no evidence of disease (NED).

for ovarian cancer after primary cytoreductive surgery. Results from high -dose chemotherapy trials supported by PBSCT in patients with recurrent disease has suggested the usefulness of such aggressive treatment. Furthermore, recent and preliminary data suggest that PBSCT is better than ABMT in supporting high-dose chemotherapy for treatment of ovarian cancer and offers certain technical and clinical advantages. The advantages of high-dose chemotherapy supported by PBSCT had less bone marrow damage and relatively low morbidity, especially by using hematopoietic growth factors.The feasibility of such an approach was tested in three clinical trials for untreated advanced ovarian cancer patients, showing 70.8-81.8% response rate (31-32). Finally we must make sure whether such high dose-chemotherapy supported by PBSCT is effective to obtain not only high response rate but also the long term survival in refractory ovarian cancer patients.

SUMMARY

Cisplatin for treatment of ovarian cancer has special entity because this anticancer agent is highly sensitive and the dose escalation correlates to increased response rate, increased duration of response and increased time to progression. Same phenomena can not be recognized in other gynecological tumors such as cervical cancer and endometrial cancer. Recent in-vitro investigations might support that solid tumors with high sensitivity to cisplatin such as epithelial ovarian cancer, germ cell tumor and testicular carcinoma have inducibility of apoptosis by cisplatin. We need to define whether very high dose escalation beyond ordinary dose of cisplatinum analogs can contribute to the long term survival as first line chemotherapy in patients with minimum residual tumor after maximal cytoreduction. More intensified cisplatin containing regimen as salvage therapy demonstrates considerable response, if the tumor showed sensitivity to cisplatin in prior chemotherapy , the residual tumor is minimum and treatment free interval is over 6 or 12 month. The longer interval of drug free, the higher response rate can be resulted in. In our clinical trials, so called JP regimen (consisted of carboplatin iv and cisplatin iv) and so called EP regimen (consisted of cisplatin ip and etoposide ip) showed satisfactory response rates as second line chemotherapy. High dose chemotherapy supported by PBSCT may be of clinical use for ovarian cancer as well as breast cancer, lymphoma and germ cell tumor.

REFERENCES

1. Ozols, R.F., and Young, R.C. Chemotherapy of ovarian cancer *Semin. Oncol.*, 11: 251-263, 1984.
2. Advanced Ovarian Cancer Trialists Group. Chemotherapy in advanced ovarian cancer: an overview of randomized clinical trials. *Br. Med. J.*, 303: 884-893, 1991.
3. Omura, G., Blessing, J. A., Ehrlich, C. E., Miller, A., Yordan, E., Creasman, W. T. and Homesley, H. D. A randomized trial of cyclophosphamide and doxorubicin with or without cisplatin in advanced ovarian carcinoma. *Cancer* 57: 1725-1730, 1986.
4. Decker, D. G., Fleming, T.R., Malkasian, G. D. Jr., Webb, M. J., Jeffries, J. A. and Edmonson, J. H. Cyclophosphamide plus cisplatinum in combination: Treatment program for stage III or IV ovarian carcinoma. *Obstet Gynecol* 60: 481, 1982.
5. Neijt, J.P., ten Bokkel Huinink, W.W., van der Burg M.E., van Oosterom, A. T., Vriesendorp, R., Kooyman, C. D., van Lindert, A. C., Hamerlynck, J. V., van Lent, M., van Houwelingen, J. C. et al. Randomized trial comparing combination chemotherapy regimens (Hexa-CAF vs CHAP-5) in advanced ovarian carcinoma. *Lancet* 2: 594-600, 1984.
6. Omura, G., Bundy, B., Berek, J., Curry, S., Delgado, G. and Mortel, R. Randomized trial of cyclophosphamide plus cisplatin with or without doxorubicin in ovarian carcinom: a Gynecologic Oncolgy Group study. *J. Clin. Oncol.* 7: 457-465, 1989.
7 Neijt, J.P., ten Bokkel Huinink, W.W., van der Burg, M. E., van Oosterom, A. T., Willemse, P. H., Heintz, A. P., van Lent, M., Trimbos, J. B., Bouma, J., Vermorken, J. B. et al. Randomized trial comparing two combination chemotherapy regimens (CHAP-5 vs CP) in advanced ovarian carcinoma. *J. Clin. Oncol.* 5: 1157-1158, 1987.
8. Conte, P.F., Bruzzone, M., Chiara, S., Sertoli, M. R., Daga, M. G., Rubagotti, A., Conio, A., Ruvolo, M., Rosso, R., Santi, L. et al. A randomized trial comparing cisplatin plus cyclophosphamide versus cisplatin, doxorubicin and cyclophosphamide in advanced ovarian cancer. *J. Clin. Oncol.* 4: 965-971, 1986.
9. Bruzzone, M., Repetto, L., Chiara, S. et al. A randomized trial comparing PC vs PAC chemotherapy in epithelian ovarian cancer: 7 years follow-up. *Proc Am. Soc. Clin. Oncol.*9: 610, 1990.
10. Gruppo Interegionale Cooperativo Oncologico Ginecologia. Randomized comparison of cisplatin with cyclophosphamide/ cisplatin and with cyclophosphamide/doxorubicin/cisplatin in advanced ovarian cancer. *Lancet* 2: 353-359,1987.

11. Bertelsen, K., Jakobsen, A., Andersen, J. E., Ahrons, S., Pedersen, P. H., Kiaer, H., Arffmann, E., Bichel, P., Boestofte, E., Stroyer, I.et al. A randomized study of cyclo-phosfamide and cisplatinum with or without doxorubicin in advanced ovarian carcinoma. *Gynecol. Oncol.* 28: 161-169,1987.
12. The Ovarian Cancer Meta-Analysis Project. Cyclophosphamide plus cisplatin versus cyclophosphamide, doxorubicin, and cisplatin chemotherapy of ovarian caricinoma: a meta-analysis. *J. Clin. Oncol.* 9: 1668-1674, 1991.
13. Levin, L., Hryniuk, W. M. Dose intensity analysis of chemotherapy regimens in ovarian carcinoma. *J. Clin. Oncol.* 5: 756-767, 1987.
14. Gill, I., Muggia, F.M., Terheggen, P.M., Michael, C., Parker, R.J., Kortes , V., Grunberg, S., Christian, M.C., Reed, E., den Engelse, L. Dose-escalation study of carboplatin (day 1) and cisplatin (day 3): tolerance and relation to leukocyte and buccal cell platinum-DNA adducts. *Ann.Oncol.* 2: 115-121, 1991.
15. Parker, R. J., Gill, I., Tarone, R., Vionnet, J., A., Grunberg, S., Muggia, F., Reed, E. Platinum-DNA damage in leukocyte DNA of patients receiving carboplatin and cisplatin chemotherapy, measured by atomic absorption spectometry. *Carcinogenesis* 12: 1253-1258, 1991.
16. Reed, E., Gupta-Burt, S., Katz, D., Poirier, M. C. Platinum-DNA adduct measured at autopsy in multiple human tissues. *Proc. Am. Assoc. Cancer Res.* 30: 276, 1989.
17. Ozols, R. F., Rubin, S. C., Dembo, A.J. and Robboy, S. *Epithelial Ovarian Cancer; Principles and Practice of Gynecologic Oncology.* J. B. Lippincott Company, Philadelphia, 731-781, 1992.
18. McGuire, W. P. Dose intensity in ovarian cancer. American Society of Clinical Oncology Educational Book, pp31-36, *American Society of Clinical Oncology*, 1993.
19. McGuire, W. P., Hoskins, W. J., Brady. M. F., Homesley, H. D. and Clarke-Pearson, D. L. The Gynecologic Oncology Group (GOC). A phase III trial of dose-intense (DI) versus standard dose (DS) cisplatin (CDDP) and cytoxan (CTX) in advanced ovarian cancer(AOC). *Proc Am. Soc. Clin. Oncol.* 11: 226, 1992.
20. Kaye, S. B. High dose cisplatin (100 mg/sm) is more effective than low dose (50 mg/sm) in combination with cyclophosphamide (750 mg/sm) for the treatment of advanced ovarian cancer. *Proc. Int. Gynecol. Cancer Soc.* 3: 170, 1991.
21. Pecorelli, S., Marsoni, S., Belloni, C.et al. Controlled clinical trial of two different dose intensity induction regimens in advanced ovarian cancer patients. *Proc. Int. Gynecol. Cancer Soc.* 3: 215, 1991.
22. Lund, B., Hansen, M., Hansen, O. P. and Hansen, H. H. High-dose platinum consisting of combined carboplatin and cisplatin in

previously untreated ovarian cancer patients with residual disease. *J. Clin. Oncol.* 7: 1469-1473, 1989.
23. Piccart, M. J., Nogaret, J. M., Marcelis, L., Longree, H., Ries, F., Kains, J. P., Gobert, P., Domange, A. M., Sculier, J. P. and Gompel, C. Cisplatin combined with carboplatin: A new way of intensification of platinum dose in the treatment of advanced ovarian cancer. *J. Natl. Cancer Inst.* 82: 703-707, 1990.
24. Lund, B., Hansen, M., Hansen, O. P. and Hansen, H. H. Combined high-dose carboplatin and cisplatin, and ifosfamide in previously untreated ovarian cancer patients with residual disease. *J. Clin. Oncol.* 8: 1226-1230, 1990.
25. Trump, D., L., Grem, J. L., Tutsch, K. D., Willson, J. K., Simon, K. J., Alberti, D., Storer, B. and Tormey, D. C. Platinum analog combination chemotherapy: cisplatin and carboplatin: a phase I trial with pharmacokinetic assessment of the effects of cisplatin administration on carboplatin excretion. *J. Clin. Oncol.* 5: 1281-1289, 1987.
26. Dittrich, C., Sevelda, P., Baur, M., Marth, C., Hudec, M., Vavra, N., Grunt, T., Fazeny, B. and Salzer, H. In vitro and in vivo evaluation of the combination of cisplatin and its anlogue carboplatin for platinum dose intensification in ovarian carcinoma. *Cancer* (Phila.) 71: 3082-3090, 1993.
27. Hardy, J. R., Wiltshaw, E., Blake, P. R., Harper, P., Slevin, M., Perren, T. J. and Tan, S. Cisplatin and carboplatin in combination for the treatment of stage IV ovarian carcinoma. *Ann. Oncol.* 2: 131-136, 1991.
28. Waterhouse, D. M., Reynolds, R. K. and Natale, R. B. Combined carboplatin and cisplatin. Limited prospects for dose intensification. Cancer (Phila.) 71: 4060-4066, 1993.
29. Reed, E., Janik, M., Bookman, M. et al. High-dose chemotherapy and rGM-CSF in refractory ovarian cancer. *Proc. Am. Soc. Clin. Oncol.* 9: 157,1990.
30. Markman, M., Blessing, J. A., Major, F. and Manettta, A. Salvage intraperitoneal therapy of ovarian cancer employing cisplatin and etoposide. A Gynecologic Oncology Group Study. *Gynecol.Oncol.* 50: 191-195, 1993.
31. Benedetti Panici, P., Scambia, G., Baiocchi, G., Greggi, S., Battaglia, F., Salerno, G., Menichella, L., Pierelli, L., Foddai, M.A., Paoloni, A., Serafini, R., Mango, G., Bizzi, B., Manucuso, S. High-dose (HD) chemotherapy (CT) and autologous peripheral stem cell (APSC) support in advanced ovarian cancer (AOC). *Proc. Am. Soc. Clin. Oncol.* 10: 195, 1991.

32. Juttner, C. A., Daby, M.L.J., To., L. B. et al. Autologous PBSC transplantation in stage III and IV ovarian cancer. *Int. Cell. Clon.* (suppl 1): 145, 1992.

CHAPTER 20

INTRAPERITONEAL CHEMOTHERAPY IN THE MANAGEMENT OF PATIENTS WITH OVARIAN CANCER[1]

Tsuneo Noda[*], Yasuhiko Kiyozuka[**], Susumu Adachi[***]
[*]Department of Obstetrics and Gynecology, Seirei Mikatabara General Hospital, [**]The Second Department of Pathology, Kurume University of Medicine, [***] Department of Obstetrics and Gynecology, Hyogo College of Medicine

INTRODUCTION

In many cases, ovarian carcinoma remains limited to the peritoneal cavity throughout the majority of its natural course. One of the most important factors in a successful therapeutic strategy for ovarian cancer is control of the disease during its intraperitoneal stage.

According to a basic pharmacologic principal it is conceivable that increased anticancer drug delivery to a tumor increases response rate and survival (1-3).

In this regard, instilling chemotherapeutic agents directly into the peritoneal cavity of patients with cancerous peritonitis may expose individual free-floating tumor cells as well as small tumor nodules to higher levels of anti-tumor agents than those achived with systemic administrration.

Treatment by the intraperitoneal route (ip) is not a new concept. In 1955, Weissberger et al. (4) described the use of intraperitoneal nitrogen mustard for patients with malignant ascites and noted improved control. In these days, while malignant pleural fluid and ascites could be successfully controlled by intracavital sclerosing therapies (5-7), local side effects (particularly severe pain) were often observed. In the late 1970s, Dedrick and his colleagues(8) reported that the peritoneal cavity received significantly greater exposure to anticancer agents by the direct intraperitoneal instillation of these agents than by administration of same agents to the systemic circulation, showing an elegant pharmacokinetic rationale for peritoneal drug

---

[1] Address for reprints: Department of Obstetrics and Gynecology, Seirei Mikatabara General Hospital, 3453, Mikarabara-Chou, Hamamatu-City, Shizuoka 437-16, Japan

administration. His mathematical model demonstrated two to three log increase in abdominal cavity drug concentration compared to systemic delivery of the same agent (8). In the 1980s, a number of investgators have demonstrated the benefits and limitations of intraperitoneal drug administration in the chemotherapy of ovarian cancer (9-12).

Many questions regarding optimal drug and dosing schedule remain unanswered. One such question is whether the higher peritoneal drug concentrations achievable with intraperitoneal chemotherapy will improve both clinical response rates and survival in ovarian cancer.

BASIC PHARMACOKINETICS OF INTRAPERITONEAL CHEMOTHERAPY

The rationale for ip-therapy rests on the pharmacologic aspects of direct intracavital administration of antineoplastic agents. It is useful and easy to think of peritoneal drug administration in terms of a two- or three-compartment model (8)(13-18).

The drug is administered directly into the peritoneal cavity which is considered the first compartment. In a three-compartment model, following ip instillation, drugs are absorbed into the blood, the second compartment, and distributed to all other tissues in contact with the bloodstream which constitute the third compartment.

When the drug was directly administered into the peritoneal cavity, its concentration will gradually fall as the drug enters into the systemic circulation.

The cavity / plasma concentration ratio shows the inverse relation of the clearance for the two compartments. A greater concentration difference indicates a smaller the clearance from the cavity and a greater the clearance from the systemic circulation . Thus the ideal agent is one that leaves the cavity very slowly but is promptly removed from the plasma once it reaches the systemic blood stream. The advantage of ip-treatment is indicated by the cavity / plasma AUC ratio.

Total drug exposure is estimated by integrating the area under the curve (AUC). Moment analysis is a good way to assess the bioavailability and pharmacodynamics of drugs. The indices of moment analysis are calculated; the AUC is the zero-order moment, the mean residence time (MRT) is the primary moment, and the variance of residence time (VRT) is the second moment (14,15).

Markman et al. (19,20) performed phase I trials of many agents (cisplatin, carboplatin, mitoxantrone,and taxol) administered by the intraperitoneal route, and showed that ip administration could obtain 10-1,000-fold higher concentration of drug in the peritoneal cavity than systemic iv administration .

ABSORBING ROUTES

The peritoneal cavity is covered with a single layer of flattened cells that constitute the peritoneal membrane. The greatest part of the surface of the peritoneal cavity consists of the visceral peritoneum, the omentum, and the mesentery. These structures drain into the portal circulation. The parietal peritoneum drains direcly into the systemic circulation (21). In the abdominal cavity there are many lymphatic networks, one of which exists on the undersurface of the diaphragms and communicates directly with the peritoneal cavity by specialized pores or "stomata" (22).

Agents administered directly into the peritoneal space can reach the plasma by 3 routes. First, the drug may be absorbed into the portal circulation and pass through the liver before it reaches the systemic circulation. Second, it may enter the capillaries of the parietal peritoneum so that drain directly into the systemic circulation. Finally, it may be absorbed into the peritoneal lymphatics and reach the venous circulation via the thoracic duct.

Kraft et al. (23) performed an interesting study in which radioactive sodium sulfate placed into the peritoneal cavity of a dog appeared in the portal vein within seconds following instillation, with significantly lower concentration in the inferior vena cava initially, and an appearance in the thoracic duct lymph minutes later. In a rat model, similar pharmacokinetics were demonstrated using several drugs including progesterone, caffeine, glycine, and glucose (24). From these studies, the portal circulation of ip-administered antineoplastic agents is the main pathway. Some agents may be metabolized while pass through the liver by portal circulation.

Lymphatic flow is less than portal circulation flow (25,26). Torres et al. (27) described significant absorption via the lymphatics only for compounds with molecular weights of 1,000 or more.

FACTORS INFLUENCING PERITONEAL CLEARANCE

Molecular weight of drug, lipid solubility and ionization

Many investigators have demonstrated that as the molecular weight of a chemotherapeutic agent increases the absorption through the peritoneal membrance decreases (23,24,27). As showing in Figure 1, Mayers et al. (28) described the clear correlation between the molecular weight of a drug and the peritoneal clearance. Apart from the molecular weight, the lipid solubility and the ionnization of the drug itself are important determinants of peritoneal clearance. As lipid solubility increases the absorption also increases. Drugs that are largely unionized at physiologic pH are absorbed more rapidly than drugs that are highly ionized (16).

Thus, the ideal drug for ip therapy would be one with low peritoneal clearance such as

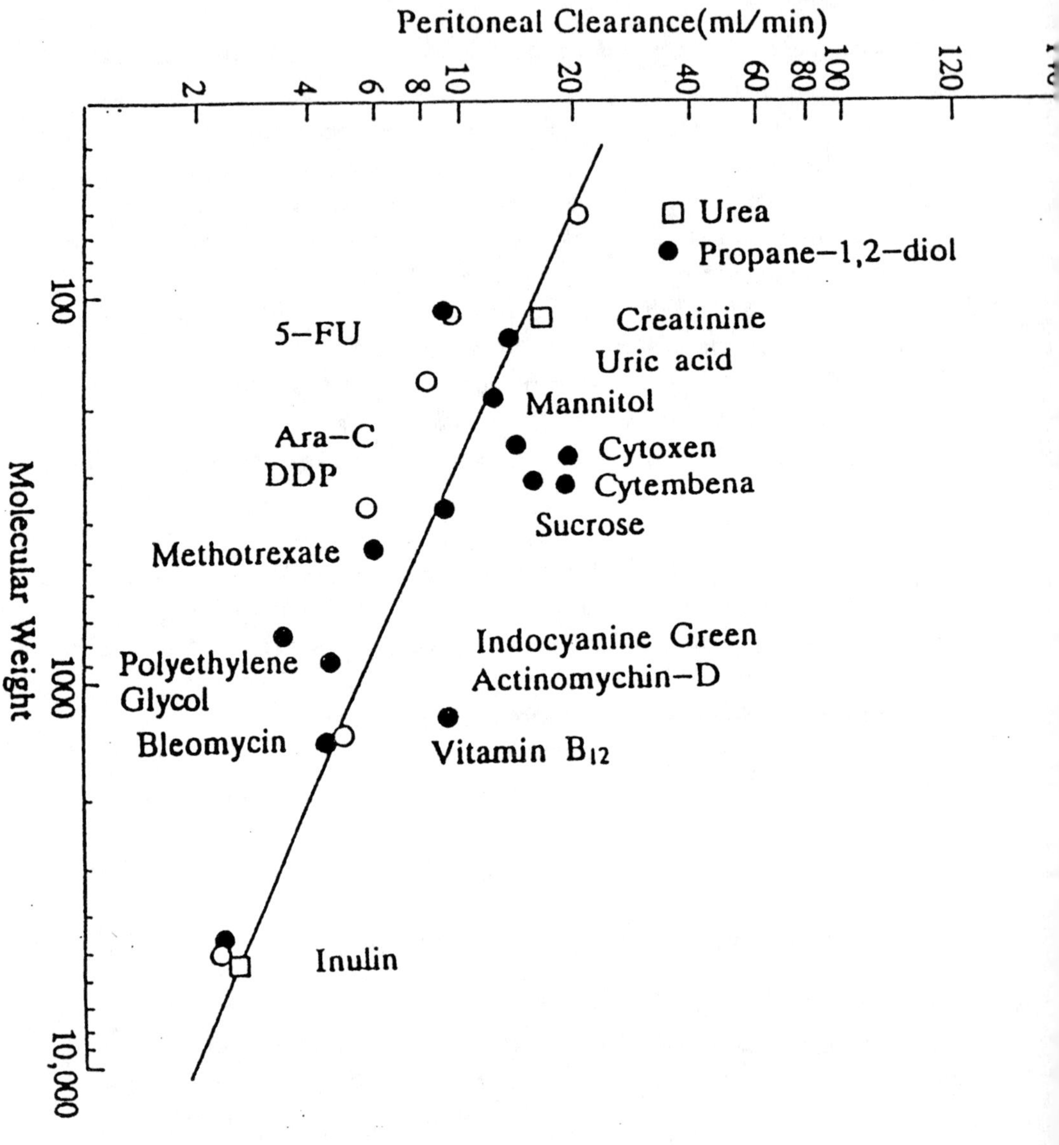

Fig. 1. Correlation between molecular weight of drug and peritoneal clearance

(Mayers CE, et al: Pharmacology of intraperitoneal chemotherapy. Cancer Invetigat 1:395- 407, 1983.)

relatively high molecular weight, hydrophilic and highly ionized at physiologic pH .

Solution volume for ip therapy

Intraperitoneal chemotherapy requires optimal peritoneal cavity distribution of the drug . All areas of the abdominal space should be filled with the drug-containing fluid. Most candidates for ip therapy will have received one or more surgical procedure befor beginning this treatment. Adhesion formation, which such surgery will result in, can significantly interfere with fluid and drug distribution. Despite the use of large volumes of drug-containing fluid there are defect areas (e.g., behind mechanical and tumor adhesions) that may not come in contact with this fluid.

To obtain good result from ip therapy, drug-containing fliuid must be distributed to all involved areras. Many studies have clearly demonstrated that a small volume of drug-containing fliuid placed into the peritoneal cavity is not evenly distributed. However, many investgators enphasized that if volumes large enough to distend the peritoneal cavity are instilled, the fluid distribution can be markedly improved (29-33). Small volumes of drug-containing fluid are inadequate to improve the fluid distribution despite position changes and abdominal massage. Rosenhein et al. (32) described 99Tc-sulfur colloid distribution in all 4 quadrants when scanned immediately after an intraperitoneal instillation in 2 liters of normal saline. Howell et al. (12) recomended more than 2 liters in order to produce adequate drug distribution in the intraperitoneal space. However in patients with a body surface area of less than 1.5m2, especially in Japanase, it may be necessary to treat with a lower volume . One additional advantage of large volumes is the avoidance of extremely high concentration pockets of drug capable of producing serious toxicity.

Braly et al. (34) showed that patients with excellent fluid distribution by CT scan were more likely to have a complete response to ip therapy, whereas patients with suboptimal fluid distribution were more likely to have progressive disease or partial response. This finding confirms the importance of completelly bathing the tumor nodules on peritoneal surfaces with drug containing fluid.

Cancerous Peritonitis

The patients with advanced cancerous peritonitis have large volume ascites, which contains large amount of protein, capable of inactivating cisplatin. This inactivation can significantly influence absorption into capillaries and the ultimate clinical activity of the drug. Large ascites increases the abdominal pressure (hydropic pressure). When ip administration of anticancer agents to patients with large ascites was made, this pressure will help these drugs enter through peritoneal membrane into the systemic circulation. The resulting plasma concentration of the drug may be higher than expected and side effects may appear.

Since pelvic and paraaortic lymphnode metastases may strongly influence lymphatic flow, drug absorbtion into the peritoneal lymphatics following ip chemotherapy may be reduced in patients with such lymphnode metastases.

The drug permeability of the peritoneal membrane may depend on not only the severity of cancerous peritonitis but also the sclerosing effect of prior ip chemothearpy. Thickened peritoneum may be the barrier to drug diffusion into capillaries.

It is important to consider these factors that can potentially influence tissue or tumor drug penetration and plasma or intraperitoneal drug concentrations. Because individual patients have different clinical conditions, we should be aware of the pharmacodynamics of intraperitoneally administrated drugs and have access to clinical pharmacological evaluations for each patient (14,15,35).

DRUG PENETRATION

It is important to know how many layers the drug must be able to penetrate once the drug comes in contact with the tumor mass. Unfortunately, a lot of studies demonstrated that tissue diffusibility and penetration of chemotherapeutic agents were poor(36-38). Ozols et al.(39-41) examined the penetration of a fluorescent drug doxorubicin in murine ovarian cancer and reported that the fluorescene was observed only in the outermost 4-6 cells of the tumor after ip dosing. However, the relationship between fluorescene and achievement of tumor kill was unclear. The limited penetration of drugs into tumor tissue has been examined both in vitro and in vivo in several experimental systems using several anticancer agents with known activity against ovarian cancer(42-44).

The geneal conclusion of such studies has been that the direct penetration of the drugs into tissue is extremely limited, ranging from several cell layers to perhaps 1 to 3 milimeters from the tumor surface. In one experimental system using cisplatin, the relative advantage of ip administration (compared to systemic iv administration) seemed to be limited to 0.1 to 1 mm tumor mass(44).

TECHNICAL ASPECTS OF IP-THERAPY

Intraperitoneal chemotherapy requires laparotomy for catheter or port placemen. Because ip therapy was often performed repeatedly for the patients with ovarian cancer, a Tenchoff Catheter, originally designated for peritoneal dialysis, was often utlized(45). For the past several years, many physicians have been using a totally implanted peritoneal access device (Port-a-Cath, Pharmacia Deltec, Inc.), which was placed in a subcutaneous pocket. Once the Port-a-Cath was placed, the peritoneal cavity can be accessed by inserting a 19-gauge (Huber) needle through the skin. This Port-a-Cath subcutaneous delivery system is best tool for repeated administration of chemotherapeutic agents. Drainage of the drug solution may be poor. At the UCSD Cancer Center, Pfeifle et al. (46) described that only 7% of ip cisplatin in two liters of saline could be drained from the peritoneal cavity after a 4-hr of ip administration.

In our hospital, we have used two types of catheters according to the stage and the size of the residual tumor at operation. One was a silicone nephrostomy catheter as a temporary catheter, which was used in the patient with 3 or 4 performance status. These patients were not operable and received by these silicone nephrostomy catheters using a peel-away introducer (Cook. Co., Ltd.) under B-scope guidance and local anesthesia(Fig. 2). Another was the Port-a-Cath, which was surgically implanted under general anesthesia. Patients with large ascites received the drug as a bolus through this apparatus, while patients without ascites did the drug diluted in 500-2000ml of physiological saline. No drainage was undertaken after ip therapy. For postoperative catheter care, 4 ml of saline with 1ml of heparine (1000IU) was injected once a week during hospitalization and once every 2-4 week during outpatient treatment(47)(48). A specimen from the irrigation fluid was used must for routine cytologic analysis. However, we recognize that a negative cytologic evaluation from the irrigation fluid may not be correlated to tumor response becouse of the limited sample from the peritoneal cavity(34).

TRIALS OF SINGLE-AGENT INTRAPERITONEAL CHEMOTHERAPY

Since the early 1980s, the peritoneal pharmacokinetics of a number of active chemotherapeutic agents have benn investigated and several effective agents have benn identified(8, 49).

Cisplatin

Cisplatin has been shown to be one of the most effective drugs currently available for the treatment of ovarian cancer(50. 51), and has been administered as a single agents and in combination regimen as a first line chemotherapy regimens. It has been used in the salvage (second-line) setting, too. (52-55). Hequet et al. (56) showed that cisplatin had more affinity in tumor tissue than carboplatin.

We investigated the in vitro cytotoxic effects of CDDP on cisplatin-resistant (SHIN-3) and -sensitive (MN-1) ovarian cancer cell lines (57, 58) using the MTT assay. MN-1 cells had IC50 values of 1mcg/ml at 4 hours and 5mcg/ml at 1hours (Fig.3), while the IC50 values of SHIN-3 cells to cisplatin were 4mcg/ml at 24 hours, 20mcg/ml at 4 hours and

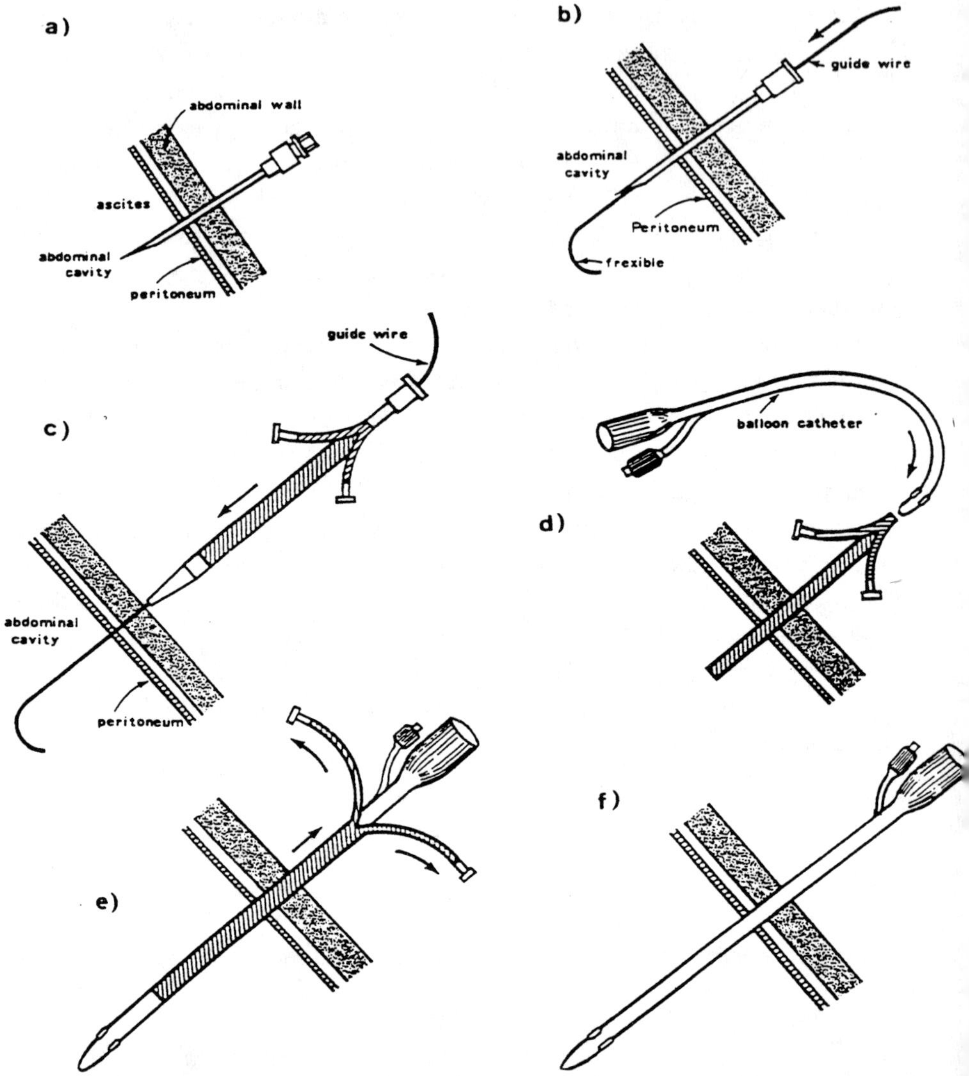

Fig. 2. Simple pericentesis using a peel-away introducer (Cook. Co., Ltd.)

a) Special 18-gauge needle is advanced toward the abdominal cavity.

b) Introduction of the guide wire through the the needle into the abdominal space.

c) Introduction of the peel-away introducer through the guide wire.

d) After removing the introducer and guide wire, introduction of the balloon catheter through the peel-away sheath.

e) Removing the peel-away sheath.

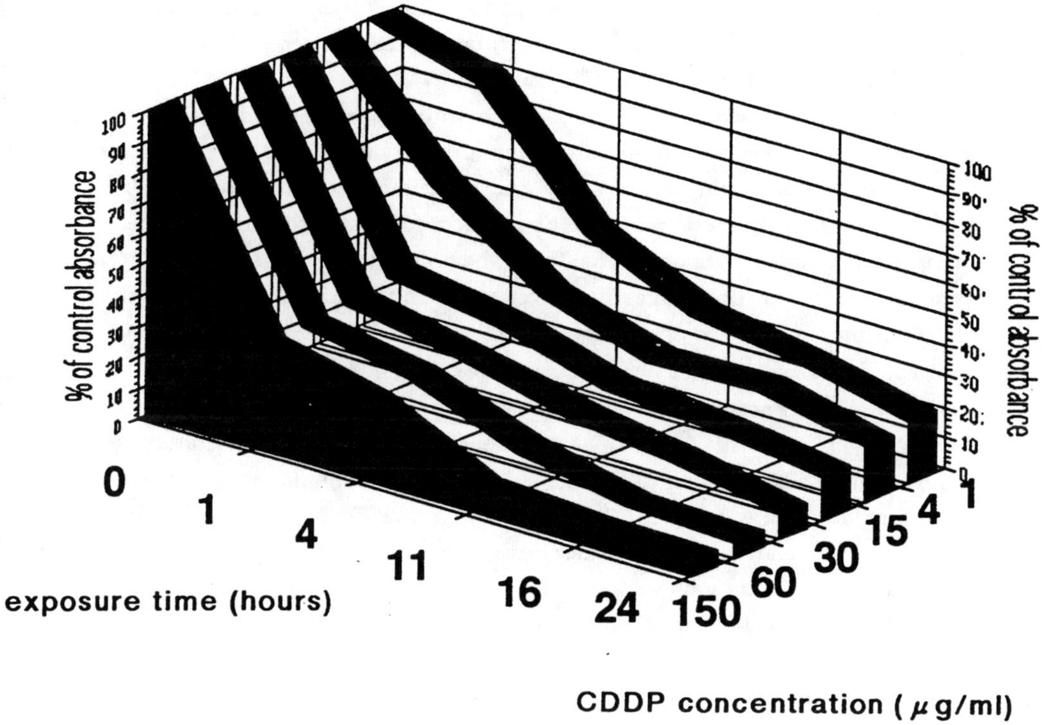

Fig. 3. Inhibitory effects of cisplatin on MN-1 cell proliferation.

40mcg/ml at 1 hours (Fig.4). From these data, a concentration-dependant growth inhibition of cisplatin was demonstrated in both SHIN-3 and MN-1.

Becouse of these reasions, cisplatin seemed to be a useful drug for intraperitoneal therapy, The efficacy and safety of intraperitoneally administered cisplatin has been examined by several investigators(49, 59, 60).

Understanding the pharmacokinetics of ip cisplatin is very important with regard to not only the manifestation of the effects but also the side effects. We examined the kinetics of cisplatin in the ascites and plasma after ip cisplatin (bolus 100mg/body administration in 500ml saline without systemic thiosulfate protection) by the compartment model and moment analysis. One hour after ip cisplatin (100mg/body), the concentrations of platinum in ascites were as high as 100mcg/ml, while total platinum in the serum was detected one hour after ip cisplatin, and thereafter serum platinum showed a prolonged biologic elimination phase (β-half life)(Fig.5). At 24 hours after ip cisplatin, the concentrations of platinum in the ascites were 4-13times higher than those in serum. The AUC , MRT (mean residence time), and VRT (variance of residence time) showed obviously high values and a direct effect on the tumor cells in the abdomonal cavity was expected. The AUC, MRT, and VRT of free-CDDP, having entered the systemic circulation, showed values nearly equal to or higher than those by intravenous administration (iv), and effects on the tumor blood vessels have been demonstrated. Cases of ovarian cancer had various level of peritoneal clearance(Clp), depending on the severity of their carcinomatous peritonitis. The Clp had a greater influence on the peak plasma concentration and the AUC of free Pt in serum. In particular, the peak plasma concentration produced by ip cisplatin was 40-80% of the plasma concentration produced by iv cisplatin. The mean peritoneal / plasma AUC ratio is 8-75 (median 24)(Markmann described 12) indicating a substantial pharmacologic advantage for this route. Meanwhile cisplatin demonstrated a low AUC-ratio, ip cisplatin has direct effects in the abdominal cavity and anti-tumor effects from the vascular side of the tumor. These findings indicate that high-dose ip cisplatin is possibly effective and useful for advanced ovarian cancer, producing only very mild side effect(14,15,35,48).

Markman et al. (49, 61) showed that despite the limited pharmacokinetic advantage for the intraperitoneal delivery of cisplatin, the peritoneal cavity is exposed to 10 to 20 times more drug than the systemic compartment following intraperitoneal administration.

Early clinical trials using cisplatin at standard doses (50-150mg/m2) have demonstrated the safety and efficacy of ip therapy. Cohen et al. (62) treated 35 patients with minimal residual disease at second-look surgery, using single agent cisplatin at a dose of 50mg/m2 every 3 weeks. Of the 35 patients, 30% entered a pathologically documented complete remission. Hacker et al. (63) described a starting dose of 120mg/m2 of ip

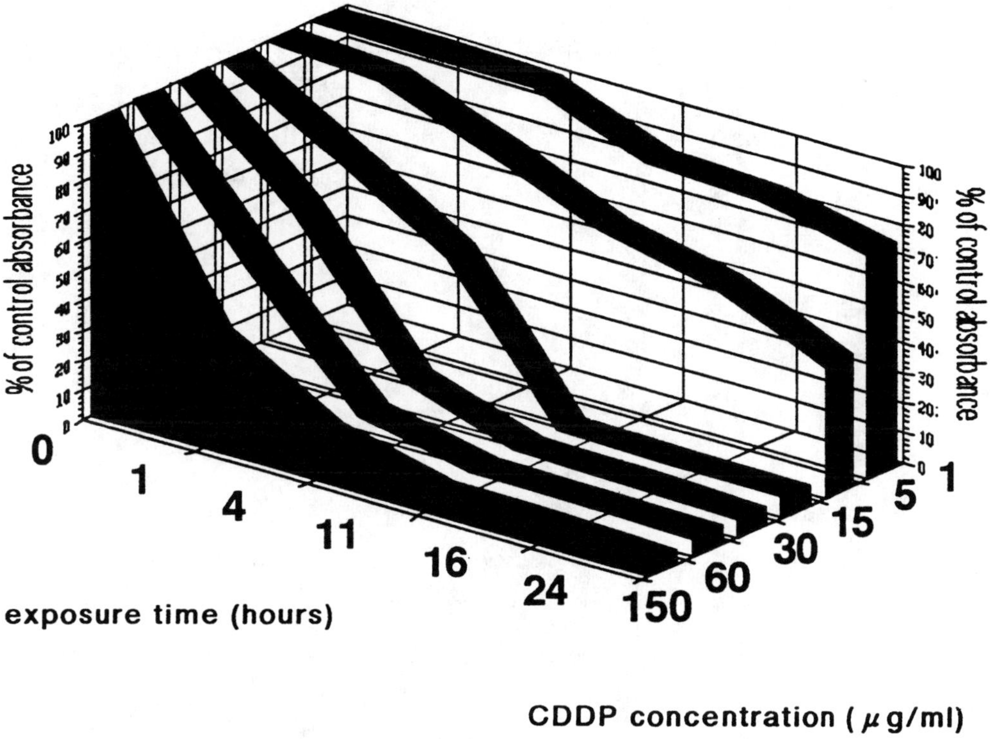

Fig. 4. Inhibitory effects of cisplatin on SHIN-3 cell proliferation.

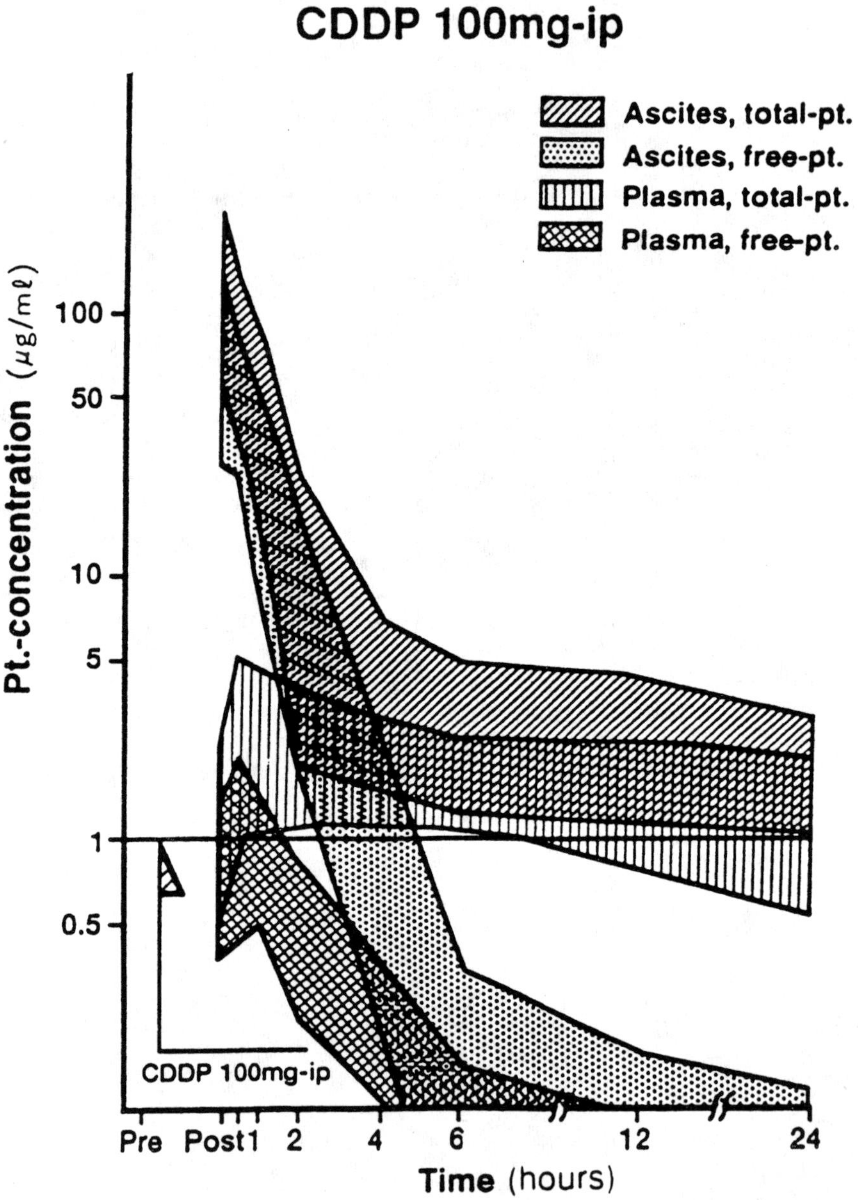

Fig. 5. Curves of platinum concentration in ascites and plasma after ip cisplatin.

cisplatin with dose escalation of 30mg/m2 every 2 weeks given to 18 patients previously treated with a systemic cisplatin-containing regimen without a complete remission. Four (27%) patients achieved a complete response and 2 (13%) achieved a partial response.

In addition, a number of clinical trials have confirmed that the intraperitoneal instillation of cisplatin is associated with minimal local toxicity (pain, adhesion formation).

2-Channel chemotherapy

This is a good opportunity to use systemically administered neutraizing agents for the ip-delivered drug. Whether the addition of neutraizing agents will be advantageous or disadvantageous for the chemotrherapy will depend on the pharmacokinetic characteristics of these drugs. Unfortunately, once the antagonist will be injected intravenouly, it will begin to diffuse into the peritoneal cavity, and may interferes with the cytotoxic effect of the anticancer agent.

Thiosulfate, an agent used clinically for many years for cyanide poisoning, has been shown experimentally to protect against platinum-induced nephrotoxicity (12, 64). Cisplatin and thiosulfate react to form a covalent bond resulting in a complex that is neither cytotoxic nor nephrotoxic. Some investigators hypothesized that the neutralization reaction is slow in the plasma but rapid (28 times faster) in the kidney(65, 66). When cisplatin and thiosulfate are administered ip and iv respectively, there is little neutralization of cisplatin in the plasma but excellent protection of the kidneys.

The use of sodium thiosulfate as a renal protective agent has allowed a significant dose escalation of cisplatin. Howell et al. (67) treated 17 patients with intraperitoneal tumors were treated with ip cisplatin and iv sodium thiosulfate. Cisplatin was started at a dose of 90mg/m2 in a 2 L treatment volume as a 4-hour dwell and escalated in 45 mg/m2 increments. Sodium thiosulfate was administered as a 7.5g/m2 rapid iv push loading dose followed by a 12-hr continous infusion at 2.13g/m2/hr. The dose of cisplatin was successfully escalated to 270 mg/m2 without evidence of clinical nephrotoxicity. At this dose the mean area under the peritoneal curve was twice that achieved with ip cisplatin given without thiosulfate($P<0.05$ analysis of variance) and more than 56 times greater than the tumor area under the curve reported for cisplatin after a maximum tolerated iv dose(17).

In our institute we have treated with CDDP-ip (50-150mg/body) bolus administration without systemic thiosulfate protection, becouse ip cisplatin is considered to affect intraperitoneal tumors through systemic circulation as well as directly and compared with iv cisplatin, ip cisplatin without thiosulfate elicited only mild nousea, myelosuppression and no significant changes of renal function(15, 35, 48).

Carboplatin

Meta analysis results have also shown that cisplatin can be replaced by carboplatin without loss of efficacy. Carboplatin has also been explored for intraperitoneal use in patients with ovarian cancer(68, 69). The pharmacokinetics of ip carboplatin, comparing with ip cisplatin, are very interesting, due to the difference of affinity to the tissue and protein(58).

We studied in vitro kinetics of carboplatin at the time of the ip administration using with a 2-compartment model and moment analyses. A bolus of 200-450mg/body (148-292mg/m2) carboplatin with 500ml saline was administered into the abdominal cavity. The shift of platium to systemic circulation depended on the peritoneal clearance. Cmax in blood was seen one hour after ip in patients with a normal peritoneum, and between 4 and 6 hours after ip in patients with carcinimatous peritonitis (Fig.6). The level was lower in the latter group. The non-binding rate of platinum with protein in ascites at the time of the ip administration was correlated with the carboplatin concentration in the ascites. The non-binding rate was 80% or more both in the ascites and in the blood within 4 hours after ip. The high nonbinding rate appeared to prolong the presence of the free-platinum in the ascites and plasma, especially in patients with carcinomatous peritonitis. The AUC level in blood was equal to or higher than that observed when the same dose was administered iv. The level of free-platinum and AUC in the abdominal cavity were 2 to 5 times higher than those in plasma in patients with a normal peritoneum, and 7 to 14 times higher in patients with carcinomatous peritonitis. Clinical effects included a reduction of pleural effusion in a patient and complete disappearance of ascites in another patient. The main side effect was myelosuppression. Ip carboplatin resulted in AUC levels in blood comparable to or higher than those achieved with iv carboplatin (70). The mean peritoneal / plasma AUC ratio wasis 2-14 (median 7)(70). Ip carboplatin has a substantial pharmacologic advantage because of direct effects in the abdominal cavity and anti-tumor effects from the systemic circulation(70).

The major advantage of ip carboplatin over cisplatin is the less toxicity. Patients who have experienced unacceptaable cisplatin-associated toxicity, particularly neurotoxicity, can reasonably be treated with ip carboplatin. But this ip-therapy is limited by the development of bone marrow suppression, principally thrombocytopenia(70).

Etoposide

Recently, etoposide, a semisynthetic podophyllotoxin derivative, has been gaining importance in both primary and salvage therapy for ovarian cancer(71, 72). This epipodophyllotoxin may exert its cytotoxic effects, in part, by interfering with the

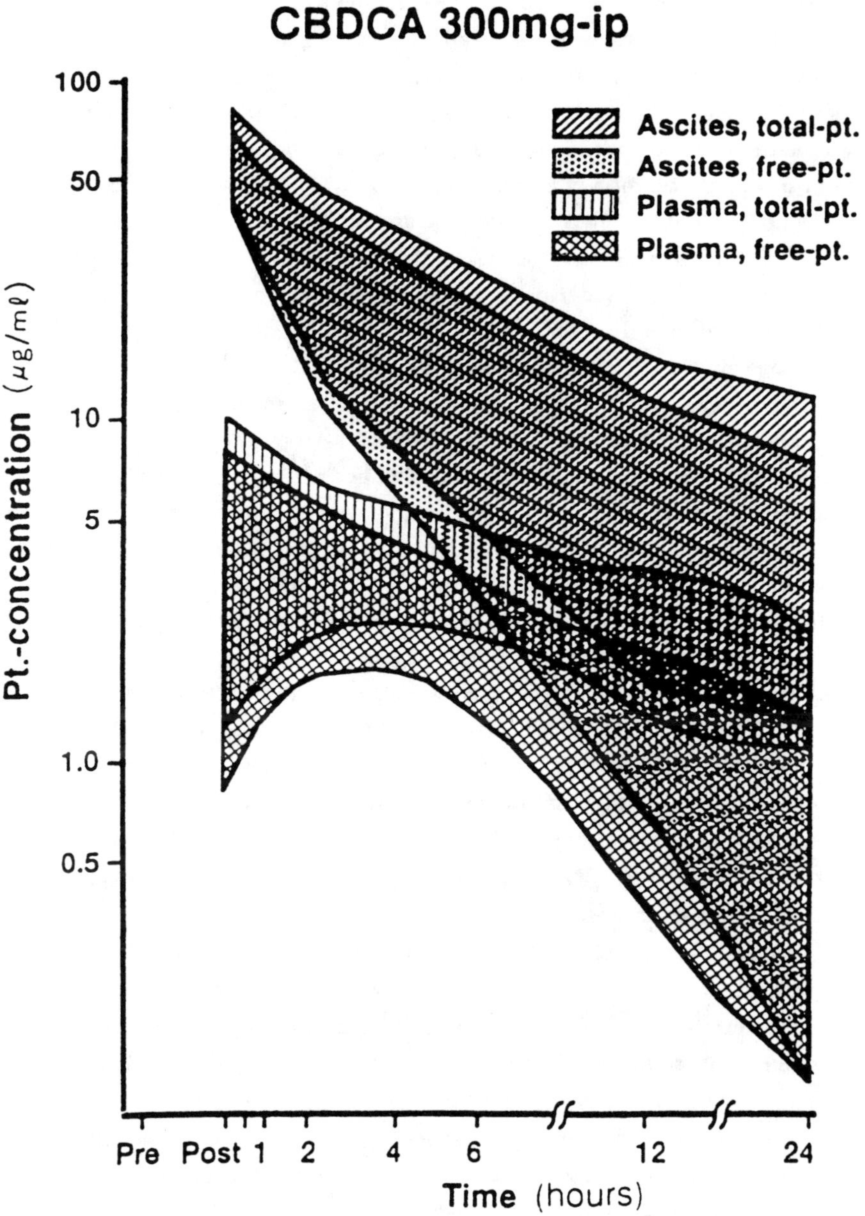

Fig. 6. Curves of platinum concentration in ascites and plasma after ip carboplatin.

scission-reunion reaction in DNA double strand of topoisomerase II(71, 72, 73). Although it has not yielded universally favorable results as a single agent, it appears to be useful when administered in combination with cicplatin or carboplatin (73, 74, 75).

We investigated the bioavailability and pharmacokinetics of ip etoposid in patients with carcinomatous peritonitis. Etoposide was administered intraperitoneally as rapidly as possible with dilution of 500ml of physiological saline when ascites was not found and without dilution when considerable ascites (>500ml) was found via exploratory laparotomy or pericentesis. The peak etoposide level in the ascites was 80mcg/ml. Twelve hours after intrapertoneal administration, more than 10mcg/ml of etoposide was still found in ascites. The serum level after ip administration of 100 mg etoposide was approximately 4mcg/ml within 30 minutes, and 1mcg/ml of etoposide was still found in serum after 24 hours. The etoposide levels in ascites and serum after 300 mg-ip were higher than those after 100 mg- ip (Fig. 7). When the peritoneum was unaffected, the area under the curve (AUC) of etoposide in ascites was low, and the peritoneal clearance (Clp) was high. In contrast, in advanced carcinomatou peritonitis, the AUC in ascites was high and the Clp was low. The AUC of etoposide in the ascites of patients with carcinomatous peritonitis was more than five-fold greater than that of patients with an unaffected peritoneum, while MRT (mean residence time) was 15-fold, and VRT (variance of residence time) was 300-fold greater. The AUC ratio in an unaffcted peritoneum was 4.1, and that in carcinomatous peritonitis ranged from 17.8 to 27.1. The AUC, MRT and VRT of etoposide transported into the blood were slightly higher in advanced cases than in those with an unaffcted peritoneum. In this study, only total etoposide levels were measured. Free etoposide (the active anticancer form) was not measured; however, a high intraperitoneal concentration of etoposide after 100 mg-ip should be sufficient to kill free malignant cells in the abdominal cavity(76). As shown in Fig.8, the anticancer effects via the vascular system of the tumor after 100 mg-ip administration are comparable to the effects after intravenous or oral administration(76, 77). The considerable variation in ascites and serum concentration observed among the cases may be a result of the stage of carcinomatous peritonitis. When the peritoneum was unaffected and there was no ascites, the Kel of etoposide from the abdominal cavity was large and Clp was high, indicating good transport of etoposide into the bloodstream . Consequently, the AUC of etoposide in peritoneal fluid was low. In contrast, in cases of advanced carcinomatous peritonitis, the Kel of etoposide from the abdominal cavity and the Clp were low. The AUC of etoposide in the ascites in advanced carcinomatous peritonitis was large and the anticancer effect of the drug in the abdominal cavity was intensified. In more advanced cases, the elimination phase of etoposide in blood was not observed. Therefore, the AUC of serum etoposide was also increased. This observation indicates not only a good effect via the vascular system but also a reduced potential for side effects such as bone-marrow suppression. Drugs

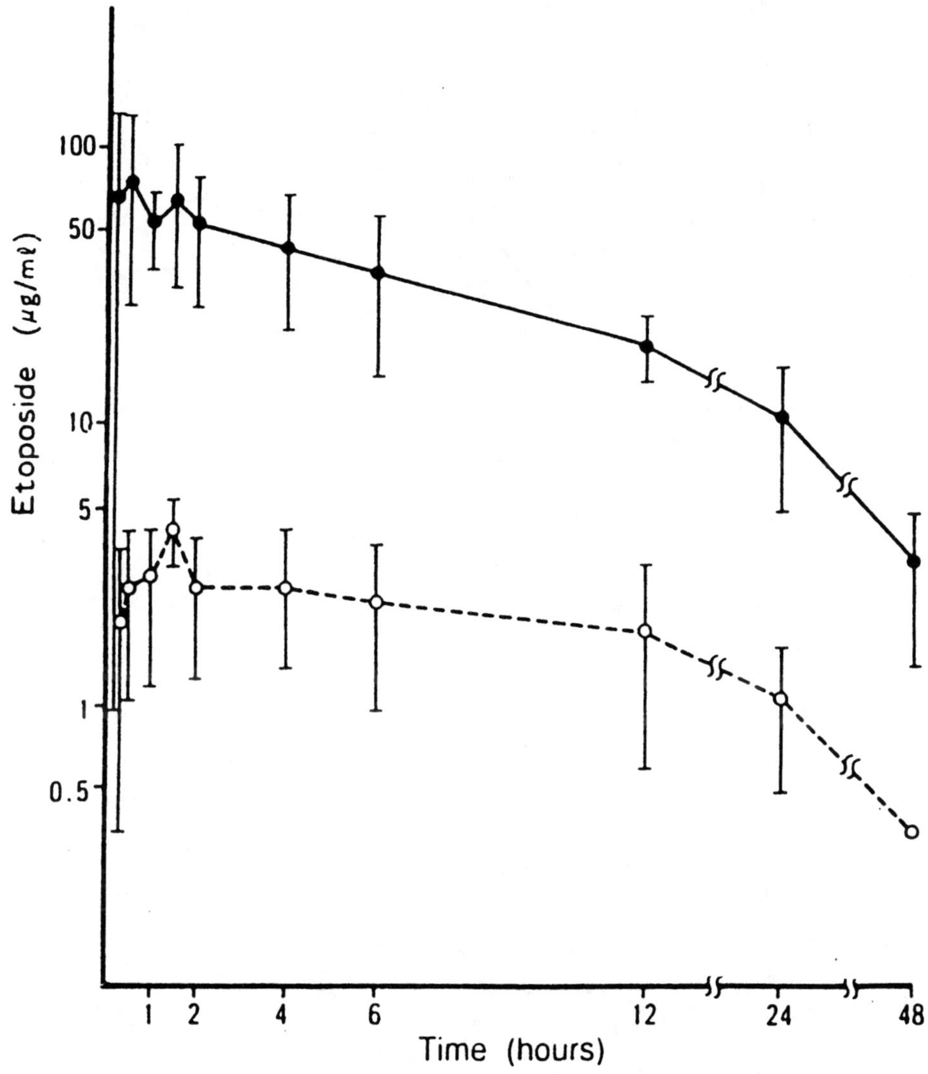

Fig. 7. Concentration curves for etoposide in ascites and plasma after intraperitoneal administration of 100mg etoposide. The data represent the mean±S.D. from five patients.

●—● : Etoposide in ascites. ○···○ : Etoposide in plasma.

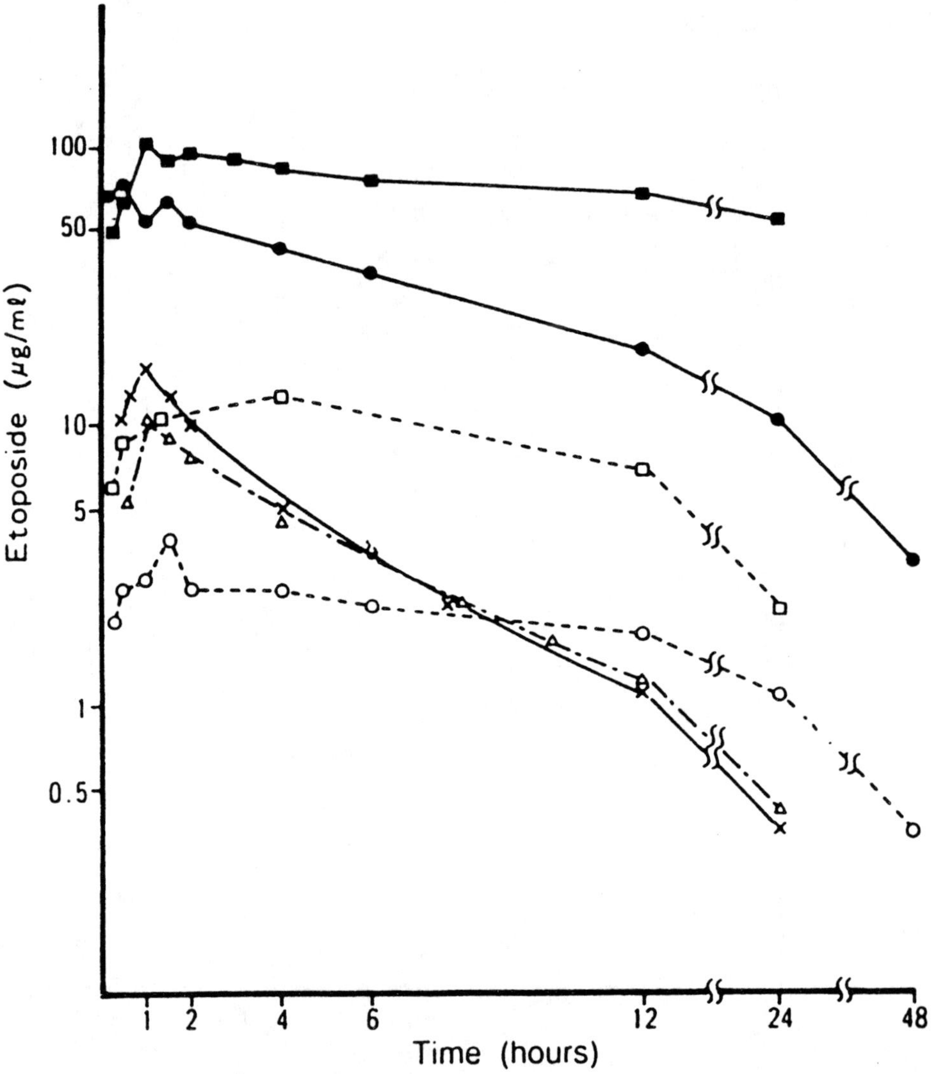

Fig. 8. Concentration curves of etoposide in ascites and plasma.
■—■ : Etoposide in ascites (300mg-ip). ●—● : Etoposide in ascites (100mg-ip).
□···□ : Etoposide in plasma (300mg-ip). ×—× : Etoposide in plasma (100mg-ip).
△···△ : Etoposide in plasma (160mg/m2 p.o.) [Pfeffer M. et al. 1987 (77)]

with a higher AUC ratio are considered to be more suitable for intraabdominal administration. However, in the present study, the AUC ratio of etoposide was low even in carcinomatous peritonitis (76). These findngs indicate that intraperitoneal etoposide has not only a direct anticancer effect in the abdominal cavity but also an indirect effect via the vascular system to the tumor.

Etoposide is a cell-cycle phase-specific drug, and the magnitude of its effect relies on the duration of exposure above a certain concentration (78,79). In small-cell lung cancer, the clinical effect of etoposide is largely dependent on a long-duration exposure to more than 1mcg/ml of the drug. An administration schedule that accounts for this fact is therefore necessary (80,81). The better effective schedule for intraperitoneal administration of etoposide may be 100 mg/day-ip for five days, rather than a single bolus intraperitoneal administration.

5-Fluorouracil

5-fluorouracil (5-FU) has a long history of ip-drug delivery for the purpose of preventing the reaccumulation of ascites (82). Pharmacokinetic studies of ip 5-FU have been performed at the NCI (83-85). Pancytopenia and mucositis were the dose-limiting toxicities, and bacterial and chemical peritonitis were also observed. In Italian study, the AUC ratio for the peritoneal cavity to plasma ranged from 120 to 1,350 (86). A phase □ trial of ip 5-FU in patients with refractory ovarian carcinoma has demonstrated a response rate of only 7% in a group of pretreated patients (87).

Doxorubicin

Several groups have studied the intraperitoneal administration of doxorubicin (ADR) both experimentally and clinically (39,40,41,88,89). The mean peritoneal cavity level of ADR during the 4-hour drip infusion was 166 times higher than the mean blood level, with a peak peritoneal to plasma concentration ratio of 474. Abdominal pain was the dose-limiting toxicity, occurring along with ascites and adhesion formation at ADR concetrations of greater than $36\mu M$ (40mg in 2 L)(89). Bone marrow depression was mild at the doses administered. This drug is suitable for intrathoracic instillation due to its sclerosing effect, but is not suitable for intraperitoneal administration due to such adhesion formation.

Mitoxantrone

Mitoxantrone was designed to alleviate the cardic toxicity of adriamycin. In Japan the indications for this drug are acute leukemia and breast cancer. Mitoxantrone has demonstrated significant activity against ovarian cancer in vitro (90). Mitoxantrone produces a profound cytotoxic effect against ovarian cancer cells at concentrations of the agent achievable following intraperitoneal instillation but not of systemic delivery

(90). Markman et al. (91) in a phase □ trial of mitoxantrone in refractory ovarian cancer demonstrated surgically-defined activity, including responses in patients previously failed to treat with intraperitoneal cisplatin. The AUC-ratio of this drug was 1,400.

Unfortunately, the drug produced excessive local toxicity (abdominal pain and bowel obstruction) at the doses administered in this trial (20mg/m2 or 30mg/m2) and its use cannot be recommended at the present time in the standard management of patients with ovarian cancer (91).

Mytomycin C

Intraperitoneal administration of mytomycin C has been used for the patients with advanced gastric cancer (92). Unfortunately, this drug produced excessive local toxicity (abdominal pain and bowel obstruction) at the mild doses administered in the treatment of carcinomatous peritonitis and its use cannot be recommended at the present time (93).

Enocitabine (BH-AC)

King et al.(94) showed that intraperitoneal instillation of Cytarabine was effective for the patients with ovarian carcinoma. N4-behenoyl-1-β-D- arabinofuranosylcytosine (BH-AC) is an analogue of Cytarabine (Ara-C) (95).

In our study, the patients with cartinomatous peritonitis were treated with the intraperitoneal administration of BH-AC, and the pharmacokinetics of ip BH-AC were studied. Immediately after ip administration, the concentration of Ara-C delivered from BH-AC in ascites was as high as 103 ng/ml. At 24 hours, more than 10ng/ml was detected in the ascites. Ara-C plasma levels were very low (<1ng/ml). These findings indicate that BH-AC is suitable drug for ip-therapy, because this drug revealed low peritoneal and high plasma clearances (AUC-ratio=100-1,000) (96).

Additional trials are needed with regard to the benefit, side effects and survival aspects of this drug.

Melphalan (L-phenylalaninemustard)

Melphalan is an alkylating agents, and is used for patients with myeloma in Japan. Howell et al.(97) reported that intraperitoneal chemotherapy with melphalan was effective for ovarian cancer and the dose limiting factor of the drug was severe myelosuppression (thrombocytopenia).

The AUC-ratio of this drug was 65.

Taxol

Taxol showed an important dose-response relationship against several tumor cell lines

(98). This drug appears to be a most promising and interesting agent for intraperitoneal administration based upon its pharmacokinetic properties and its documented activity in ovarian cancer (99). The major pharmacokinetic advantages following regional delivery of the drug depend on its large bulky structure and hepatic metabolism (100). Since lymphatic absorptions following ip-therapy is significant only for bulky or high molecular weight compounds, taxol may be absorbed into the peritoneal lymphatics and effective for lymphnode metastasis. A phase I trial of intraperitoneal taxol has confirmed that the dose-limiting toxicity was abdominal pain (20).

Further exploration of optimal dosing and scheduling for intraperitoneal taxol is currently in progress.

MULTIAGENT THERAPY

Goldie and Goldmann (101) proposed that the optimal method for reducing the risk of tumor resistance was administration of multiple noncross-resistant drug combinations early in the treatment program. Combination chemotherapy has the advantage of a synergistic effect between the administered drugs. For example cytarabine has been shown to markedly enhance the cytotoxicity of cisplatin in a concentration-dependent manner and combination ip-chemotherapy of these agents might be the optimal method for refractory ovarian carcinoma (102-104).

The combination of cisplatin and etoposide may be an interesting treatment protocol. In an in vivo murine model etoposide demonstrated significant synergy with cisplatin (105). Some clinical trials have documented excellent activity of this combination in testicular, small cell, and ovarian carcinoma when administered systemically (106-107).

When this combination was given via the ip route, Zimm et al.(108) demonstrated a significant pharmacologic advantage for ip etoposide. Kirman et al.(109) performed a phase II trial in patients with minimal residual disease (<2cm) by ip-chemotherapy of cisplatin and etoposide with iv administration of sodium thiosulfate.

Further studies of optimal dosing and scheduling for intraperitoneal etoposide are currently in progress.

INTRAPERITONEAL DRUG DELIVERY TO OVERCOME DRUG RESISTANCE

The use of intraperitoneal chemotherapy in the management of ovarian cancer may have the potential advantage to overcome drug resistance by significantly increasing exposure to the cytotoxic agent in the peritoneal space. If a tumor is highly resistant to first line with cisplatin-based systemic chemotherapy, it is very unlikely that the second line therapy with ip cisplatin will significantly improve tumor cell kill. Conversely, if a cancer mass shows sensitivity to intravenous cisplatin-based chemotherapy, cisplatin-based ip chemotherapy may lead to better cell kill than the iv chemotherapy because of increased direct exposure to cisplatin.

To assess the efficacy of ip cisplatin for ovarian cancer, we investigated the in vitro cytotoxic effects of cisplatin against a platinum-sensitive cell line MN-1 (58), a platinum-resistant cell line SHIN-3 (57) and a spheroid (colony) formation of SHIN-3 cells as micro-metastasis model using the MTT assay. The IC90 of platinum for MN-1 cells was 2mcg/ml after exposure for 24 hours (AUC: 48 mcg/ ml/h), while that for SHIN-3 was 20mcg/ml after exposure for 11 hours (AUC: 220 mcg/ml/h). The IC90 for SHIN-3 colonies was 500mcg/ml after exposure for 4 hours (AUC: 2,000 mcg/ml/h) (Fig.8). Since the clinical 24-hr AUC obtained with ip 100mg cisplatin is about 100 mcg/ml/h, it appears that total cell kill of single cells can be achieved by ip cisplatin even for platinum-resistant ovarian cancer. However, it is impossible to achieve total cell kill against platinum-resistant micro-metastases even by ip cisplatin (110).

Many investigators have showed that second-line intarperitoneal cisplatin or carboplatin-based therapy was reasonable treatment for patients with small volume residual ovarian cancer (microscopic disease or tumor nodules< 0.5 to 1 cm) who previouly demonstrated a response to systemic cisplatin or carboplatin therapy (111-115).

SIDE EFFECTS

Ip cisplatin affects intraperitoneal tumors directly as well as through the systemic circulation. Typical cisplatin-associated adverse effects, such as renal toxicity, myelosuppression, and gastrointestinal symptoms, are lower in intraperitoneal administration than in intravenous administration. In addition, this low side effect rate probably depends on the somewhat lower total dose and peak cisplatin levels in the systemic compartment following regional drug delivery.

Toxicities associated with intraperitoneal drug delivery can be local or systemic. Local toxicities of intraperitoneal administration include abdominal swelling by the delivered fluid volume, abdominal pain by the direct inflammation or irritation, or bowel dysfunction by a chemical peritonitis or mechanical obstruction due to adhesion. Both cisplatin and carboplatin produce minimal local toxicity (69,116,117). Thus, it is possible to escalate the intraperitoneal dose and concentration of these agents until the point at which systemic toxicities (e.g. marrow suppression, nephrotoxicity, neurotoxicity) become dose limiting.

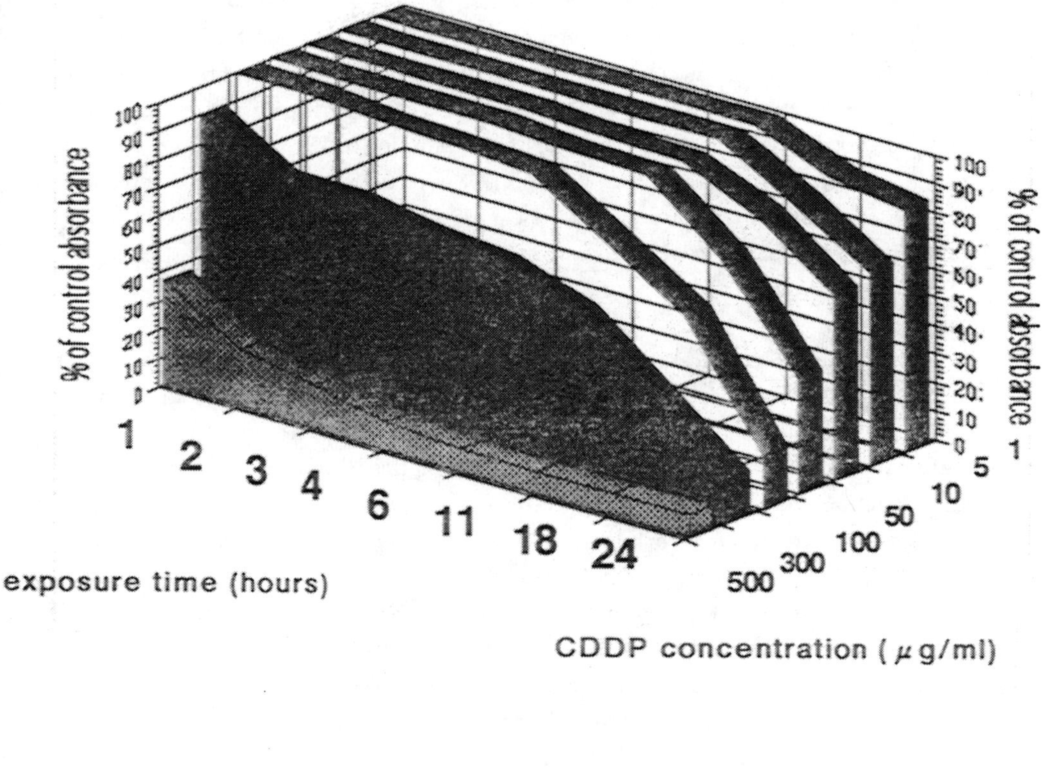

Fig. 9. Cell growth inhibition by cisplatin in SHIN-3 micrometastasis model.

However, ip- chemotherapy requires catheter placement at the time of laparotomy. We investigated the complications of catheters in an intraperitoneal administration route. The subjects were 84 patients, 39 with temporary catheters and 45 with an implantable port and catheter system. Twenty-seven percent of the temporary catheter patients experienced complications consisting of infection (8%), inflow obstruction (3%), leakage (5%), and severe pain (3%). A total of 22% of patients with an implantable port and catheter system experinced complications including inflow obstruction (9%), infection (2%), leakage (4%), and extrusion (7%). Fortunately, no serious complications were observed at our laboratory, and the complication incidence seemed to be lower, compared to that of other laboratories (118).

Infection

Septic complications of ip-therapy were rare and all episodes of peritonitis responded to antibiotics. Patients were diagnosed as peritonitis if they were febrile and had a positive peritoneal fluid culture. After diagnostic evaluation and appropriate cultures, these patients were treated with intravenous antibiotics including an aminoglycoside if renal function was adequate (34,119,120). Gram positive organisms were usually the cause of infection. In our laboratory the use of the completely subcutaneous portal delivery system has reduced the incidence of infection.

If patients received with ip-therapy had bacterial infections, active antibiotics should be administered intravenously for 7 days. If the cultures become negative and the patient remains afebrile, oral antibiotics can be substituted in a 14-day course. However, if fever persists and cultures remain positive, or if there is an obvious tunnel infection, removal of catheter is required.

Chemical peritonitis and intraperitoneal recurrence

Complications from this form of therapy are usually due to either catheter failure or peritonitis. Catheter failure is most commonly due to the formation of fibrous sheath around the outside of the catheter. In this situation the fluid flows in quite readily but will not drain properly due to a check valve mechanism. Peritonitis can be due either to an infecting organism or to the irritative properties of the agents administered.

We evaluated the correlation between the intraperitoneal adhesion and cycles of intraperitoneal chemotherapy in patients who underwent second and third-look operations following cisplatin intraperitoneal chemotherapy (Table 1). The severity of adhesion did not correlate with a number of cycles. Most chemical adhesions were made up of fibrous membranes that were easily dissected at the second-look laparotomy. Many areas with severe adhesions which could not be dissected easily, were the sites of recurrence in the abdominal cavity (Table 2). From these findings, we conclude that all suspicious areas of adhesions must be biopsied.

Table 1. Correlation between Adhesion at S.L.O. and Cycles of Intraperitonea Chemotherapy

	IP (cycles)		
adhesion	0-1	2-4	5 or more than
no adhesion	43% (3/ 7)	71% (12/17)	25% (2/ 8)
mild adhesion	14% (1/ 7)	12% (2/17)	38% (3/ 8)
severe adhesion	43% (3/ 7)	17% (3/17)	38% (3/ 8)
total	7	17	8

Table 2. Correlation between Adhesion at S.L.O. and Tumor Recurrence

adhesion	no evidence of disease	microscopic tumor (<2cm)	macroscopic tumor (2>cm)
no adhesion	77% (14/18)	60% (3 / 5)	0% (0/ 9)
mild adhesion	17% (3/18)	20% (1/ 5)	22% (2/ 9)
severe adhesion	6% (1/18)	20% (1/ 5)	78% (7/ 9)
total	18	5	9

INDICATION FOR I.P.THERAPY

The most appropriate clinical situations for intraperitoneal therapy in the management of ovarian cancer are those with only microscopic intraperitoneal disease or very small tumor nodules (< 0.5cm. maximum tumor diameter) following systemic therapy or secondary surgical debulking (19,121). Of great importance, responses to intraperitoneal cisplatin are essentially limited to patients whose tumors have previously exhibited cisplatin-sensitivity. Several non-randomized retrospective reports have suggested that salvage intraperitoneal chemotherapy in small volume residual ovarian cancer was very effective (111)(122).

A SWOG-GOG-ECOG intergroup conducted a phase III randomized trial of ip cisplatin versus iv cisplatin with iv cyclophosphamide to determine the effect of regional cisplatin administration on survival, and pathological complete response rates, and to compare the toxicities between the two regimens. In this newest report, all patients received at least a bilateral oophorectomy, total abdominal hysterectomy, omentectomy and resection of all tumor masses and had <2cm residual tumor. Within 4 weeks, 6 courses of ip cisplatin (100mg/m2) with iv cyclophosphamide (600mg/m2) or iv cisplatin (100mg/m2) with cyclophosphamide (600mg/m2) were started at 3 week intervals. Median survival for living patients was 51months in the ip-arm and 44 months in the iv-arm. Pathologically proven complete response in patients undergoing second-look surgery was documented in 31% in the iv-arm and 40% in the ip-arm ($p=0.1$). Patient survival in the ip-arm (median=51 months) was significantly longer (Cox two-sided $p=0.03$) than that in the iv-arm (median= 41months). They concluded that the ip-administration of 100mg/m2 cisplatin combined with cyclophosphamide-iv was associated with superior patient survival, less clinical hearing loss and less myelosuppression in patients with stage III ovarian cancer (123). This study was the first phase III randomized trial of ip cisplatin versus iv cisplatin, and proved that ip cisplatin in patients with small volume residual tumor was associated with better survival and less side effects.

The degree of systemic drug exposure following intraperitoneal administration is a very important factor. The dose limiting toxicities of drugs delivered by the intraperitoneal route will be either systemic side effects (ie, marrow suppression, mucositis, etc) or local side effects (ie, abdominal pain, bowel obstruction, etc). If systemic side effects limit the amount of the drug that can be delivered into the peritoneal cavity, the systemic exposure will approximate that achieved with intravenous administration of the drug. Conversely, if local side effects of the agent limit the amount that can be delivered into the peritoneal cavity, the systemic exposure may be far less than that attained following intravenous administration of the drug.

Therefore, the delivery of cytotoxic agents to the tumor by capillary flow following intraperitoneal administration will be greatly influenced by the agents selected. For example, the intraperitoneal administration of cisplatin or carboplatin result in minimal local toxicity, because systemic side effects limit the amount of drug that can be delivered into the peritoneal cavity.

Because the extent of systemic exposure to cisplatin and carboplatin following regional delivery should, at least theoretically, approximate that attained following intravenous adoministration of the agents, we would like to emphasize that ip cisplatin and ip carboplatin have not only a direct anticancer effect in the abdominal cavity but also indirect effects via the systemic circulation.

The appropriate indication for intraperitoneal therapy in the management of ovarian cancer could expand other clinical situations. Ip-chemotherapy as an initial frontline approach has several potential applications for the patients with small volume residual stage III disease following optimal tumor debulking, the patients with stage I-II disease where the risk of unrecognized microscopic disease involving free-floating cancer cells in the upper abdomen is substantial, and the patients with limited tumor volume remaining following several courses of initial systemic chemotherapy. The ip-delivery of chemotherapeutic agents could become a part of in vivo sensitivity tests if suppression of ascites occured (Table 3). Although it is highly unlikely that free surface diffusion will kill a large fraction of tumor when large masses are present, if drugs are used at near-maximal tolerated doses, then the combination of drug delivery by capillary flow (from absorbed drug) and free surface diffusion may still be more effective than iv-treatment alone. It is also possible that repeated courses of ip-therapy may result in sequential layers of tumor destruction.

At second-look laparotomy this technique can be applied in patients with minimal residual or no residual disease who are suspected of having free-floating cancer cells following initial systemic therapy (Table 4).

CONCLUSION

Accurate surgical staging and aggressive debulking followed by intensive chemotherapy with cisplatin-containing regimens have become the standard treatments for most patients with ovarian cancer (124,125). Although these combination modality approaches have produced a large number of complete responses, the anticipated marked improvement in long-term survival or cure has not been documented (126,127).

Ip-chemotherapy is one of these combination modality approaches. However, several important issues may remain to be resolved before this intracavital treatment approach can become the standard therapy. Carefully designed controlled clinical trials such as

Table 3. Purpose of IP-Therapy - At First Look Operation-

Stage I	Total kill of free-floating cancer cells
Stage II~III	Total kill of small volume residual tumor
Stage IIIc~IV	1) Suppression of ascites 2) Dose up (low perontoneal clearance due to carcinomatous peritonitis) • direct effect in the abdominal cavity • systemic effect from the vascular side 3) *in vivo* sensitivity test
⇒ in combination with tumor reduction and lymphadnectomy	

Table 4. Purpose of IP-Therapy - At Second Look Operation-

Cytology positive	Total kill of free-floating cancer cells in ascites
Nodules ≤ 0.5 cm.	Total kill of small volume residual tumor
Nodules ≥ 0.5 cm.	1) Suppression of ascites 2) Dose up (low perontoneal clearance due to carcinomatous peritonitis) • direct effect in the abdominal cavity • systemic effect from the vascular side 3) *in vivo* sensitivity test
⇒ in combination with tumor reduction	

studies of the SWOG-GOG-ECOG intergroup (123) will need to be conducted to define the role of this treatment technique in the therapy of tumors confined to body cavities.
Future studies will need to examine new drugs (including biologicals) and drug combinations, and critically evaluate the clinical utility of this approach, compared to alternative therapeutic strategies.
When new drugs were identified, their effectiveness in the ip route will also need to be evaluated. Some agents may be especially usefull in the ip route, if effective concentrations would be achievable.
However, ip-therapy may not be able to replace iv-systemic treatment with anticancer agents. It is most important to evaluate not only the characteristics of anticancer agents but also the individual patients with their various clinical conditions, before decision of treatment strategy with anticancer drugs.

Reference

1. Frei E III and Canellos GP: Dose: A critical factor in cancer chemotherapy. Amer J Med 69: 585-594, 1980.
2. Goldman AJ and Goldie JH: Impact of dose-intense chemotherapy on the development of permanent drug resistance. Semin. Oncol 14(4 suppl. 4): 29-33, 1987.
3. Murray N: The importance of dose and dose intensity in lung cancer chemotherapy. Semin. Oncol 14(4 suppl. 4): 20-28, 1987.
4. Weissberger AS, Levine B, Storaasli JP: Use of nitrogen mustard in treatment of serous effusions of neoplastic origine. JAMA 159: 1704-1707, 1955.
5. Green HL: Hemisulfer mustard in the palliation of patients with metastatic ovarian carcinoma. Obstet Gynecol 13: 383-393, 1959.
6. Kottmeier HL: Treatment of ovarian cancer with thio-tepa. Clin Obstet Gynecol 11: 447-448, 1968.
7. Suhrland LG, Weissberger AS: Intracavitary 5-fluorouracil in malignant effusion. Arch Intern Med 116: 431-433, 1965.
8. Dedric RL, Myers CE, Bungay PM, et al: Pharmacokinetic rationale for peritoneal drug administration in the treatment of ovarian cancer. Cancer Treat Rep 62: 1-9, 1978.
9. Ozols RF, Corden BJ, Jacob J, et al: High-dose cisplatin in hypertonic saline. Ann Intern Med 100: 19-24, 1984.
10. Alberts DS, Young L, Mason N, et al: In vitro evaluation of anticancer drugs against ovarian cancer at concentrations achievable by intraperitonral administration. Semin Oncol (suppl 4) 12: 38-42, 1985 .
11. Dedric R L: Theoretical and experimental basis of intraperitoneal chemotherapy. Semin Oncol (Suppl. 4)12: 1-6, 1985.
12. Howell SB, Pfeifle C E, Wung WE, et al: Intraperitoneal cisplatin with systemic thiosulfate protection, Ann Int Med 97: 845-851, 1982.

13. Collins JM: Pharmacokinetic rationale for regional drug delivery. J Clin Oncol 2: 498-504, 1984

14. Oku M, Noda T, Kiyozuka Y, et al: Pharmacokinetic analysis of intraperitoneal cisplatinum administration. J Jpn Soc Cancer Ther 23: 657-664, 1988 (in Japanese).

15. Noda T, Oku M, Kiyozuka Y,et al: Intraperitoneal high-dose cisplatinum chemotherapy (CDDP-ip) in patients with carcinomatous peritonitis. Jpn J Cancer Chemother 14: 1025-1032, 1987 (in Japanese).

16. Markman M: Intraperitoneal "bell bath" chemotherapy. Cancer Chemotherapy by infusion. Second Edition. Kokich JJ. ed. Chicago, IL, Precept Press, pp 552-574, 1990.

17. McClay EF and Howell SB: A review: intraperitoneal cisplatin in the management of patients with ovarian cancer. Gynecol Oncol 36: 1-6, 1990.

18. Surbone A. and Myer CE: Regional the rapies. in "New directions in cancer treatments (ed. Magrath, I)",Springer Verlag, Berlin. pp166-190, 1989.

19. Markman M: Intraperitoneal chemotherapy. Semin Oncol 18: 248-254, 1991.

20. Markman M, Rowinsky E, Hakes T, et al: Phase I trial of intraperitoneal taxol: A Gynecologic Oncology Group study. J Clin Oncol 10: 1485-1491, 1992.

21. Dedrick RL, Flessner MF, Collins JM, et al: Is the peritoneum a membrane? Am Soc Artificial Int Organs 5: 1-8, 1982.

22. Leak LV, Rahil K: Permeability of the diaphragmatic mesothelium: the ultrastructural basis for "stomata". Am J Anat 151: 577-594, 1978.

23. Kraft AR, Tompkins RK, Jesseph JE: Peritoneal electrolyte absorption: analysis of portal, systemic venous and lymphatic transport. Surgery 64: 148-153, 1968.

24. Lukas G, Brindle SD, Greengard P: The route of absorption of intraprtitoneally administered compounds. J Pharmacol Exp Ther 178: 562-566, 1971

25. Bolman JK, Cain JC, Grindlay JH: Techniques for the collection of lymph from liver, small intestine, or thoracic duct of the rat. J Lab Clin Med 33: 1349-1352, 1948.

26. Reininger EJ, Saperstein LA: Effect of digestion on distribution of blood flow in the rat. Science 126: 1176, 1957.

27. Torres IJ, Litterst CL, Guarino AM: Transport of model compounds across the peritoneal membrane in the rat. Pharmacology 17: 330-340, 1978.

28. Mayers CE, et al: Pharmacology of intraperitoneal chemotherapy. Cancer Invetigation 1: 395-407, 1983.

29. Tully TE, Goldberg ME, Loken MK: The use of 99Tc-sulfur colloid to assess the distribution of 32P chromic phosphate. J Nucl Med 15: 190-191, 1974.

30. Taylor A, Baily NA, Halpern SE,et al: Loculation as a contraindication to intracavitary 32P chromic phosphaate therapy. J Nucl Ned 16: 318-319, 1975.

31. Vider M, Deland FM, Maruyama Y: Loculation as a contraindication to intracavitary 32P chronic phosphate therapy. J Nucl Med 17: 150-151, 1976.

32. Rosenhein N, Blake D, McIntyre P A, et al: The effect of volume on the distribution

of substances into the peritoneal cavity. Gynecol. Oncol 6: 106-110, 1978.
33. Dunnick NR, Jones RB, Doppman JL, et al: Intraperitoneal contrast infusion for assessment of intraperitoneal fluid dynamics. A J R 133 , 221-223, 1979.
34. Braly P, Doroshow J, Hoff SRN: Technical aspects of intraperitoneal chemotherapy in abdominal carcinomatosis. Gynecol Oncol 25: 319-333, 1986.
35. Noda T, Saitoh S, Ando Y, et al: Intraperitoneal (Ip) high-dose cisplatinum (CDDP) chemotherapy in patients with advanced ovarian cancer. J Jpn Soc Cancer Ther 20: 797-807, 1985 (in Japanese).
36. Levin VA, Patlak CS, Landahn MD: Heuristic modelling of drug delivery to malignant brain tumors. J Pharmacokinet Biopharm 8: 257-296, 1980.
37. West GW, Weichselbau R, Little JB: Limited penetration of methotrexate into human osteosarcoma spheroids as a proposed model for solid tumor resistance to adjuvant chemotherapy. Cancer Res 40: 3665-3668, 1980.
38. Durand RE: Flow cytometry studies of intracellular Adriamycin in multicell spheroides in vitro. Cancer Res 40: 3665-3668, 1980.
39. Ozols R F, Locker G Y, Doroshow J H, et al: Pharmacokinetics of adriamycin and tissue penetration in murine ovarian cancer. Cancer Res 39: 3209-3214, 1979.
40. Ozols RF, Grotzinger KR, Fisher RI, et al: Kinetic characterization and response to chemotherapy in a transplantable murine ovarian cancer. Cancer Res 39: 3202-3208, 1979.
41. Ozols RF, Locker GY, Doroshow JH, et al: Chemotherapy for murine ovarian cancer: a rationale for IP therapy with adriamycin. Cancer Treat Rep 63: 269-273, 1979.
42. West GW, Weichselbau R, Little JB: Limited penetration of methotrxate into human osteosarcoma spheroids as a proposed model for solid tumor resistance to adjuvant chemotherapy. Cancer Res 40: 3665-3668, 1980.
43. Nederman T, Carlsson J: Penetration and binding of vinblastine and 5-fluorouracil in cellular spheroides. Cancer Chemother Pharmacol 13:131-135, 1984.
44. Los G, Mutsaers PHA, van der Vijgh WJF, et al: Direct diffusion of cis-diamminedichloroplatinum(II) in intraperitoneal rat tumors after intraperitoneal chemotherapy. A comparison with systemic chemotherapy. Cancer Res 48: 3380-3384, 1989.
45. Tenchoff H, Schechter H: A bacteriologically safe peritoneal access device. Trans Am Aac Artif Intern Organs 14: 181-187, 1968.
46. Pferifle CE, Howell SB, Markman M, et al: Totally implantable system for peritoneal access. J Clin Oncol 2: 1277-1280, 1984.
47. Adachi S, Noda T, Ito K,et al: Complication associated with CDDP intraperitoneal chemotherapy. Asia-Oceania J Obstet Gynaecol 20: 7-12, 1994.
48. Noda T, Adachi S,Yamamoto T et al: Intraperitoneal (I.P.) chemotherapy in the management of ovarian cancer -Pharmacokinetics and methods of sequential I.P.

chemotherapy. Jpn J Cancer Chemother 17: 1561-1568, 1990 (in Japanese).
49. Markman M, Hakes T, Reichman B, et al: Intraperitoneal therapy in the management of ovarian carcinoma. Yale J Biol Med 62: 393-403, 1989.
50. Pasando JM, Come SE, Parker LM, et al: cis-Diamminedichloroplatinum (CDDP) therapy of advanced ovarian cancer. Proc Amer Assoc Cancer Res 20: 328, 1978.
51. Thigpen T, LaGasse L, Bundy B: Phase II trial of cisplatinum in treatment of advanced ovarian adenocarcinoma. Proc Amer Assoc Cancer Res 20: 84. 1979.
52. Markman M, Reichman B, Hakes T, et al: Responses to second-line cisplatin-base intraperitoneal therapy in ovarian cancer: influence of a prior response to intravenous cisplatin. J Clin Oncol 9: 1801-1805, 1991.
53. Reichman B, Markman M, Hakes T, et al: Intraperitoneal cisplatin and etoposide in the treatment of refractory/recurrent ovarian carcinoma. J Clin Oncol 7: 1327-1332, 1989.
54. Markman M, Hakes T, Reichman B, et al: Intrperitoneal cisplatin and cytarabin in the treatment of refractory ovarian carcinoma. J Clin Oncol 9: 204-210, 1991.
55. Howell SB, Kirmani S, Lucas WE, et al: A phase II trial of intraperitoneal cisplatin and etoposide for primary treatment of ovarian epithelial cancer. J Clin Oncol 8: 137-145, 1990.
56. Hequet B, Leroy A, Lefebvre JL, et al: Uptake of platinum compounds in human tumors, in vitro study. Bull Cancer (Paris) 43: 535-541, 1986.
57. Kiyozuka Y, Imai S, Noda T, et al: Establishment and characterization of human ovarian serous cystadenocarcinoma cell line (SHIN-3) which produces CA 125 and TPA in vitro. J Jpn Soc Clin Cytol 27: 926-935, 1988 (in Japanese).
58. Yoshida M, Kiyozuka Y, Imai S, et al: Establishment and characterization of human ovarian mucinous cystadenocarcinoma cell line (MN-1) and its subline MN-1A, MN-1B. J Jpn Soc Cytol 32: 1-8, 1993 (in Japanese).
59. Casper ES, Kelsen DP, Alcock NW, et al: IP cisplatin in patients with malignant ascites: pharmacokinetic evaluation and comparison with the IV route. Cancer Treat Rep 67: 235-238, 1983.
60. Pretorius RG, Hacker NF, Berek JS, et al: Pharmacokinetics of IP cisplatin in refractory ovarian carcinoma.Cancer Treat Rep 67: 1085-1092, 1983.
61. Markman M: Intracavital chemotherapy. CRC Critical Reviews in Oncology / Hematology 3: 205-233, 1985.
62. Cohen C: Surgical considerations, in Gastrointestinal Tumor Study Group Workshop on Intraperitoneal Therapy, Orlando FL, March 1985.
63. Hacker NF, Berek JS, Pretorius G, et al: Intraperitoneal cis-platin as salvage therapy for refractory epithelial ovarian cancer. Obstet. Gynecol 70: 739-764, 1987.
64. Howell SB, Taetle R: Effect of sodium thiosulfate on cis- dichlorodiammineplatinum (II) toxicity and antitumor activity in L1210 leukemia. Cancer Treat Rep 64: 611-616,

1980.
65. Shea M, Koziol JA, Howell SB: Kinetics of sodium thiosulfate, a cisplatin neutralizer. Clin Pharmacol Ther 35: 419-425, 1984.
66. Pfeifle CE, Howell S B, Felthouse R D, et al: High dose cisplatin with sodium thiosulfate protection. J Clin Oncol 3: 237-244, 1985.
67. Howell SB, Pfeifle CL, Wung WE, et al: Intraperitoneal cis-Diamminedichloroplatinum with systemic thiosulfate protection. Cancer Res 43: 1426-1431, 1983.
68. Speyer JL, Beller U, Colombo N, et al : Intraperitoneal carboplatin: Favorable results in women with minimal residual ovarian cancer after cisplatin therapy. J Clin Oncol 8: 1335-1341, 1990.
69. Pfeiffer P, Bennedack O, Bertelsen K: Intraperitoneal carboplatin in the treatment of minimal residual cancer. Gynecol Oncol 36: 306-311, 1990.
70. Ito K, Itani Y, Huruki K, et al: Usefulness of intraperitoneal carboplatin administration - Pharmacokinetic Analysis- . Acta Obst Gynaec Jpn 44: 1180-1186, 1992 (in Japanese).
71. Chambers SK, Chambers JT, Kohorn EI, et al: Etoposide(VP-16-213) plus cisdiamminedichloroplatinum as salvage therapy in advanced epithelial ovarian cancer. Gynecol Oncol 27: 233-240, 1987.
72. Dottino PR, Goodman HM, Kredentser D, et al: Clinical trial etoposide and cisplatin as salvage therapy in advanced ovarian carcinoma. Gynecol Oncol 27: 350-356, 1987.
73. Barlow JJ, Lele SB: Etoposide (VP-16) plus cisplatin (DDP): A new active chemotherapeutic combination in patients with stage III-IV ovarian adenocarcinoma. J Surg Oncol 32: 43-45, 1986.
74. Delena M, Lorusso V, Romito S: Cisplatin plus etoposide as second-line treatment in advanced ovarian carcinoma. Cancer Treat Rep 70: 893-895, 1986.
75. Goldie JH, Durand RE: Interaction of etoposide and cisplatin in a vitro tumor system. Cancer Treat Rep 71: 673-679, 1988.
76. Noda T, Adachi S, Ito K, et al: Pharmacokinetic study of intraperitoneally administered etoposide against peritonitis carcinomatosa. J Nara Med Ass 45: 301-310, 1994.
77. Pfeffer M, Nardella PA, Van Harken DR, et al: The absolute oral bioavailability and pharmacokinetics of etoposide, in "Etoposide (VP-16)". 1st. ed., Academic Press Inc., New York, pp127-140, 1984
78. Dombernowsky P, Nissen NI: Schedule dependency of the antileukemic activity of the podophyllotoxin derivative VP-16-213 (NSC 141540) in L1210 leukemia. Acta Path Microbiol Scand 81: 715-724, 1973.
79. Kalwinsky DK, Look AT, Ducore J, et al: Effects of the epipodophyllotoxin VP-16-213 on cell cycle traverse, DNA synthesis, and DNA strand size in cultures of human

leukemic lymphoblasts. Cancer Res 43: 1592-1597, 1983.

80. Slevin ML, Clark PI, Joel SP, et al: A randamized trial to evaluate the effect of schedule on the activity of etoposide in small-cell lung cancer. J Clin Oncol 7: 1333-1340, 1989.

81. Slevin ML, Clark PI, Joel SP, et al: A randomized trial to examine the effect of more extened scheduling on etoposide administration in small cell lung cancer (SCLC). Proc Am Soc Clin Oncol 8: 236, 1989.

82. Suhrland LG, Weisberger AS: Intracavital 5-fluorouracil in malignant effusions. Arch Intern Med 116: 431-433, 1965.

83. Speyer JL, Sugarbaker PH, Collins JM, et al: Portal levels and hepatic clearance of 5-fluorouracil after intraperitoneal administration in humans. Cancer Res 41: 1916-1922, 1981.

84. Speyer JL, Collins JM, Dedrick RL, et al: Phase I pharmacologic studies of 5-fluorouracil administration intraperitoneally. Cancer Res 40: 567-572, 1980.

85. Speyer JL, Myers CE: The use of peritoneal dialysis for delivery of chemotherapy to intraperitoneal malignancies. Cancer Res 74: 264-269, 1980.

86. Demicheli R, Jirillo A, Bonciarelli G, et al: Pharmacological data and techinical feasibility of intraperitoneal 5-fluorouracil administration. Tumori 68:437-441, 1982.

87. Ozols RF, Myers CE, Young RC: Intraperitoneal chemotherapy (editorial). Ann Intern Med 101: 118-120, 1984.

88. Litterst CL, Collins JM, Lowe MC, et al: Local and systemic toxicity resulting from large-volume IP administration of doxorubicin in the rat. Cancer Treat Rep 66: 157-161, 1982.

89. Ozols RF, Young RC, Speyer JL, et al: Phase I and pharmacological studies of Adriamycin administered intraperitoneally to patients with ovarian cancer. Cancer Res 42: 4265-4269. 1982.

90. Alberts DS, Surwit EA, Peng YM, et al:Phase I clinical and pharmacokinetic study of mitoxantrone given to patients by intraperitoneal administration. Cancer Res 48: 5874-5877, 1988.

91. Markman M, George M, Hakes T, et al: Phase 2 trial of intraperitoneal mitoxantrone in the management of rfractory ovarian carcinoma. J Clin Oncol 8: 146-150, 1990.

92. Hagiwara A, Takahashi T, Lee R, et al.: Selective delivery of high levels of mitomycine C to peritoneal carcinomatosis using a new dosage form. Anticancer Res 6: 1161-1164, 1986.

93. Monk BJ, Surwit EA, Alberts DS, et al.: Intraperitoneal mitomycine C in the treatment of peritoneal carcinomatosis following second-look surgery. Semin Oncol 15: 27-31, 1988.

94. King ME, Pfeifle CE, Howell SB: Intraperitoneal cytosine arabinoside therapy in ovarian carcinoma. J Clinical Oncology 2:662-669, 1984.

95. Ueda T, Nakamura T, Ando S, et al: Pharmacokinetics of N4-behenoyl-1-β-D-arabinofuranosylcytosine in patients with acute leukemia. Cancer Research 43: 3412-3416, 1983.

96. Noda T, Oku M, Kiyozuka Y, et al: Pharmacokinetics of N4-behenoyl-1-β-D-arabinofuranosylcytosine after intraperitoneal administration. Jpn J Cancer Chemother 15: 2929-2935, 1988 (in Japanese).

97. Howell SB, Pfeifle CE, Olshen RA: Intraperitoneal chemotherapy with melphalan. Ann Intern Med 101: 14-18, 1984.

98. Rowinsky EK, Donehower RC, Jones RJ, et al: Microtubule changes and cytotoxicity in leukemic cell lines treated with taxol. Cancer Res 48: 4093-4100, 1988.

99. McGuire WP, Rowwinsky EK, Rosenshein NB, et al: Taxol: a unique antineoplastic agent with significant activity in advanced ovarian epithelial neoplasms. Ann Intern Med 111: 273-279, 1989.

100. Monsarrat B, Mariel E, Crois S, et al: Taxol metabolism. Isolation and identification of three major metabolites in rat bile. Drug Med Disp 18: 895-901, 1990.

101. Goldie JH, Goldmann AJ, Gudauskas GA: Rationale for the use of alternating noncross-resistant chemotherapy. Cancer Treat Rep 66: 439-449, 1982.

102. Bergerat JP, Drewinko B, Corry P, et al: Synergistic lethal effect of cis-dichlorodiammineplatinum and 1-beta-D-arabinofuranosylcytosine. Cancer Res 41 :25-30, 1981.

103. Markman M, Howell SB, Luca WE, et al: Combination intraperitoneal chemotherapy with cisplatin, cytarabine and doxorubicine for refractory ovarian carcinoma and other malignancies principally confined to the peritoneal cavity. J Clin Oncol 2:1321-1326, 1984.

104. Markman M, Cleary S, Lucas W, et al: Ip chemotherapy employing a regimen of cisplatin, cytarabine and bleomycin. Cancer Treat Rep 70: 735-760, 1986.

105. Schabel FF Jr, Trader MW, Laster WR Jr, et al: cis-Dichlorodiammineplatinum (II): Combination chemotherapy and cross resistance studies with tumor of mice. Cancer Treat Rep 63: 1459-1473, 1979.

106. Williams SD, Einhorn LH: Etoposide salvage therapy for refractory germ cell tumors; an update. Cancer Treat Rev 9(Suppl A): 67-71, 1982.

107. Evans WK, Shepard FA, Feld SR, et al: VP-16 and cisplatin as first-line therapy for small-cell lung cancer. J Clin Oncol 3: 1471-1477, 1985.

108. Zimm S, Cleary SM, Lucas WE, et al: Phase I / Pharmacokinetic study of intraperitoneal cisplatin and etoposide. Cancer Res 47: 1712-1716, 1987.

109. Kirmani S, Zimm S, Cleary SM, et al: Intraperitoneal cisplatin and etoposide as salvage therapy for ovarian cancer. Proc ASCO 7: 117, 1988.

110. Adachi, S. and Noda, T.: Efficacy of CDDP (P) intraperitoneal administration (ip) for ovarian cancer. IJGOA L 46(Suppl 1): 202, 1994.

111. Howell SB, Zimm S, Markman M, et al: Long term survival of advanced refractory ovarian carcinoma patients with small-volume disease treated with intraperitoneal chemotherapy. J Clin Oncol 5: 1607-1612, 1987.
112. Menczer J, Ben-Baruch G, Modan M, et al: Intraperitonealcisplatin chemotherapy versus abdominopelvic irradiation in ovarian carcinoma patients after second-look laparotomy. Cancer 63: 1509-1513, 1989.
113. Hoskins WJ, Rubin SC, Dulaney E , et al: Influence of secondary cytoreduction at the time of second-look laparotomy on the survival of patients with epithelial ovarian carcinoma. Gynecol Oncol 34: 365-371, 1989.
114. Copeland LJ, Gershenson DM, Wharton JT, et al: Microscopic disease at second-look laparotomy in advanced ovarian cancer. Cancer 55: 472-478, 1985.
115. Podratz KC, Schray MF, Wieand HS, et al: Evaluation of treatment and survival after positive second-look laparotomy. Gynecol Oncol 31: 9-21, 1988.
116. Markman M, Cleary S, Howell SB, et al: Complications of extensive adhesion formation following intraperitoneal chemotherapy. Surg Gynecol Oncol 112: 445-448, 1986.
117. Speyer JL, Beller U, Colombo N, et al: Intraperitoneal carboplatin: favorable results in women with minimal residual ovarian cancer after cisplatin therapy. J Clin Oncol 8: 1335-1341, 1990.
118. Adachi S, Noda T, Ito K, et al: Complication associated with CDDP intraperitoneal chemotherapy. Asia-Oceania J Obstet Gynaecol 20: 7-12, 1994.
119. Brenner OE: Intraperitoneal chemotherapy. A review. J Clin Oncol 4: 1135-1147, 1986.
120. Kaplan RA, Markman M, Lucas WE, et al: Infectious peritonitis in patients receiving intraperitoneal chemotherapy. Am J Med 78: 49-53, 1985.
121.Markman M, Reichman B, Hakes T, et al: Responses to second-line cisplatin-based intraperitoneal therapy in ovarian cancer: influence of a prior response to intravenous cisplatin. J Clin Oncol 9: 1801-1805, 1991.
122. Markman M, Reichmann B, Hakes T, et al: Impact on survival of surgically-defined favorable responses to salvage intraperitoneal chemotherapy in small volume residual ovarian cancer, J Clin Oncol 10: 1479-1484, 1992.
123. Alberts PY, Liu EV, Hannigan R, et al: Phase III study of intraperitoneal (IP) cisplatin (CDDP)/ intravenous (IV) cyclophosphamide(CPA) vs IV CDDP/IV CPA in patients(PTS) with optimal disease stage III ovarian cancer. Proc Am Soc Clin Oncol 14: 273, 1995.
124. Hacker NF, Berek JS, Lagasse LD, et al: Primary cytoreductive surgery for epithelial ovarian cancer. Obstet Gynecol 61: 413-420, 1983.
125. Griffiths CT, Parker LM, Fuller AF: Role of cytoreductive surgical treatment in the management of advanced ovarian cancer. Cancer Treat Rep 63: 235-240, 1979.

126. Bell DR, Woods RL, Levi JA: Advanced ovarian cancer: A prospective randomized trial of chlorambucil vs combined cyclophosphamide and cis- diamminedichloro-platinum. Aust NZ J Med 12: 245-259, 1982.
127. Omura GA, Ehrlich CE, Blessing A: A randomized trial of cyclophosphamide plus adriamycin with or without cis-platinum in ovarian carcinoma. Proc Amer Soc Clin Oncol 1: 104, 1982.

Index

—D—